Dental Care for Children with Special Needs

Travis M. Nelson • Jessica R. Webb
Editors

Dental Care for Children with Special Needs

A Clinical Guide

Springer

Editors
Travis M. Nelson
Department of Pediatric Dentistry
University of Washington
Seattle, WA
USA

Jessica R.Webb
Children's Village
Yakima, WA
USA

ISBN 978-3-030-10482-5 ISBN 978-3-030-10483-2 (eBook)
https://doi.org/10.1007/978-3-030-10483-2

Library of Congress Control Number: 2019931880

This Springer imprint is published by the registered company Springer Nature Switzerland AG
The registered company address is: Gewerbestrasse 11, 6330 Cham, Switzerland

We would like to dedicate this book to all those who have taught us, mentored us, inspired us, and allowed us the privilege of caring for their children with special needs. We are forever grateful to our patients and their families, our instructors, and our colleagues who have educated us and shaped our philosophy of care.

Jessica would also like to dedicate this book to her sisters, Jocelyn and Amy DeBord, her first and best teachers on this topic.

Preface

Providing dental care to children with special healthcare needs (CSHCN) is a unique and challenging experience. It also offers the most interesting and rewarding professional encounters many of us will ever experience. This patient population has historically experienced barriers to care that have resulted in inequality and poor oral health outcomes. The objective of this short book is to better equip clinicians to address the needs of this special population and reduce overall care disparities. It is intended to serve as a resource for students in training and experienced dental providers alike. While there are a number of high-quality texts that cover specific genetic disorders and details of medical and dental treatment, the focus of these pages is different. Our intent is to provide clinicians with a better understanding of the culture of disability, improve interactions with patients and families, and offer practical tools that expand the clinician's ability to care for this patient population. We hope that the concepts within this text will enable providers to grow in their own comfort and familiarity with CSHCN and increase the amount and quality of care that they are able to deliver.

Seattle, WA, USA — Travis M. Nelson
Yakima, WA, USA — Jessica R. Webb

Acknowledgments

We wish to thank each of the authors who has contributed to this project. It was an honor to work with such a fine group of professionals, and we are grateful to them for sharing their expertise.

Contents

Abbreviations

AAC	Augmentative and alternative communication
AAPD	American Academy of Pediatric Dentistry
AAP	American Academy of Pediatrics
ABA	Applied behavior analysis
ADA	American Dental Association
ADHD	Attention deficit hyperactivity disorder
AI	Amelogenesis imperfecta
AIN	Atomized intranasal
ANC	Absolute neutrophil count
ART	Atraumatic/alternative restorative treatment
ASA	American Society of Anesthesiologists
ASD	Autism spectrum disorder
ASDA	American Society of Dentist Anesthesiologists
BAHA	Bone-anchored hearing devices
BRONJ	Bisphosphonate-related osteonecrosis of the jaws
CAMBRA	Caries management by risk assessment
CDC	Centers for Disease Control and Prevention
CHD	Congenital heart disease
CHX	Chlorhexidine gluconate
CMC	Children with medical complexities
CMS	Center for Medicare and Medicaid Services
CMT	Congenitally missing teeth
CNS	Central nervous system
CPAP/BiPAP	Continuous positive airway pressure/bilevel positive airway pressure
CPP-ACP	Casein phosphopeptide-amorphous calcium phosphate
CSHCN	Children with special healthcare needs
CT	Computerized tomography
CWF	Community water fluoridation
DDE	Developmental defects of enamel
DE	Dental erosion
DEJ	Dentin-enamel junction
DSM-5	Diagnostic and Statistical Manual of Mental Disorders
EAPD	European Academy of Pediatric Dentistry

ESRD	End-stage renal disease
FDA	Food and Drug Administration
GA	General anesthesia
GERD	Gastroesophageal reflux disease
GIC	Glass ionomer cement
GO	Gingival overgrowth
HSCT	Hematopoietic stem cell transplant
HOME	Hand over mouth exercise
ICF	International Classification of Functioning, Disability, and Health
ID	Intellectual disability
IDEA	Individuals with Disabilities Education Act
IEP	Individualized Education Program
IN	Intranasal
INR	International normalized ratio
ITR	Interim therapeutic restoration
MCHB	Maternal and Child Health Bureau
MH	Malignant hyperthermia
MHAUS	Malignant Hyperthermia Association of the United States
MIH	Molar incisor hypomineralization
MIPS	Medical immobilization/protective stabilization
MRI	Magnetic resonance image
MTHFR	Methylenetetrahydrofolate reductase
OT	Occupational therapy
OTC	Over the counter
PCP	Primary care provider
PEB	Post-eruptive enamel breakdown
PPM	Parts per million
RMGI	Resin-modified glass ionomer
SADE	Sensory adapted dental environment
SBE	Subacute bacterial endocarditis
SCDA	Special Care in Dentistry Association
SDF	Silver diamine fluoride
SES	Socio-economic status
SHCN	Special healthcare needs
SIB	Self-injurious behavior
SMART	Silver modified atraumatic restorative technique
SN	Supernumerary teeth
SSB	Sugar-sweetened beverages
SSC	Stainless steel crown
TIVA	Total intravenous anesthesia
TMD	Temporomandibular disorders
TMJ	Temporomandibular joint
VNS	Vagus nerve stimulator
VP	Ventriculoperitoneal
WHO	World Health Organization

List of Editors and Contributors

Editors

Travis M. Nelson, DDS, MSD, MPH Department of Pediatric Dentistry, University of Washington, Seattle, WA, USA

Jessica R. Webb, DDS, MSD, MA Children's Village, Yakima, WA, USA

Contributors

Marc B. Ackerman, DMD, MBA Boston Children's Hospital, Boston, MA, USA

Carolyn R. Baylor, PhD, CCC-SLP Department of Rehabilitation Medicine, University of Washington, Seattle, WA, USA

Department of Speech and Hearing Sciences, University of Washington, Seattle, WA, USA

Marcio A. da Fonseca, DDS, MS Department of Pediatric Dentistry, College of Dentistry, University of Illinois at Chicago, Chicago, IL, USA

Kimberly M. Espinoza, DDS, MPH Department of Oral Medicine, University of Washington, Seattle, WA, USA

Lisa J. Heaton, PhD Department of Oral Health Sciences, University of Washington, Seattle, WA, USA

Joseph P. Kelly, DDS, MSD, MPH Department of Dentistry, Seattle Children's Hospital, Seattle, WA, USA

Evelina Kratunova, MDSc, DChDent Department of Pediatric Dentistry, College of Dentistry, University of Illinois at Chicago, Chicago, IL, USA

Elizabeth A. Palmer, DMD, MS Department of Pediatric Dentistry, Oregon Health and Science University School of Dentistry, Portland, OR, USA

Marilynn L. Rothen, RDH, MS Department of Oral Health Sciences, University of Washington School of Dentistry, Seattle, WA, USA

Elise W. Sarvas, DDS, MSD, MPH Division of Pediatric Dentistry, Department of Developmental and Surgical Sciences, University of Minnesota, Minneapolis, MN, USA

Barbara L. Sheller, DDS, MSD Department of Dentistry, Seattle Children's Hospital, Seattle, WA, USA

Leah I. Stein Duker, PhD, MA, OTR/L Chan Division of Occupational Science and Occupational Therapy, University of Southern California, Los Angeles, CA, USA

James W. Tom, DDS, MS Herman Ostrow School of Dentistry, University of Southern California, Los Angeles, CA, USA

Janice A. Townsend, DDS, MS The Ohio State University, Columbus, OH, USA

Nationwide Children's Hospital, Columbus, OH, USA

Overview of Disability

Jessica R. Webb

Introduction

Dental providers have the responsibility to care for all patients, including those with disabilities. Providing care to children with disabilities is a cornerstone of pediatric dentistry, so much so that the American Academy of Pediatric Dentistry includes children with special needs in its definition of the profession:

> Pediatric Dentistry is an age-defined specialty that provides both primary and comprehensive preventive and therapeutic oral health care for infants and children through adolescence, including those with special health care needs. [1]

Pediatric dentists are uniquely trained to care for all children, including those with complex dental needs, those who are the most vulnerable, and those who require behavioral strategies. For these reasons, caring for children with special needs is clearly at the core of what pediatric dentists do and important to those for whom pediatric dentists exist to serve. Additionally, many children with special needs can be well cared for by dental providers that are not pediatric dentists. These individuals are often very involved in providing care to patients with special needs as they transition to adulthood. The aim of this book is to give clinicians an understanding of disability and provide practical strategies to aid all dental providers in delivering quality care to this population.

The number of children with disabilities is rising due to improvements in medical technology and treatment. Medical advances have facilitated the survival of children who previously would have passed away, which sometimes means survival with a disability. Also, children with complex disabilities are able to live much longer thanks to modern medicine. As with all children, providing dental care to this population requires that dental providers take a holistic view of the child and family,

J. R. Webb (✉)
Children's Village, Yakima, WA, USA
e-mail: Jessica.DeBord@nyulangone.org

T. M. Nelson, J. R. Webb (eds.), *Dental Care for Children with Special Needs*,
https://doi.org/10.1007/978-3-030-10483-2_1

not just the teeth. Much of what clinicians are taught in training about people with special needs is about the medical conditions themselves, dental implications inherent to those medical conditions, and the dental management of those medical and dental conditions. This foundation is, of course, critical to providing safe and appropriate quality care to children with special needs. Understanding medical conditions and their impact is critical. However, it is just the beginning of providing comprehensive care, and in isolation this approach medicalizes these children. The unintended consequence may be that the patient is not viewed as a person, but instead she is reduced to her conditions and teeth.

In the modern era, healthcare practice is increasingly focused on data, performance measures, and outcomes. This requires accurate and thorough documentation of patient symptoms, diagnoses, and treatments. While this is necessary, we risk reducing children to the characteristics of their condition rather than a unique individual with particular strengths and areas of need. It is the duty of the dental provider to work to understand each child, especially those with disabilities.

Children with special needs, like all children, are all unique in their personalities, interests, family situation, strengths, and challenges. Each has a diagnosis, which provides clues about medical, dental, and behavioral management; however, the reality is that every patient is an individual. One child with autism or cerebral palsy may have needs that are entirely different from another child with the same diagnosis. It is a joy, privilege, and challenge to discover each child and develop an individual approach to deliver dental care that promotes a lifetime of oral health. It is the aim of this book to provide clinicians with everyday strategies to better achieve that goal.

Definitions

Special Needs

The Maternal and Child Health Bureau (MCHB) defines children with special healthcare needs (CSHCN) as those who:

> have or are at increased risk for chronic physical, developmental, behavioral or emotional conditions and who also require health and related services of a type or amount beyond that required by children generally. [2]

It is estimated that between 15% and 20% of US children under 18 meet that definition, affecting almost a quarter of families [2, 3]. The American Academy of Pediatric Dentistry expounds upon that definition by stating that:

> Special health care needs include any physical, developmental, mental, sensory, behavioral, cognitive, or emotional impairment or limiting condition that requires medical management, health care intervention, and/or use of specialized services or programs. The condition may be congenital, developmental, or acquired through disease, trauma, or environmental cause and may impose limitations in performing daily self-maintenance activities or substantial limitations in a major life activity. Health care for individuals with

> special needs requires specialized knowledge, as well as increased awareness and attention, adaptation, and accommodative measures beyond what are considered routine. [4]

Disability

Impairment results from a functional or structural problem that causes a physical, mental, or sensory difference. Disability is a broader term that encompasses the impairment as well as its effect on activity, participation, and opportunity [5, 6]. The World Health Organization (WHO) defines the phenomenon of disability as:

> The interaction between the person's body and the social and physical environment in which that person lives [5].

Approximately 15% of the world's population has a disability, and this number is increasing as people are able to live longer with chronic conditions [7]. Within the context of disability, *associated conditions* are those that are a consequence of the primary condition [8]. For example, periodontal disease and intellectual disability are conditions associated with trisomy 21. *Secondary conditions* are those that are related to the primary diagnosis but are frequently known and preventable, such as obesity in those with intellectual disabilities [7]. *Comorbid conditions* are those that occur in addition to the primary diagnosis, but are not related, such as autism spectrum disorder (ASD) and attention-deficit/hyperactivity disorder (ADHD) [7].

It should be noted that the term disability is preferred over special needs by some individuals within this community. The term special needs reinforces the assumption that people with disabilities are "other," "different," or "special," rather than being a person who happens to have a disability. The idea is that by making them and their needs seem exceptional, it emphasizes their differences. There is also a school of thought that suggests all children have unique needs based on their individual personality and circumstances and that those with disabilities simply fall into that continuum. Providers should be aware of the issues with common terms. We have chosen to use the term special needs in this book because it is most frequently used in the healthcare setting, given the MCHB and AAPD definitions [2, 4].

Intellectual and Developmental Disabilities

Developmental disabilities are defined as:

> a group of conditions due to an impairment in physical, learning, language, or behavior areas. These conditions begin during the developmental period, may impact day-to-day functioning, and usually last throughout a person's lifetime [9].

Approximately 15% of US children between ages 3 and 17 have a developmental disability [9]. Intellectual disability, formerly termed "mental retardation," is defined by the American Academy of Intellectual and Developmental Disabilities as:

a disability characterized by significant limitations in both intellectual functioning and in adaptive behavior, which covers many everyday social and practical skills. This disability originates before the age of 18. [10]

Models of Disability

Various models describe multiple ways to conceptualize disability. Some are descriptive and capture the way that disability has been viewed historically. Others are somewhat aspirational in describing how disability ought to be viewed. They are relevant to clinicians in that learning about the models of disability helps each of us understand how we view disability. The models may show us ways that we unknowingly perpetuate negative conceptions of disability and they can offer a guide to reframe the concept of disability in a more thoughtful way.

Moral Model

The moral model of disability is predicated on the belief that disability is a punishment resulting from moral failings or sins of the person or family with the disability. This results in judgment and stigma surrounding disability [6, 11]. This model is not utilized in healthcare, but is a construct that a healthcare provider may encounter in working with families or the community.

Medical Model

The medical model views disability as a medical condition resulting from variation in typical species function [6, 12]. This removes the moral judgment surrounding disability [6]. However, this view carries with it the assumption that disability is a pathological condition that should be treated or cured [6, 11]. It leaves little room for individuals who have developmental and lifelong disabilities that are not going to be cured. It views them as tragedies or failures of medicine, rather than people of value and worth.

This conceptualization also played a role in the eugenics movement where people with disabilities were targeted for sterilization in an attempt to reduce the perpetuation of intellectual disabilities or what was at the time termed "feeblemindedness." [13] The idea of disability as something that can be eliminated with medical intervention stems from the notion that these are medical conditions in need of cure. The traditional medical model recognizes a disease as something that must be targeted and killed [14]. Unlike some medical conditions, lifelong disabilities cannot be treated nor are they a pathology that can be cured. The challenge with this model is that it creates the perception that disability ought to be fixed and, when it is not, medicine has failed. This carries over into societal attitudes that people with disabilities ought to be treated and fixed, that their disabilities are failures, or that they are somehow less valuable than those without disabilities.

Rehabilitation Model

The rehabilitation model of disability recognizes that people with disabilities require services, therapies, and interventions (e.g., assistive technology). It states that if those services are adequate, individuals with disabilities can compensate enough to allow for appropriate functioning [15]. The value in this model is that it advocates for appropriate services for people with disabilities. However, the criticisms of this model are that it views the person with the disability in a more deficit-based approach, it is similar to the medical model in looking for therapy and interventions to "treat" the disability, and it does not capture the effect of societal norms and attitudes on the lived experience of disability.

Social Model

The social model of disability holds that a person may have a given impairment; however the social views, attitudes, and public policies are largely what make the condition disabling [6, 11, 16]. This model calls for us to respect and value people with disabilities, accepting them as they are, rather than viewing them as in need of fixing. Proponents of this model view disability as diversity and argue for acceptance and inclusion of people with disabilities in society. One of the challenges in making healthcare decisions for children with disabilities is that parents and clinicians frequently carry negative attitudes and medicalized views about disability. Familiarity with the social model facilitates more informed decision-making and can result in improved outcomes for patients [16].

Minority Model

The minority model holds that people with disabilities are discriminated against because they are not considered to be "able-bodied." This concept has been termed "ableism." Similar to the social model, the minority model holds that attitudes and bias of society are the problem, not individual impairments [6, 11]. This model contends that disability ought to not have a negative connotation associated with it and that disability can, in fact, be a point of pride. It recognizes disability as diversity that should be valued and celebrated in the same manner as race, culture, gender, and sexual orientation.

Disability Paradox

The concept of the "disability paradox" reflects the fact that most people associate disability with ill health, a state that is incompatible with a quality and fulfilling life [17]. While others may not perceive that they lead a satisfying existence, people with disabilities rate their own quality of life much higher than others do for them.

Indeed, most rank their quality of life as equivalent to the nondisabled [17, 18]. This "paradox" provides evidence that providers should form conceptions of disability based upon firsthand knowledge of individuals with disabilities, rather than developing negative attitudes that are not based in authentic experiences [17].

Biopsychosocial Model

The WHO developed the International Classification of Functioning, Disability, and Health (ICF) as a method of categorizing disability. The ICF recognizes that disability relates to the function of the condition or impairment within the physical and social context in which a person lives [19]. Rather than focusing on a diagnosis, the ICF aims to integrate the key components of both the medical and social models of disability. It looks at the health and function of the person as well as the impact of the contextual factors of the environment, social conditions, and personal situations and the impact of those factors on functioning [15]. This is considered to be a biopsychosocial approach. The ICF considers the health condition, body structure and function, activity, participation, environmental factors, and personal factors (Fig. 1). This provides a more accurate picture of what is actually disabling and aims to capture the dynamic experience of disability. Under the ICF, depending on the various domains, individuals with the same diagnosis may experience different levels of disability. Someone who is more medically complex may be considered less disabled than another individual if she is able to engage in activities and meaningfully participate.

The challenge with the ICF is its ability to be used practically in a clinical setting. It is conceptually accepted and praised for its biopsychosocial approach but

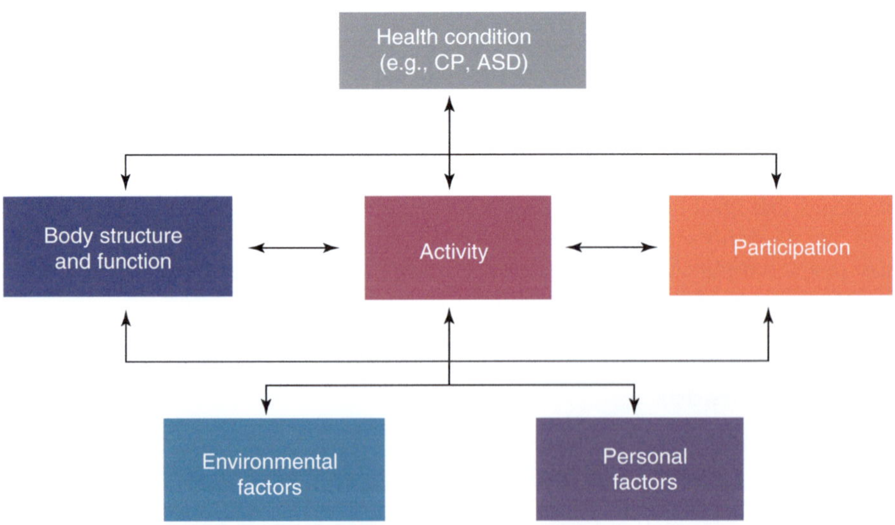

Fig. 1 Rosenbaum & Gorter adaptation of the ICF (WHO, 2001)

can be cumbersome to use [20, 21]. Rosenbaum and Gorter offer an adaptation of the ICF that they call the "F-words" (Table 1, Fig. 2). It captures the conceptual components of the ICF, but is more practical for children with disabilities than the standard ICF classification [22]. The F-words and the corresponding components of the ICF that they capture are:

The other two "F-words" that Rosenbaum and Gorter refer to are "fixing" and "future" [22]. They caution against the perception that children with disabilities need to be fixed [22]. Additionally, due to the multitude of factors at play, fixing is typically not possible with childhood disabilities [22]. Furthermore, they highlight the importance of allowing children with disabilities to adapt to the environment, their bodies, and their abilities in the way that works best for them, rather than forcing notions of how typically developing children use their bodies and progress [22]. Early on they encourage clinicians to think positively about the child's future growth and progress [22].

Table 1 Rosenbaum & Gorter F-words [22]

"F-word"	ICF
Function	Activity Participation
Family	Environment
Fitness	Body structure and function
Fun	Personal factors
Friends	Personal factors Participation

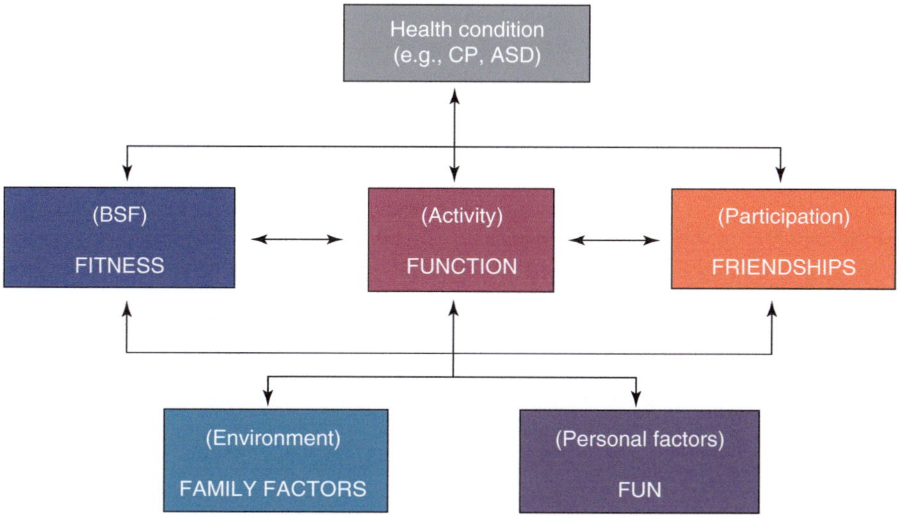

Fig. 2 Rosenbaum & Gorter F-words and the ICF

Understanding a patient's diagnosis and the medical and dental implications of that diagnosis is a necessary prerequisite to quality care. The next step is learning more about a child's overall well-being and the disabling effects of her health condition. The F-word framework is a quick and effective way to get a sense of the child within a broader context. The concept of "fixing" reminds us that we may need to do things differently for our patients with disabilities. Rather than expect patients to visit the dentist or do homecare in the same way as other children, we should determine what adaptations we can make to the dental experience or homecare to better suit the patient. We can recognize that the patient's ability to visit the dentist or her homecare routine may be unique, but are normal for her. The idea of "future" reminds us that the children we treat will someday be adults, and it is our job to prepare them to have the life skill of being able to successfully receive dental care as an adult.

Clinicians often view completion of treatment as the mark of success, but it is more prudent to keep in mind the long-term goal. Children with disabilities grow to become adults. Adults who are able to manage their own oral hygiene, accept assistance from others, and cooperate for routine dental care have a huge advantage in being able to access care and prevent dental disease. The oral health disparities faced by people with disabilities are tremendous and multifactorial. There is no single solution, but the more clinicians are able to help children with disabilities learn to accept dental care, the better their opportunities for access and oral health will be in the future.

Disability Language

Person-First and Identity-First Language

In the medical model of disability, people are defined by their condition. Terminology used to describe individuals with disability reflected that model in language. For example, a patient with a diagnosis of Down syndrome may have been referred to as "a Downs child." In contemporary practice, the goal is to use *person-first language*. Person-first language recognizes the patient as a person before their medical condition. This approach reflects respect for a person's humanity and her value as an individual. Using person-first language, the patient would be referred to as "a child with Down syndrome," rather than "a Downs child." Condition-focused terminology and terminology with negative connotations perpetuate detrimental attitudes about people with disabilities. For example, stating that a person "is wheelchair bound" or "suffers from cerebral palsy" indicates that a person may have a poor quality of life. Adopting a more patient-focused approach, instead, refers to the individual as "a person who uses a wheelchair" or "a person with cerebral palsy" [6, 11, 15, 23].

Historically, the term "mental retardation" was used for people with intellectual disabilities. While it may still be used in popular language and in clinical discussions, this term is no longer appropriate. It has been replaced with *intellectual disability*. This is not only the case in the medical community, but with the ratification of Rosa's Law, all federal documents must replace the term "mental retardation" with intellectual disability [24, 25].

Every patient is entitled to be considered a person first, but many people with disabilities see their disability as part of their identity. It is something they are proud of and an integral part of who they are. The minority model of disability, the disability rights movement, and the disability studies discipline recognize that this sentiment can be reflected using identity-first language [15, 23]. Individuals who choose to be identified by their disability may prefer alternate terminology. For example, people with autism may self-identify as "autistic." Similarly those who identify as part of the Deaf community prefer to be referred to as "Deaf." The capitalized "D" reflects pride in Deaf culture, as opposed to deaf with a lower case "d" which refers to a condition without the cultural implications. Proponents of identity-first language believe that person-first language separates them as a person from their disability. They feel this reinforces the idea that there is something stigmatizing about that disability, necessitating the desire to dissociate from it [15].

In the healthcare literature, person-first language is more frequently utilized for children with disabilities than for those without disabilities (e.g., "typically developing child" or "nondisabled children" [23]. Proponents of identity-first language argue that there should be parity between children with disabilities and those without disabilities. They feel the appropriate choice would be to treat all children equally, including in the way to which they are referred [23]. Some have argued that, while the intention of person-first language is theoretically sound, it may have been an overcorrection for previously used problematic language in describing people with disabilities [15, 23].

Language Pitfalls

Language can unintentionally reinforce problematic attitudes about disability. Euphemistic terms, such as "differently abled" or "handicapable," are perceived as patronizing. Use of euphemisms may be reflective of an underlying attitude that there is something inherently wrong or tragic about disability. Another example involves categorizing people with disabilities and those who love them as exceptional. This seemingly positive language is actually indicative of negative attitudes about disability. This attitude reinforces that disability is terrible to live with and surviving with it or loving someone with a disability is a superhuman accomplishment [26]. Extolling a parent for loving a child with a disability implies that the parent had to overcome a tremendous hurdle to care for their child, rather than recognizing that loving a child with a disability is as easy and natural as the love between any parent and child.

As discussed previously, "special needs" is a term that is used widely throughout healthcare when referring to children with disabilities; however, this language has been criticized for implying that children with disabilities are different from other children and that it is euphemistic to refer to them as "special." It is also problematic to view those with disabilities as inspirational. Identifying people with disabilities as an inspiration reflects a tacit attitude of superiority. People with disabilities can lead lives that are as full and meaningful as anyone else, and they do not exist to make people without disabilities feel better about themselves or to act as a gratitude reminder for others. Stella Young articulates this concept very well in her TED Talk, "I'm not your inspiration, thank you very much" [26].

There is also an insider/outsider distinction in language surrounding disability. Some people with disabilities have adopted terms that are otherwise considered offensive. For example, individuals with physical disabilities may refer to themselves or others with similar conditions as "crips," "quads," or "gimps" [15]. While acceptable when used by individuals who have these types of physical impairments, this terminology is inappropriate when used by nondisabled outsiders (Table 2). It should not be adopted by the nondisabled, in spite of the fact that one may hear those with disabilities using it [15].

Reconciling Models of Disability and Terminology

The language used to describe disability is intertwined with and reflective of the various models of disability [15]. Derogatory terms are reflective of a moral model that held that those with disabilities were inferior. The language of the medical model reflects an emphasis on the perceived deficit where people are referred to as simply their diagnosis. Person-first language is reflective of the social model whereby the person's humanity and individuality are emphasized and their disability is, literally, secondary. Identity-first language is reflective of the minority model of disability where diversity is valued and people identify their disability as an integral part of who they are.

The language of the moral and medical models has been dismissed as inappropriate in contemporary society. However, tension between the language of the social model (person-first language) and the minority model (identity-first language) can cause providers to be confused about appropriate terminology. At this time, the preferred approach is to default to person-first language in clinical interactions. When circumstances and relationships allow, ask a person how they prefer to be addressed. An understanding of the different paradigms in disability-related language facilitates awareness and allows providers to be more sensitive to how a person prefers to refer to herself. In turn, this understanding also prepares providers for such a conversation when the opportunity presents itself.

Disability and Health

The WHO defines health as "as state of complete physical, mental and social well-being and not merely the absence of disease or infirmity" [31]. There has been a long-standing and widespread perception that disability is equivalent to illness and is incompatible with health, but this is not the case [18]. People with disabilities may have health conditions that contribute to poor health, but disability by

Table 2 Communication Themes that may Contribute to Ableism in Dental Practice. Courtesy of Espinoza K, Heaton L, Baylor C, 2018

Theme	Examples	Rationale
Pity	"I feel so bad for her." "She suffers from autism." "The patient is a 14 year old boy afflicted with cerebral palsy."	Pity often implies tragedy that one is less than human due to a disability and therefore needs sympathy. Disability advocates have long spoken out about the problematic nature of pity [27]. The terms "suffers from" and "afflicted with" imply tragedy as well. In the medical record, it is more appropriate to list/name the diagnosis without this subjective terminology
Awe and inspiration	"You're such an inspiration." "You're such a good parent; I don't know how you do it." "What a special girl." "You've overcome so much!"	While well-deserved praise is generally appreciated, congratulatory remarks for basic everyday activities are likely to be perceived as condescending [28]. Praising and being inspired by "overcoming" a disability can send a message that disability makes one less than and that inspiration comes from overcoming this less than status [29]
Denial and minimization	"There's no way you're disabled." "She looks normal to me." "I don't see disability."	Children with disabilities will have varying levels of how important disability is to their self-identity. This will change over time as a child ages. Denial of one's personal identity or experience of disability can feel paternalistic that the provider cannot trust and/or does not respect the expertise of a disabled person about their own body and environmental circumstances [30]. Additionally, the claim that one does "not see disability" can send the message that they are not seeing the whole person and/or their unique needs
Assumptions and generalizations	"He has cerebral palsy; he won't be able to understand you." "All people with disabilities want…" "Autistic patients are really hard to treat."	There is considerable diversity among people with disabilities, including among those with the identical diagnoses. Generalizations about people with disabilities can lead to incorrect assumptions about their abilities [30]. One should not assume that one type of disability implies another type of disability (such as a physical disability implying an intellectual disability)
Infantilization	"Are you ready to get your teethies cleaned today?"	Acting as if people with disabilities are younger than they actually are, such as speaking in baby talk when not age appropriate, can be seen as condescending and denying of full personhood [30]

definition does not mean that the person is unhealthy [7]. There is increasing recognition that, while some disabilities are associated with conditions that negatively impact health, disability is not the same as illness and disabled people can be perfectly healthy [18]. Additionally, health is not simply the absence of disease; rather it is indicative of complete well-being. Well-being for people with disabilities has been widely overlooked. A more robust notion of health and well-being can be conceptualized as we move away from the medical model, seeing people with disabilities as more than their conditions.

People with intellectual disabilities experience poorer health than their nondisabled peers, and those discrepancies are readily apparent early in their lives [32]. The MCHB created measures for assessing the quality of health services that CSHCN have access to, yet less than 20% achieve the standards of high-quality care [3]. This is important not only for the well-being of children, but it is particularly critical given the well-established connection between childhood health and health in adulthood [3].

Social Determinants of Health

Social determinants of health are the socioeconomic conditions that influence health. These include factors such as education, income, housing, the social and physical environment, and access to healthcare [33]. Social determinants of health play a significant role in health inequities [34]. They affect cognitive, social, and emotional development in children [33]. Social determinants are associated with an increase in developmental disabilities due to the profound influence that social determinants have on child development [33]. The effects not only impact childhood health but have subsequent implications throughout adulthood [35]. Children with intellectual disabilities are more likely to experience low socioeconomic status (SES), a known social determinant of health [32]. Low SES has been shown to account for a 20–50% increase in the risk of poor mental and physical health in children with intellectual disabilities [32]. The social determinants of health also lend credence to the importance of family-centered care in improving the health of children with disabilities individually and in mitigating health disparities more broadly [33].

Barriers & Disparities

Disparities refer to differences in health status that result from discrimination, lack of access, or systematic exclusion from services. Disparities are not associated with biological factors [8]. The United Nations Convention on Rights of Persons with Disabilities calls for the "highest attainable standard of health" for people with disabilities [36]. In 2002, nearly two decades ago, the Surgeon General of the United States released the report *Closing the Gap*, outlining the disparities encountered by those with intellectual disabilities and calling for improvements and broad systematic improvement to combat those disparities [37]. Unfortunately, they still exist.

Barriers to healthcare for people with disabilities include financial barriers such as lack of insurance coverage, high out-of-pocket expenses, and high deductibles [38]. These financial barriers to healthcare disproportionately financially burden CSHCN and their families due to their significant healthcare needs [38]. Other barriers include lack of access to healthcare services, physical barriers, and limited knowledge of or experience with disability on the part of healthcare providers [18]. Compared to nondisabled people, people with disabilities are less likely to find a healthcare provider that can meet their needs. They are also more likely to report being treated poorly by a healthcare provider or being denied care [7]. These barriers result in people with disabilities having poor access to care and unmet healthcare needs [7].

Transition

Transition can be difficult for children and adolescents with special needs. Small transitions may involve changing from one activity or setting to another during the course of the day. More significant life transitions such as changing schools, living situations, or healthcare providers can be even more challenging. One major challenge that all CSHCN face is transition from pediatric to adult medical and dental care. One of the goals of the MCHB is to ensure that both families and providers facilitate transition of children with disabilities to adult providers and services [2]. Each patient's experience with this process is different. Some adolescents feel it is appropriate to transition to an adult dental provider, as the pediatric dental environment can be infantilizing [39]. However, both parents and clinicians find it difficult to find adult dental providers who are comfortable caring for patients with special needs and accept Medicaid insurance [39, 40]. While dentists agree that transitioning adolescents with special needs from pediatric to adult care is important, both providers and families view pediatric and general dentists as key in facilitating the transition of adolescents with special needs to adult dental care [39, 40].

Disability and Oral Health

People with intellectual disabilities have poorer oral health when compared to the general population, and they have more untreated dental disease. Interestingly, those with moderate to severe intellectual disabilities have better oral hygiene than those with mild intellectual disabilities [41]. This is likely due to increased assistance received by those with moderate and severe intellectual disabilities [41]. These findings are particularly concerning given that approximately 85% of people with intellectual disabilities have mild intellectual disabilities [42].

Dental care is routinely reported as the greatest unmet need among CSHCN [43, 44]. These disparities are further impacted by SES. CSHCN who are enrolled in Medicaid are less likely to receive preventive dental care than those with private insurance, and they have higher caries rates [43, 45]. Frequently, parents do not realize that preventive dental care is needed [43–45]. Behaviors and sensory sensitivities of CSHCN are frequently barriers to providing homecare and to establishing a dental home [44]. CSHCN who are uninsured and have more complex needs are even less likely to receive dental care [45]. Dentists report that Medicaid does not reimburse at levels that are commensurate with the additional time required to care for children with complex special needs [45]. It has been established that unmet dental needs for children with special needs are lower when Medicaid reimbursement rates are higher, reflecting the implications of inadequate reimbursement on access [45].

Dental care is clearly an unmet need for children with disabilities. Dental providers are able to mitigate this need, but they are also well positioned to help children with disabilities and their families in meaningful ways beyond simply providing dental care. Dental providers touch on the topics of diet, hygiene, behavior, and routines, all of which can deeply affect children with disabilities and their families. Sharing this knowledge with children and families provides support for improved oral health and overall well-being.

Recommendations to Improve Access

There are multiple potential avenues to improve oral health and access for children with disabilities.

- Integrate oral health promotion and screening into the community [41].
- Partner with early intervention programs to help connect children with a dental home and share the need for early preventive dental care [44].
- Advocate for increased Medicaid reimbursement for medically complex children [38].
- Increase healthcare provider experience with people who have disabilities [17].

Challenges to Research with People with Disabilities

People with intellectual disabilities have had atrocities committed against them in the name of research. Examples include the Willowbrook Hepatitis Study and the Vipeholm Study. In the Willowbrook Study, institutionalized residents of the Willowbrook School were intentionally infected with hepatitis to understand its course and evaluate potential treatments [46]. In the Vipeholm Study, people with intellectual disabilities were intentionally fed various forms of carbohydrates, including sticky toffee between meals, to gain information about the caries process [47]. Many of the studies where people with intellectual disabilities were subject to this type of abuse were conducted to benefit the nondisabled.

Today, regulation through the institutional review board process has largely eliminated those abuses, but people with intellectual disabilities are often not meaningfully included in research to benefit those with intellectual disabilities.

This leaves a lack of evidence regarding best practices for care of this population. Quality research is needed to understand the health status of people with disabilities and inform best practices for diagnosis, treatment, and prevention. Existing best practices for those without disabilities are applied, but they do not always translate to this population. For example, in dentistry, altered recall intervals, preventive protocols, or behavioral approaches may better suit the needs of people with intellectual disabilities, but the evidence base is limited. Many clinical research studies are conducted under ideal clinical conditions, with compliant patients and long-term follow-up. When working with people with intellectual disabilities, it is frequently not possible to conduct research with this level of control.

There are a multitude of challenges in conducting research with individuals with intellectual disabilities. Challenges include identifying and sampling this population, consent for treatment, cooperation, compliance with protocols, and follow-up. Given the difficulty in identifying and accessing this population, it is challenging to accurately determine their health status. Enrollment is also hampered by an inability of many patients to provide consent. There are guidelines for consent with other vulnerable populations, such as those with Alzheimer's disease; however, they do not exist for those with intellectual disabilities [48].

It is difficult to make progress in mitigating barriers and disparities without data and a more accurate and comprehensive understanding of health status, barriers, and outcomes for people with disabilities [7]. This has led to a call by the WHO to increase health research focused on people with disabilities [7].

Current oral health data suggest that CSHCN receive less preventive care, less restorative care, and more extractions, and they have higher rates of gingivitis and periodontal disease [41]. This clearly reflects that our current practices are inadequate to meet the unique needs of this population. To fully understand the oral health status of people with intellectual disabilities and develop best practices that will result in meaningful improvements in their oral health, efforts must focus on fully inclusive participation in good quality, ethical research.

Key Concepts in Caring for Children with Special Healthcare Needs

Neurodiversity

Neurodiversity is the concept that humans vary considerably in neurological function and processing, and this variety is desirable like other forms of diversity. This perspective contrasts with the view that neurological differences are problematic deficiencies that need to be fixed. Instead, neurological differences are embraced and celebrated as part of humanity [49]. For example, people with intellectual disabilities or people with autism whose brains may function differently than those who are neurotypical should be valued for their unique perspectives and contributions.

Strengths-Based Approach

The strengths-based approach to care of CSHCN focuses on understanding the strengths of individuals and families and builds upon those to achieve positive outcomes. It seeks to understand, support, and leverage the competencies of people with disabilities. This contrasts with a deficit-based approach, where the focus is limitations. The deficit-based approach is rooted in the medical model, where the focus is on correcting impairments [50]. When working with children with disabilities and their families in the dental setting, a strengths-based approach is ideal. Members of the dental team should seek out areas of child and family success and competency and build from there.

Patient- and Family-Centered Care

A core tenet in the care of CSHCN is patient- and family-centered care. Historically this concept was known as family-centered care, but the term has been modified to reflect an emphasis on including the child in the partnership in a developmentally appropriate manner [51]. Patient- and family-centered care views the relationship between the provider and the family as a partnership [51, 52]. Just as teeth do not exist independently from children, children do not exist independently from families. Therefore, it is critical to include the families of children with disabilities in their care. Families know the child best and are an invaluable resource in understanding CSHCN. They have a keen knowledge of the child's medical and dental history, motivations, strengths, and challenges. Professionals come and go in the lives of CSHCN, but families are with them the majority of the time, and those relationships endure even as the child ages into adulthood [51]. Furthermore, the care that the family provides every day has much more of an impact than what clinicians do during an appointment once every 6 months. For a healthcare intervention to be meaningful, the family must be included.

The best way to foster a lifetime of oral health for a child with disabilities is to develop good practices and healthy attitudes in childhood. To promote lifelong habits, it is crucial to engage the family early in life and to support them as the primary influence on their child. Families that are well supported and informed are more capable of providing an excellent foundation for their child.

The core concepts of patient- and family-centered care are:

- Treating patients and families with dignity and respect
- Sharing complete and unbiased information
- Allowing patients and families to participate in care and decisions
- Collaborating with patients and families in the delivery of care and in facility and program design, professional education, and policy development [52]

Providers have the most meaningful impact through the inclusion and support of the family. Patient- and family-centered care has been shown to improve outcomes, overall satisfaction, healthcare experiences, and resource utilization, and it decreases healthcare costs [51].

Team Care

Given the vast and varied needs of CSHCN, team care is a common approach for healthcare delivery in this population [53]. The benefits of providing care in a team model are increased quality of care, decreased error and duplication of services, increased cost-effectiveness and efficiency, provision of both medical and psychosocial components of healthcare, improved family convenience and satisfaction, increased collaboration, development of innovative approaches and solutions, and increased professional development for those on the team [53]. *Multiple disciplines* is the general term for a team approach to medical care. There are four types of teams under that umbrella term [53]. The types of teams are unidisciplinary/intradisciplinary, multidisciplinary, interdisciplinary, and transdisciplinary [53]. The terms multidisciplinary and interdisciplinary are commonly used interchangeably.

Unidisciplinary or intradisciplinary teams are those with multiple members, all of whom are from the same discipline, but they may collaborate together. An example would be multiple dental providers working together as a team. This could be a group pediatric dental practice where providers collaborate to share skills and expertise, a general dentist and a hygienist who work together to care for patients with disabilities, or dentists from various specialties working together. That could involve a pediatric dentist, an orthodontist, and an oral surgeon collaborating to provide care to a child with a special need.

Multidisciplinary teams are those where there are professionals of different disciplines. Team members may evaluate the patient together or create a care plan together, but each member continues to work in her own discipline and assess and treat independently [53]. Typically, these teams are hierarchical with someone from a given discipline, usually a physician, being the lead [53]. These teams are viewed as additive, equivalent to the sum of the disciplines that comprise them [53]. This is a common way for cleft lip and palate or craniofacial teams to function.

Interdisciplinary teams aim to be more interactive than multidisciplinary teams [53]. They are more egalitarian than hierarchical between disciplines [53]. Assessment and treatment are typically coordinated between members of the team, and all members of the team share their unique perspectives from their disciplines with the goal of generating a care plan that is agreed upon by the team and the responsibility of the entire team to execute [53]. These types of teams are ideally more than the sum of their individual components because of the inherent collaboration [53]. Interdisciplinary teams are relatively uncommon but may exist in a clinic focused on a given condition, such as Down syndrome, cleft lip and palate, or a craniofacial team [53].

Transdisciplinary teams are the most integrated team model. In transdisciplinary teams, the team members think outside the confines of their own discipline and aim to work together to formulate new approaches and solutions to complex challenges

[53]. Key components of transdisciplinary teams are *role release*, the recognition that another team member may be better suited for a given task, and *role expansion*, the acquisition of new expertise that expands the knowledge and skills set of a provider beyond her discipline and previous training [53]. Transdisciplinary care in the context of children with developmental disabilities is an aspirational goal and has not been studied.

A helpful metaphor in understanding these types of teams is fruit in different forms. A unidisciplinary team is a fruit bowl of a single type of fruit, such as a bowl of oranges. Each discipline is contained and similar to those by which it is surrounded. A multidisciplinary team is a fruit bowl with a variety of fruits: oranges, apples, strawberries, and pineapple. There are a variety of types of fruit, or disciplines, and they are together, but each is still distinct and can be taken in or out without much consequence. An interdisciplinary team is a fruit salad, where the skins and peels have been removed like the boundaries between disciplines. There is a melding of flavors of the fruit and juices, the various types of fruit are still readily identifiable, but they meld and enhance one another. Similarly the disciplines are still identifiable and operating in their own discipline, but barriers are broken down, and they are enhancing each other and far more comingled. A transdisciplinary team is like a smoothie, the boundaries between types of fruit are gone, as are those between disciplines with role release and role expansion. The fruit is so well integrated that they are no longer identifiable as their component parts or even as fruit. The sum of the parts is beyond enhancing each other, but it has created a new entity; it is now a smoothie not resembling the fruit from which it was made. In a transdisciplinary team, boundaries between professions are gone, and a new entity is derived from the disciplines that compose it [54].

Universal Design

The impact of disability on a person is not singularly a result of her condition. It is the relationship between the condition and her social and physical environment. Universal design is the concept wherein the products and the environment are created and designed to be accessible to the greatest number of people. This minimizes the disabling effects of a condition [55]. The key components of universal physical or social design are [55, 56]:

- Equitable use—useful for people with diverse abilities.
- Flexibility—accommodates range of preferences and abilities.
- Simple and intuitive use—can be understood by people of all abilities.
- Perceptible information—communicates information regardless of sensory abilities.
- Tolerance of error—minimizes adverse consequences of unintended actions.
- Low physical effort—can be used easily with minimal fatigue.
- Size and space for approach and use—useful for a variety of body sizes, postures, and levels of mobility.

Universal design is distinct from accessibility. Accessibility tends to focus on improving physical access, predominately for wheelchair users. Making environments more physically accessible is certainly a large step in the right direction, but proponents of universal design would argue that it does not go far enough. One limitation of accessibility is that it does not typically maximize use for all people [55]. It is predominantly focused on physical access and not thoughtful about products and environments being usable by individuals with diverse abilities. For example, while a movie theater may be physically accessible to someone who uses a wheelchair, the electronic ticket purchasing system may not be clear and easy to use for someone with a visual impairment or an intellectual disability. Another limitation of accessibility is that it tends to promote separateness of people with disabilities [55]. Accessibility is routinely focused on separate entrances, seating areas, or the use of specialized equipment and modifications. These require the person with the disability to be physically and consequently socially segregated. They may also create the need to use the product or environment differently. Utilizing the example of the movie theater, there may be seats designated as accessible to those who utilize wheelchairs, but they are in a certain area with a certain configuration. A person who uses a wheelchair can come into the theater and watch the movie, so it is considered accessible. However, movie theaters do not typically incorporate universal design. Universal design enables a person utilizing a wheelchair to experience the environment in a manner similar to others. She is able to select seat in a location she prefers that accommodates the group with whom she attends the movie. Theater design that is only wheelchair accessible may force the individual to sit in a certain section and configuration, which contributes to physical and social separation.

Alternatively, universal design promotes the inclusive use of products and the environment by people with a range of abilities without segregation or modification. Ideally, universal design is incorporated from the time a product or environment is conceived. This ensures that it is integral to the design, rather than a modification after the fact.

Universal design can be readily incorporated into a dental practice:

- Installation of lever handles instead of doorknobs as they require less dexterity to use.
- Closed captioning and large print facilitate understanding of audio and written messages.
- Headphones provide pleasant sounds or block out unpleasant ones.
- Adjustable volume and light make the experience more accommodating to those with sensory sensitivities.
- Family restrooms are beneficial to families with young children and also provide adequate room for an older child with a disability who may need assistance in toileting or who may wear diapers.
- Ramped curbs are helpful for wheelchairs, strollers, and bags with wheels.

Universal design aims to make the environment more successful for all people, whether a person in a wheelchair, a parent with a stroller, or someone wheeling a suitcase. Small design modifications can make the environment more accessible and comfortable for all.

Case-Based Scenario

Patient

Amy is a 9-year-old girl with cerebral palsy who presents for a recall dental visit. She utilizes a power wheelchair, has an intellectual disability, is hypertonic with limbs in a flexed position, and has limited fine motor skills. Here we discuss the differences between a dental visit to an accessible and a universally designed dental office.

Accessible Dental Office

Amy is scheduled on a Tuesday morning. This is not an ideal appointment for her mother, but the office only sees patients with special needs on certain days at certain times. The office is unable to obtain a current weight due to her wheelchair. She is transferred to the dental chair for her dental visit. When she needs to go to the restroom midway through her prophylaxis, she is transferred back to her wheelchair and given a key to the shared restroom down the hall in the medical office building where the dental office is located. Her mother uses the key to open the doorknob, and there is an accessible stall in the bathroom where her mother is able to assist her in using the restroom. It is challenging due to the limited space. She returns to the dental operatory and is transferred back to the dental chair. She is fatigued by the end of the appointment because of the way her body fits on the dental chair with her hypertonic flexed limbs. Amy is caries-free and will return in 6 months for her next recall.

Universally Designed Dental Office

Amy's mom is able to schedule her dental appointment for a Thursday afternoon. This works best for their family because Amy's mom doesn't work on Thursdays and did not have to take time off of work. Amy also tolerates outside-the-home activities better in the afternoon. Amy is able to independently get on the scale in her wheelchair so she can be weighed (Fig. 3). Amy is taken to an operatory with adequate room to place her wheelchair next to the dental unit and a Specialized Care Co® Stay N Place® chair cushion in the dental chair (Fig. 4). She is given the option of either staying in her wheelchair or transferring to the dental chair with the cushion, which will support her flexed limbs. She elects to stay in her wheelchair, which can recline to allow for prophylaxis and exam. When she needs to use the restroom midway through her prophylaxis, she does not need to transfer back into her wheelchair. She is able to wheel herself down the hall to the accessible family restroom located in the dental office, and she is able to independently open the door with a lever handle to let herself into the restroom (Fig. 5). The

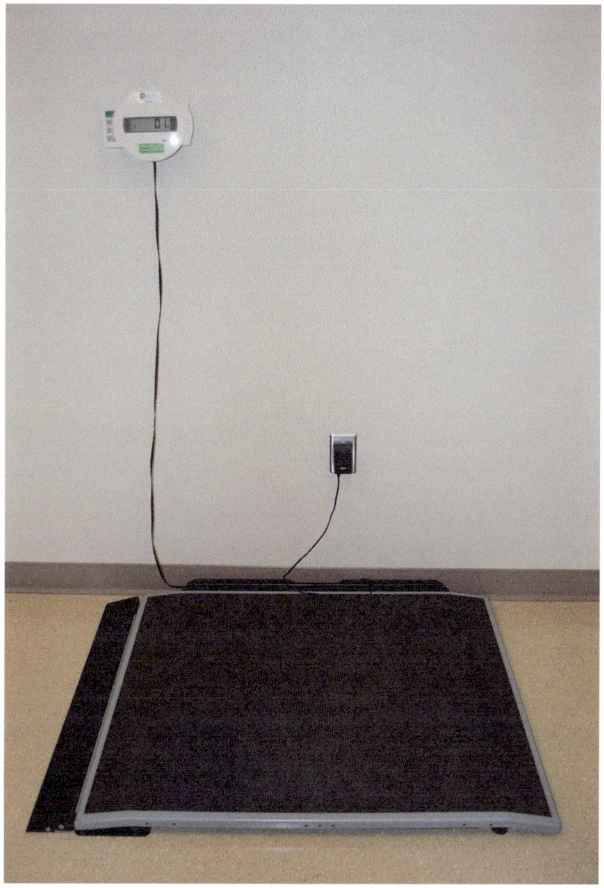

Fig. 3 Wheelchair accessible scale

single-stalled family restroom is large enough for her mom to easily assist her. Amy is able to let herself out of the restroom, return to the operatory independently, and to resume her appointment without the need to transfer again. She is comfortable throughout the appointment, since she was able to stay in her chair that provides appropriate support for her body. Amy is caries-free and will return in 6 months for her next recall.

Accessible Versus Universal Design

In the case that describes an office with accessible design, Amy is able to have a dental recall visit and access the dental office. In the case with universal design, Amy is able to utilize the dental office in a way that better meets her needs and to interact with the environment more similarly to the way someone without a

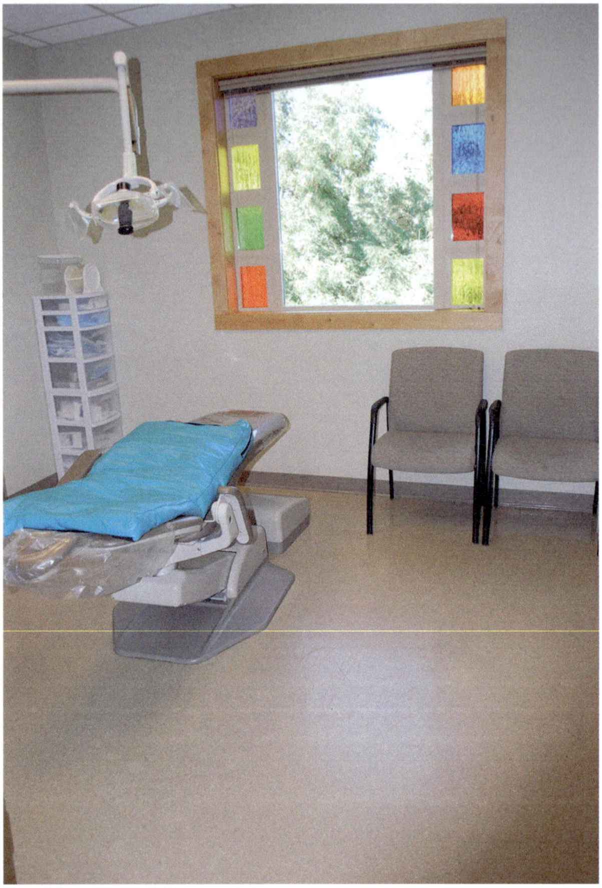

Fig. 4 Specialized Care Co® Stay N Place® chair cushion

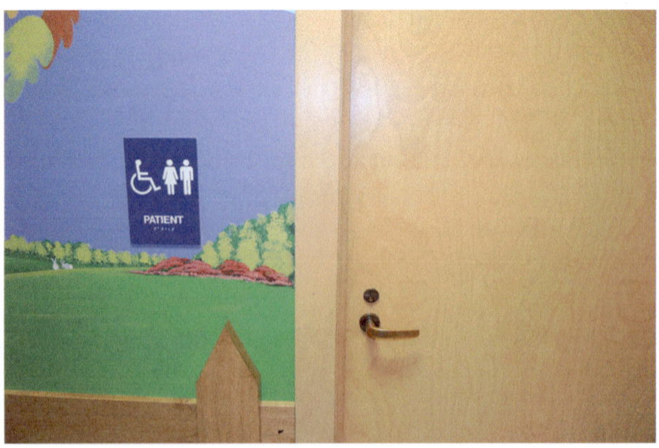

Fig. 5 Lever-style door handle

disability would. The idea behind universal design is to make the environment usable by the greatest number of people. For example, in the accessible office, Amy was able to obtain an appointment, albeit not at a preferred day and time. In the universally designed office, Amy had the opportunity to visit the dentist during the same timeframes as any other patient. A wheelchair scale allows those with and without wheelchairs to be weighed using the same space and equipment. In both offices she was able to receive a prophylaxis and recall exam, but in the universally designed office, she had the option of staying in her wheelchair or using a cushion to support her body in the dental chair. Amy is able to visit the dentist and receive dental services in both offices, but the universally designed facility better meets her needs. It allows her to be more independent and facilitates an experience that is similar to others.

Conclusion

- People with disabilities face a multitude of barriers to care and healthcare disparities. To mitigate barriers and disparities, there is a need for more research focused on this population, increased provider training, and increased focus on outreach, health promotion, and preventive services for people with disabilities.
- The contemporary medical and dental perspective is moving away from older models and beliefs about disability. Current terminology reflects a strengths-based approach and equates disability with diversity, not illness.
- Compassionate care of CSHCN requires that dental providers celebrate neurodiversity, seek out patient strengths, involve patients and families in care, embrace team care, and adopt elements of universal design in practice.

References

1. American Academy of Pediatric Dentistry. Overview. Pediatr Dent. 2017;39(6):5–7.
2. HRSA Maternal and Child Health. Children with special health care needs. https://mchb.hrsa.gov/maternal-child-health-topics/children-and-youth-special-health-needs. Accessed 10 Feb 2018.
3. Bethell CD, Newacheck PW, Fine A, Strickland BB, Antonelli RC, Wilhelm CL, Hornberg LE. Optimizing health and health care systems for children with special needs using the life course perspective. Matern Child Health J. 2014;18:467–77.
4. American Academy of Pediatric Dentistry. Definition of special health care needs. Pediatr Dent. 2017;39(6):16.
5. World Health Organization. Disabilities. http://www.who.int/topics/disabilities/en/. Accessed 6 Jan 2018.
6. Dunn DS. The social psychology of disability. 1st ed. New York, NY: Oxford University Press; 2015.
7. World Health Organization. Disability and health fact sheet. http://www.who.int/mediacentre/factsheets/fs352/en/. Accessed 6 Jan 2018.

8. Krahn GL, Hammond L, Turner A. A cascade of disparities: health and health care access for people with intellectual disabilities. Ment Retard Dev Disabil Res Rev. 2006;12:70–82.
9. Centers for Disease Control and Prevention. Facts about developmental disabilities. https://www.cdc.gov/ncbddd/developmentaldisabilities/facts.html. Accessed 6 Jan 2018.
10. American Academy of Intellectual and Developmental Disabilities. Intellectual disability definition. http://aaidd.org/intellectual-disability/definition - .WlZMuiOZNsM. Accessed 6 Jan 2018.
11. Goodley D. Disability studies: an interdisciplinary introduction. 2nd ed. London: SAGE; 2017.
12. Sisti DA. Naturalism and the social model of disability: allied or antithetical? J Med Ethics. 2015;41:553–6.
13. Baker JP, Lang B. Eugenics and the origins of autism. Pediatrics. 2017;140(2):e20171419.
14. Mukherjee S. TED Talk: Soon we'll cure diseases with a cell, not a pill. Available at https://www.ted.com/talks/siddhartha_mukherjee_soon_we_ll_cure_diseases_with_a_cell_not_a_pill. Accessed 22 Dec 2017.
15. Dunn DS, Andrews EE. Person-first and identity-first language. Am Psychol. 2015;70(3):255–64.
16. Goering S. Revisiting the relevance of the social model of disability. Am J Bioeth. 2010;10(1):54–5.
17. Albrecht GL, Devlieger PJ. The disability paradox: high quality of life against all odds. Soc Sci Med. 1999;48:977–88.
18. Shakespeare T, Iezzoni LI, Groce NE. Disability and the training of health professionals. Lancet. 2009;374(9704):1815–6.
19. World Health Organization. International classification of functioning, disability and health. http://www.who.int/classifications/icf/en/. Accessed 6 Jan 2018.
20. Dawson SL. International classification of functioning, disability, and health. In: Austin DR, McCormick BP, editors. Perspectives on recreational therapy. 1st ed. Urbana, IL: Sagamore Venture; 2017.
21. Faulks D, Norderyd J, Molina G, Phadraif CM, Scagnet G, Eschevins C, Hennequin M. Using the international classification of functioning, disability and health (ICF) to describe children referred to special care of paediatric dental services. PLoS One. 2013;8(4):e61993.
22. Rosenbaum P, Gorter JW. The 'f-words' in childhood disability: I swear this is how we should think! Child Care Health Dev. 2011;38(4):457–63.
23. Gernsbacher MA. Editorial perspective: the use of person-first language in scholarly writing may accentuate stigma. J Child Psychol Psychiatry. 2017;58(7):859–61.
24. Special Olympics. Rosa's Law. https://www.specialolympics.org/Regions/north-america/News-and-Stories/Stories/Rosa-s-Law.aspx. Accessed 10 Feb 2018.
25. Federal Register. Rosa's Law. https://www.federalregister.gov/documents/2017/07/11/2017-14343/rosas-law. Accessed 10 Feb 2018.
26. Young S. TED Talk: I am not your inspiration, thank you very much. Available at https://www.ted.com/talks/stella_young_i_m_not_your_inspiration_thank_you_very_much. Accessed 24 Feb 2018.
27. Stramondo J. How an ideology of pity is a social harm to people with disabilities. Soc Philos Today. 2010;26:121–34.
28. Chrisman WL. A reflection on inspiration: A recuperative call for emotion in disability studies. J Lit Cult Disabil Stud. 2011;5(2):173–84.
29. Harbour WS, Boone R, Heath EB, Ledbetter SG. "Overcoming" in disability studies and African American culture: implications for higher education. In: Kerschbaum SL, Eisenman LT, Jones JM, editors. Negotiating disability: disclosure and higher education. Ann Arbor: University of Michigan Press; 2017. p. 149–69.
30. Keller RM, Galgay CE. Microaggressive experiences of people with disabilities. In: Sue DW, editor. Microaggressions and marginality: manifestation, dynamics, and impact. Hoboken, NJ: Wiley; 2010. p. 241–67.

31. World Health Organization. Constitution of WHO. http://www.who.int/about/mission/en/. Accessed 10 Feb 2018.
32. Emerson E, Brigham P. Exposure of children with developmental delay to social determinants of poor health: cross-sectional case record review study. Child Care Health Dev. 2014;41(2):249–57.
33. Edwards K, Towle PO, Levitz B. Incorporating life course theory and social determinants of health into the LEND curriculum. Matern Child Health J. 2014;18:431–42.
34. World Health Organization. Social determinants of health. http://www.who.int/social_determinants/sdh_definition/en/. Accessed 10 Feb 2018.
35. American Academy of Pediatrics. Community pediatrics: navigating the intersection of medicine, public health, and social determinants of children's health. Pediatrics. 2013;131(3):623–8.
36. UN Convention on Rights of Persons with Disabilities. Article 25 – Health. https://www.un.org/development/desa/disabilities/convention-on-the-rights-of-persons-with-disabilities/article-25-health.html. Accessed 6 Jan 2018.
37. Closing the gap: a national blueprint to improve the health of persons with mental retardation. https://stacks.cdc.gov/view/cdc/21851. Accessed 20 Feb 2018.
38. Bachman SS, Comeau M, Long TF. Statement of the problem: health reform, value-based purchasing, alternative payment strategies, and children and youth with special health care needs. Pediatrics. 2017;139:S89–98.
39. Cruz S, Neff J, Chi DL. Transitioning from pediatric to adult dental care for adolescents with special health care needs: adolescent and parent perspectives – part one. Pediatr Dent. 2015;37(5):442–6.
40. Bayarsaikhan Z, Cruz S, Neff J, Chi DL. Transitioning from pediatric to adult dental care for adolescents with special health care needs: dentist perspectives – part two. Pediatr Dent. 2015;37(5):447–51.
41. Owens PL, Kerker BD, Zigler E, Horwitz SM. Vision and oral health needs of individuals with intellectual disability. Ment Retard Dev Disabil Res Rev. 2006;12:28–40.
42. Healthy Place. Mild, moderate, severe intellectual disability differences. https://www.healthyplace.com/neurodevelopmental-disorders/intellectual-disability/mild-moderate-severe-intellectual-disability-differences/. Accessed 12 Feb 2018.
43. Kenney MK. Oral health care in CSHCN: state medicaid policy considerations. Pediatrics. 2009;124:S384–91.
44. Huebner CE, Chi DL, Masterson E, Milgrom P. Preventive dental health care experiences of preschool-age children with special health care needs. Spec Care Dentist. 2015;35(2):68–77.
45. McManus BM, Chi D, Carle A. State medicaid eligibility criteria and unmet preventive dental care need for CSHCN. Matern Child Health J. 2016;20:456–65.
46. Coleman CH, Menikoff JA, Goldner JA, Dubler NN. The ethics and regulation of research with human subjects. 1st ed. Newark, NJ: LexisNexis; 2005.
47. Krasse B. The Vipeholm dental caries study: recollections and reflections 50 years later. J Dent Res. 2001;80(9):1785–8.
48. Veenstra MY, Walsh PN, Valk H, Haveman MJ, Linehan C, Kerr MP, Weber G, Salvador-Carulla L, Carmen-Cara A, Azema B, Buono S, Germanavicius A, Tossebro J, Matta T, van Hove G, Moravec D. Sampling and ethical issues in a multicenter study on health of people with intellectual disabilities. J Clin Epidemiol. 2010;63:1091–100.
49. Baron-Cohen S. Editorial perspective: Neurodiversity – a revolutionary concept for autism and psychiatry. J Child Psychol Psychiatry. 2017;58(6):744–7.
50. Niemiec R, Shogren KA, Wehmeyer ML. Character strengths and intellectual and developmental disability: a strengths-based approach from positive psychology. Educ Train Autism Dev Disabil. 2017;52(1):13–25.
51. American Academy of Pediatrics. Patient- and family-centered care and the pediatrician's role. Pediatrics. 2012;129(2):394–404.
52. Institute for Patient- and Family-Centered Care. http://www.ipfcc.org/about/pfcc.html. Accessed 20 Feb 2018.

53. Patel DR, Pratt HD, Patel ND. Team processes and team care for children with developmental disabilities. Pediatr Clin N Am. 2008;55:1375–90.
54. Hahn EA, Carrol C, and De Bord JR. Personal communication. May 2014.
55. Imrie R. Universalism, universal design and equitable access to the build environment. Disabil Rehabil. 2012;34(10):873–82.
56. Bichenbach J. Universally design social policy: when disability disappears? Disabil Rehabil. 2014;36(16):1320–7.

A Systematic Approach to Creating a Dental Home for Children with Medical Complexities

Joseph P. Kelly and Barbara L. Sheller

Introduction

The Maternal and Child Health Bureau provided the "person first" definition of children with special health-care needs or CSHCN in 1998 [1]. Within this population, there is a notable subgroup of medically fragile children with concentrated health-care needs. Their medical home encompasses coordinated multispecialty care. Children with complex medical needs with at least one chronic condition resulting in increased utilization of health services, including medications, devices, and equipment to support outpatient functioning, are the subject of this chapter [2, 3]. The prevalence of children in this category ranges from 13% to 18% [4]. There is a broad range of type and degree of medical complexity within this group. Several authors have suggested continuing the "person first" nomenclature in designating this subset of CHSCN as children with medical complexities or CMC [5].

The rate of hospitalization admissions and relative medical complexities of children with multiple comorbidities has increased over the past two decades [6]. In the not too distant past, children with extreme premature birth, severe congenital anomalies, and unstable or rare medical conditions had a limited life expectancy and were infrequent visitors to an outpatient dental clinic. At present, most medically complex children survive and live outside of an institutional setting and present with gastrostomy tubes, tracheostomies, portable ventilators, CPAP/BiPAP machines, and implanted devices such as vagus nerve and deep brain stimulators, cardiac pacemakers, and cochlear implants, among others. The rate of death among children in the age group of 1–9 years directly associated with their chronic condition is much lower than is experienced in infants and young adults and adolescents with the same condition [7]. For instance, children with hypoplastic left heart syndrome who survive infancy now have about a 90% survival rate to age 18 years [8]. Due to medical,

J. P. Kelly (✉) · B. L. Sheller
Department of Dentistry, Seattle Children's Hospital, Seattle, WA, USA
e-mail: joseph.kelly@seattlechildrens.org

T. M. Nelson, J. R. Webb (eds.), *Dental Care for Children with Special Needs*,
https://doi.org/10.1007/978-3-030-10483-2_2

surgical, and technological advances, increasing numbers of medically complex children enter a phase in their lives when dental and oral care has risen in importance to the family as the child's medical conditions become stable and chronically managed.

Like their healthy peers, CMC benefit from dental homes that are medically appropriate and family-friendly. Professionally guided oral health services for children with CSHCN-CMC may be difficult to locate and access. Most dentists receive their general training with a focus on medical problems of adults and associated precautions for their dental management. Consequently, children presenting with multiple medical concerns may have seemed beyond the capacity for inclusion in most dental practices.

A common theme voiced by parents of children with a CMC is their desire to find dental providers for their children who offer careful and appropriate treatment without creating dental fear. They want their children to enjoy clean and healthy teeth like any other child. Our ability to achieve these goals relies both on our openness to match our dental knowledge and expertise to the needs of this subgroup of children and adapting dental encounter protocols to include additional considerations for the child with medical complexities. Our role is to collaborate with the child's family and medical team to support their quality of life and to prevent oral problems or their treatment from negatively affecting his health, well-being, or medical stability [9].

This chapter offers a systematic approach to establishing family-oriented, comprehensive, coordinated, and safe delivery of dental care for the child with medical complexities. We suggest that taking an individualized strength-based approach to assessment for children with complex medical conditions offers the safest foundation for the provision of care. Additionally, we identify components of the typical dental visit that can be modified to match patient strengths.

There are multiple valuable reference texts [10, 11, 12] and online resources [13] for the dental practitioner to guide considerations when providing dental care for persons with special needs. Every dental office library should contain a variety of such resources. The breadth and depth of their coverage will augment information in this chapter. The changing reality is that children with complex medical conditions present with a constellation of challenges and seldom have a single disease entity. There may or may not be a unifying diagnosis which can be neatly packaged to help guide care decisions. We will offer some specific considerations with the intention to inform an individualized preemptive approach to standardize the dental encounter. Providing a community-based dental home is a reasonable expectation and a growing necessity for children with complex medical conditions.

Creating a Collaborative Care Network for Children with Medical Complexity

Children with unstable, complex, or extremely uncommon medical conditions often locate their dental home within a university or a children's hospital where dentistry integrates readily into a team of various medical specialists. If the institution-associated dental home is a long distance from where they live, it is beneficial for the family to have a local dental resource available to coordinate with the hospital/university dental team on an as-needed basis. Access to a brief problem-focused visit with a local dental provider is an invaluable asset for assessment of acute problems.

Most children with medical complexities do not require hospital-based preventive dental services. When appropriate, we recommend co-management of routine preventive and restorative care with hospital-associated pediatric dental specialists for needed sedated dental care. Dental providers who do not elect to acquire hospital privileges should actively collaborate with a provider who can coordinate and complete hospital-based dental treatment. This person may be a competent dental colleague in the area or an institution-based dental practicioner. Unless the patient has an uncontrolled or advanced progressively debilitating medical condition, the patient's home community is the preferred location for routine preventive recalls and simple dental procedures. A general dentist with advanced general practice training or pediatric dental specialist in their local community is the appropriate provider for children with chronic but stable medical conditions. Table 1 offers one approach to locating the place of care for children with a complex medical condition. The child's state of health combined with interim and long-term treatment

Table 1 Site of dental care selection for children with medical complexity

Medical complexity	Hospital-associated practice	Community-based practice
Oncology patients	Under active treatment	Cancer survivors
Behaviorally complex (autism, ADHD, etc.)	Physically violent, unsafe for protective stabilization	All others
Transplant patients (solid organ or hematopoietic stem cell transplant)	Pretransplant period and 6 months posttransplant	Stable and greater than 6 months posttransplant
CSHCN-CMC with dental treatment requiring sedation/GA	Consult and treat. Transfer for ongoing preventive care after completion	Dental home for preventive and simple restorative care
Hematological or bleeding disorders (Sickle cell, hemophilia, von Willebrand's, beta thalassemia, pancytopenia, etc.)	Site of care for treatment requiring medical intervention (lab tests or infusions) before or after dental procedure(s)	Dental home for preventive and simple restorative care
Seizure disorder	Medically unstable, intractable seizures	Medically stable, well controlled
Ventilator dependent	Dental home if medically fragile	Dental home if medically stable
Planned congenital heart defect surgery	Pre-surgical sedated dental care	Dental home pre- and post-surgery
Progressively debilitating medical conditions (spinal muscular atrophy, etc.)	Medically unstable	Medically stable

needs suggests the most medically appropriate and family-friendly site for dental care.

Patient Assessment

Establish a Comprehensive Baseline of Medical and Dental History

Our role as the primary dentist is to collaborate with the child's family and medical team to identify any patient ability-related risks, evaluate these with known risks of proposed treatment, and modify dental protocols so as not to affect the child's medical stability. An accurate and complete history is the foundation for the provision of safe and appropriate care. It is a prudent practice to gather baseline medical and dental information before the child with a complex medical condition arrives for his first visit. A pediatric medical history form for starting this process is available from the American Academy of Pediatric Dentistry [14]. This health history is suitably comprehensive as an entry-level screening tool. Soliciting this information in advance of the first visit facilitates adequate time on the part of the parent/caregiver to complete the form, especially if past medical history is extensive. Some parents unintentionally filter medical history information to reveal only the aspects they deem relevant to what they think a dentist needs to know to care for their child's teeth. Inadvertent omissions can occur in an interview if the questions lack clarity or if there are interruptions. A residential caregiver who accompanies a child to their appointment may not know or have ready access to the details of the medical history. The primary care provider (PCP) or medical home is a comprehensive source of information about the child's medical and social history. In addition to the report provided by the family, collaborating with the child's primary medical provider for this information will ensure full disclosure of past medical history, allergies, and medications. This first contact with the child's PCP serves as a building block toward a vital working relationship with the child's medical home.

A timely review by the dentist before the initial visit may precipitate a follow-up phone interview with the parent or medical home to better understand the status of the health condition. Differentiating past from existing medical conditions under current treatment is useful. Exploring the nature of any recently encountered medical emergencies and hospitalizations reveals additional aspects of the child's medical status. This information assists in identifying any ability-related risk factors and facilitates preparedness should an emergency associated with their medical condition occur during the dental visit.

The medical history should also include the contact information for medical specialists caring for the patient (e.g., hematology, oncology, cardiology, endocrinology, nephrology, pulmonary medicine, rehabilitation medicine). Additional information may be required to explain clinical findings. For instance, age of patient at onset of disease or initiation of therapy, exposure to therapeutic radiation, and history of chemotherapy may correlate with dental and maxillofacial growth anomalies. Multidisciplinary collaboration may be required when planning invasive dental treatments or procedural sedation.

When significant past dental history exists, include these in the list of medical diagnoses. Identify date, type, and location of dental trauma, previous dental treatment under sedation or general anesthesia (GA), and any dental condition requiring periodic follow-ups such as root canal therapy, sedative fillings, dental trauma, and silver diamine fluoride application. Carry these forward in the clinic notes as ongoing/unresolved dental conditions to prompt timely and appropriate follow-up.

Be prepared to manage all emergencies in the dental office with attention to managing an in-office emergency related to the child's known condition. The patient with a seizure disorder may have a seizure, a patient with asthma may experience breathing difficulties, and a child with diabetes may become hypoglycemic. The morning huddle with clinical staff should identify these children as potential safety concerns and prompt individualized preparedness to manage any adverse event.

Medications

- Identify all daily and as-needed prescription medications and record dosage. Include homeopathic and alternative supplements taken regularly.
- If the medication list includes a "rescue medication" such as an as-needed antiepileptic or an inhaler, inquire as to its most recent use, and record the parental report of the agent's efficacy. Encourage families to bring rescue medications to all dental appointments.
- Record the hematologist's current bleeding management plan for children with bleeding disorders. Document experience of oral bleeding in response to challenges such as exfoliating primary teeth or extractions, and note type and effectiveness of bleeding control intervention(s).
- For patients with a history of metabolic bone disease, avascular necrosis, osteoporosis, or non-ambulatory children, inquire about past or current bisphosphonate use. It is easy for both caregiver and dentist to overlook monthly, quarterly, or semiannual administration of bisphosphonates when reviewing medications taken on a daily or as-needed basis.

Allergies

- Record all medication and non-medication allergies. Inquire about and record symptoms related to the reaction.
- Attempt to differentiate adverse medication reactions from actual allergic reactions. If in doubt of an allergy to local anesthetic or a dental material, a referral to identify the allergen is indicated.

- Identify indications to avoid any commonly prescribed or over-the-counter drugs used in dentistry (e.g., ketogenic diet restrictions).

Physical Evaluation

Observe and Document

- The child's level of functioning by noting how much physical assistance is needed: use of upper body limbs and stability while sitting, standing, and walking. The Gross Motor Functioning Classification Scale of cerebral palsy [15] is helpful in assessing this ability.
- Devices required for mobility: external orthopedic appliances (braces and splints), walker, wheelchair, or stroller.
- Portable devices such as supplemental oxygen tanks with attached nasal cannula, suction, or ventilator.
- Communication method: spoken language, American Sign Language, augmentative communication (pictures or storyboard), or assistive technologies such as computers, smartphones, or another communication device.
- Hearing: unimpaired, ear tubes, hearing aids, bone-anchored hearing devices (BAHA), cochlear implants.
- Vision: normal, low visual acuity, corrective lenses, cortical vision blindness.
- General appearance of hygiene, grooming, clothing, and condition of mobility devices.
- Other medical technologies: gastrostomy/jejunostomy, central venous catheters, tracheostomy, home mechanical ventilation, supplemental oxygen, pulse oximetry, CPAP/BiPAP, vagus nerve stimulator, chest physiotherapy vest.

Laboratory Evaluation

Medical laboratory assessments to follow the CMC's health status and therapeutic response are a standard part of the medical home or specialist's history and physical report. For some conditions, it is useful for the dental provider to review laboratory values when planning invasive dental procedures or predicting the level of support that will be needed following dental treatment.

Examples

- Glycosylated hemoglobin (HbA1c) for assessing control of diabetes
- Absolute neutrophil count (ANC) for neutropenic patients for determining the need for antibiotic prophylaxis
- Platelet counts for patients with thrombocytopenia to predict bleeding vulnerability
- The international normalized ratio (INR) for patients taking anticoagulant medications to evaluate procedural bleeding risk

For some CMC, consulting with their specialist(s) may be required to understand their status and readiness to undergo proposed dental treatment.

Setting Oral Health Goals

The parents are strong advocates for their child's smile and oral health. They do not accept, nor should they, that the oral health goal for their CMC should be less than that which is commonly endorsed for the typically developing child.

Ask the child and their parent about their dental goals for the near and long term. For the CMC, the process toward achieving these goals is often incremental. Influential factors include medical fragility, intellectual or developmental disability, and behavioral challenges. Examples of goals are: to accept a dental examination adequate to answer parent/caregiver questions about the child's oral health, establish a routine or periodicity of preventive dental services, or integrate dental and medical care. Goals initiated by a medical provider may include dental clearance for a future treatment or surgery or resuming dental care after recovery from illness, treatment, or social challenges.

Alteration of Dental Protocols: Ability Influenced Decision-Making

The Americans with Disabilities Act defines a person with a disability as "a person who has a physical or mental impairment that substantially limits one or more major life activity." The term "disability" in this context is relatively dichotomous. It is useful for the dentist to think of CMC as persons with variable abilities. A child's medical or behavioral diagnoses influence the initial dental ability level in addition to their age; physical, cognitive, or behavioral development; social belief; and support systems. By identifying these aspects of a child's capacity to adapt, the type and manner of dental care delivery can be customized to remain safe. Anticipating relevant elements of the dental encounter that may challenge the child's threshold ability helps prevent the dental treatment from detrimentally affecting their health and well-being.

Individualized alterations in practice early in the dental visit can be expected for the child with affected functional abilities. For the child with a medical complexity that does not affect their functional abilities, modifications of the protocol to account for condition-related ability variance may occur at a later point in the dental encounter such as when planning invasive treatment.

Baseline Ability and Risk Assessment

There are hundreds of complex chronic diseases of childhood. Handbooks on oral health and reference manuals for specialized care in dentistry are useful adjuncts for treatment planning, but cannot be relied upon as the sole support for decision-making. Due to the current health-care trend of expanding outpatient management of complex medical conditions, there may be features of the child's medical status or support technologies that are not included in such references. Identifying the relevant features of a child's medical condition and assessing an individualized ability threshold require current resources and information. While the dentist best understands dental procedures and protocols, the child's parent and medical team may have valuable input into what modifications are required. Equipped with this knowledge, the dental office can safely and efficiently meet many of these patients' preventive and restorative needs without undue delay.

When assessing the child's ability, the ultimate oral health goals should approximate those of the typically developing child. For the child with affected functional abilities, the difference in approach may be the degree and number of adaptations required. An approach that promotes adapting the current ability safely toward the next level is most likely to satisfy the family and lead to best results.

The baseline ability assessment connected with child's medical status or support technologies includes an evaluation of condition-related procedural risks that advises which precautions or modification in protocol is necessary. Table 2 is a partial list of commonly encountered risks that should be considered before performing any dental procedure. All offices should be prepared to manage the most common medical emergencies that can occur at any time with any patient or family member in the dental office. In addition, focused emergency preparation for each encounter is recommended based on the child's medical condition.

Special Considerations for Children with Ostomies

Gastrostomies and jejunostomies are skin openings in the stomach or jejunum that are maintained by the presence of an indwelling tube commonly referred to as a PEG, G-tube, MIC-KEY, J-Tube, or G-J tube. The purpose of these ostomies is to provide access to the gastrointestinal tract for nutrition, hydration, or medications for those who cannot tolerate oral intake. Restricted oral intake may be complete or partial and may be due to oral aversion, oromotor dysphagia, or an anatomic limitation such as esophageal stricture. It is essential to differentiate the indication for the gastrostomy to determine the safest approach to the most fundamental aspects of the dental visit.

Patients who take solids and thickened liquids orally with a G-tube used for supplemental nutrition, supplemental hydration, or administration of medications may tolerate typical dental procedures. It is imperative to discuss with the parent/caregiver the optimum positioning for the examination. At a child's first dental examination, the parent may not fully understand your proposed approach and to what degree their child will tolerate it. If the child arrives upright in their stroller or caregiver's arms, it is safe to assume this is a good starting point for positioning. The child may need to be examined in an upright or very slightly reclined position with ready and frequent suctioning. Children with dysphagia and a history of aspiration pneumonia are often challenged to manage their salivary secretions efficiently; lap exams or fully reclined positions are best avoided for these patients. If copious saliva is present, it may be necessary to add an additional dental assistant dedicated only to suctioning. During scaling and polishing procedures, moistened gauze pads

Table 2 Commonly encountered conditions and related risks

Related risks	Commonly encountered conditions
Aspiration	Oromotor dysphagia, 100% gastrostomy dependence for hydration, uses thickener for thin liquids, excessive salivation, gastroesophageal reflux, cyclic vomiting, tracheotomy
Spine at risk	Atlantoaxial instability, osteogenesis imperfecta, scoliosis
Increased sensitivity to UVA/UVB, ionizing radiation	UVA/UVB exposures—xeroderma pigmentosa Routine screening dental radiographs—Fanconi anemia, Gorlin syndrome, and hereditary retinoblastoma (use sparingly); ataxia telangiectasia (avoid)
Risk related to infection [16, 17, 18]	Aggressive management of dentoalveolar infection: poorly controlled diabetes (hemoglobin A1c > 7.6), sickle cell disease, neutropenia with ANC <1000/mm^3 Antibiotic prophylaxis for invasive procedures: cardiac conditions per American Heart Association (AHA) guidelines, high-dose immunosuppression, chemotherapy with ANC <500/mm^3, hereditary hemorrhagic telangiectasia with lung AVM, during first-year post-allogeneic hematopoietic stem cell transplant Consensus about antibiotic prophylaxis for these conditions is inconclusive but recommended when treating infected sites: neutropenia with ANC 500–1000/mm^3, VA shunts, sickle cell disease, indwelling central lines, dialysis catheters, chronic immunosuppression For patients requiring antibiotic prophylaxis, use banded space maintainers with caution (consider oral hygiene, follow-up compliance, etc.); distal shoe appliances contraindicated Full-coverage restorations necessary to avoid "spontaneous dental abscess formation"—dentinogenesis imperfecta, vitamin D-resistant rickets
Risk of increased bleeding	Congenital coagulopathy: von Willebrand's disease, hemophilias, platelet function disorder, Noonan syndrome Acquired coagulopathy: idiopathic, anticoagulants, drug side effects, thrombocytopenia, hemodialysis, liver disease, some herbal supplement side effects Capillary fragility: scurvy, severe malnutrition, chronic high-dose steroid use
Medication-related risks	Osteonecrosis of the jaws: bisphosphonates, denosumab Gingival hyperplasia—Dilantin, phenobarbital, calcium channel blocker antihypertensives, cyclosporine Adrenal suppression: chronic high-dose corticosteroids Aphthous ulcers: sirolimus, everolimus, dental products containing colophony or sodium lauryl sulfate Increased bronchial secretion thickening: diphenhydramine (use with caution in asthmatics) Defects in platelet aggregation: aspirin, nonsteroidal anti-inflammatory drugs, divalproex sodium, omega-3 fatty acids, ketogenic diet, some herbal supplements
Elevated risk of in-office medical emergency	Intractable or poorly controlled seizure disorders, reactive airway disease, symptomatic cardiac disease, history of frequent aspiration, bleeding disorders, untreated moyamoya disease, sickle cell disease

(continued)

Table 2 (continued)

Related risks	Commonly encountered conditions
Risk associated with delivery of dental care	Waterline microbial aerosols—cystic fibrosis, less than 6 months post-hematopoietic stem cell transplant Sonic and ultrasonic scaler, high-speed handpiece without rubber dam isolation should be used with caution for children with dysphagia, cystic fibrosis, and moderate to severe asthma Epidermolysis bullosa: skin blistering and mucosal erosion with minor friction. Scar formation and progressively decreasing oral opening
Monopolar electrocautery [19]	Cochlear implants, some cardiac pacemakers, vagus nerve stimulators, deep brain stimulators (relative contraindication) Bleeding disorders: potential for repeat bleeding when eschar sloughs (use with caution) Implanted cardiac defibrillator (absolute contraindication)
Local anesthetic [20]	Avoid epinephrine—cardiac arrhythmias, supraventricular tachycardia/Wolff-Parkinson-White, some attention deficit hyperactivity disorder meds, pheochromocytoma, cardiac or renal disease with poorly controlled hypertension, transplanted hearts Specific local anesthetic restrictions—Brugada syndrome, glucose-6-phosphate dehydrogenase deficiency Bleeding disorders: nerve blocks contraindicated. Local infiltration, intraligamental, or intraosseous injections are acceptable Sickle cell disease: some authors recommend against local anesthesia with epinephrine to avoid prolonged injection site ischemia Benzocaine topical: contraindicated in children less than 2 years. Concern for methemoglobinemia
Nitrous oxide [21]	Neurodegenerative effects: cobalamin C disease, vegan diet, methylene tetrahydrofolate reductase deficiency, pernicious anemia, vitamin B12 deficiency Gas-filled space expansion (bronchiectasis, otitis media), pulmonary hypertension, increased intracranial pressure Sickle cell disease: intraoperative oxygen level at least 50% and 10-min posttreatment period of 100% oxygen to avoid diffusion hypoxia. For longer procedures, consider extending period of observation before discharge
Analgesic risk	Aspirin/NSAIDs—bleeding disorder, during chemotherapy, kidney disease, solitary kidney, severe asthmatics Acetaminophen—liver disease, mitochondrial disorders, during chemotherapy Opioids—respiratory depression (muscular dystrophy), histamine release (severe asthma)
High risk for general anesthesia	Mucopolysaccharidoses, cystic fibrosis, spinal muscular atrophy, mitochondrial cytopathy, cardiomyopathy, single ventricle cardiac physiology, family history of adverse reactions to GA
Restorative decision-making	Avoid placing metal restorations in patients who are on a schedule of periodic magnetic resonance imaging taken to monitor tumors or arteriopathies in the brain or head and neck region Extraction versus pulp therapy in primary teeth for children at high risk for negative medical consequences of odontogenic infection

are preferred to remove loosened debris or prophylaxis paste instead of the standard water rinse with suctioning. Hand scaling of calculus is safer than sonic or ultrasonic scaling for patients with dysphagia.

Children with dysphagia and uncoordinated swallowing are at increased risk of chronic aspiration and may have a tracheostomy tube in place. The presence of a tracheostomy allows direct access to the lower respiratory tract for periodic suctioning. When aspiration is a risk, a portable suction usually travels with the patient. The home health-care provider or parent will be adept at suctioning through the tracheostomy tube. Suctioning of the tracheostomy may be required frequently during the dental encounter when intraoral manipulation promotes additional salivation. The dental suction should be used to remove oral secretions and loosened debris. The expectation for active teamwork between the parent or caregiver and dental team should be carefully discussed before challenging the child's ability, with allowances made for coordinated oral secretion management at each encounter. In addition to your observations of verbal and nonverbal cues from the patient, invite the caregiver to share their ongoing assessment of the child's tolerance as the dental encounter proceeds. This is an essential aspect of keeping the visit within the patient's functional ability and stress threshold. Frequent short procedure breaks allow the child to catch his breath without inference and will generally extend his endurance.

Dental Radiographs

The indication for and periodicity of dental radiographs are decided based upon caries risk assessment, past caries history, stage of dental development, and current clinical findings. When obtaining diagnostic quality dental radiographs is within the child's ability, the American Dental Association (ADA) provides guidance [22]. Dentists should only order radiographs when they expect that the additional information will affect patient care. There are rare conditions when routine dental radiographs are best minimized or contraindicated. Examples of these are Fanconi anemia and ataxia telangiectasia, respectively. Negotiating a reasonable interval for screening radiographs for children who have had significant exposure of the head and neck to radiation therapy should be considered by carefully following ADA indication guidelines.

Children with chronic complex medical conditions may or may not be able to tolerate intraoral radiographs. A panoramic or lateral oblique image may be helpful in providing the radiographic information (Fig. 1). Some modern panoramic instruments can generate a suitable bitewing image taken extraorally for gross screening purposes. If circumstances dictate a reduction in radiation exposure, a secondary panoramic image can be produced from an existing cone beam computerized tomography (CT) or medical CT scan. For patients with absolute contraindication to ionizing radiation, specialized computer software may be used to "invert" a magnetic resonance image (MRI) into a diagnostic quality panoramic image. When minimal caries risk exists, investigating the etiology of eruption disturbances, predicting the timing of anticipatory extractions to improve dental arch development,

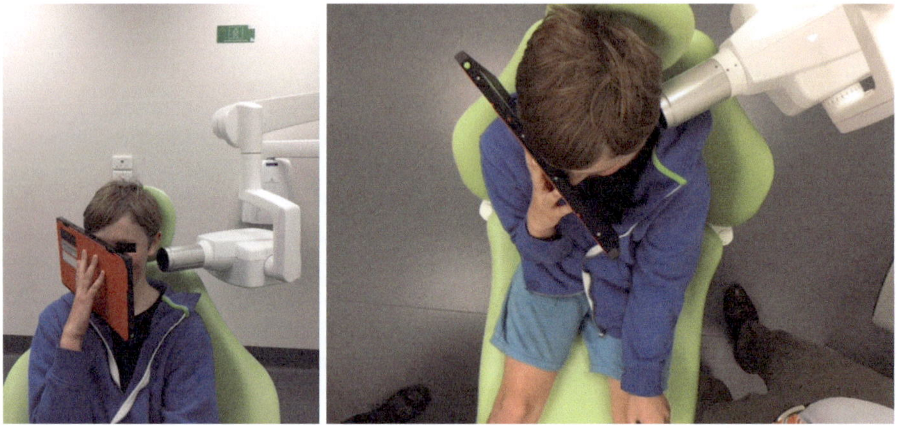

Fig. 1 Technique for taking a lateral oblique radiographic image (photos courtesy of Dr. Johan Aps)

and assessing the development of third molars are some of the more common reasons to take radiographs.

When an examination with intraoral radiographs is indicated with no additional dental treatment anticipated, and the dental examination/radiographs are only possible under hospital sedation, consider requesting to combine these brief dental procedures with sedated procedures by other medical services. Procedures are often categorized as "clean" or "sterile," indicating the level of asepsis required for infection control. Combining with "clean" procedures (e.g., botox injections for muscle spasm, placement of a NG tube) is more likely to meet with approval than with "sterile" procedures (e.g., cardiac surgery) [23]. If the radiographs are requested from a dental colleague, be sure to specify the diagnostic indication and which radiographic images are needed. When extraoral radiographic techniques are unsuccessful, and dental radiographs are only possible under sedation, consider broadening scope of the radiographic examination beyond caries diagnosis to include age-related assessment of dental development and screening for alveolar bone loss, dental anomalies, or occult pathology.

Ketogenic Diet

The ketogenic diet is commonly used an as adjunct to anticonvulsant medications for seizure control (see Chapter "Oral Hygiene and Prevention for CSHCN" for additional details). A notable potential adverse side effect of the ketogenic diet is a decrease in platelet function leading to prolonged bleeding times [24]. Provider selection of flavored medications or dental products should meet the approval of the child's nutritionist.

Special precaution should be taken when extracting loose primary teeth or scaling calculus adjacent to inflamed gingiva in patients with a seizure disorder on a ketogenic diet who also present with an aspiration risk. Assurance of adequate hemostasis before discharge is essential for these patients.

Dental Prophylaxis

Patients who are candidates for antibiotic prophylaxis should be premedicated with the appropriate antibiotic if scaling or rubber cup polishing is expected to initiate sulcular bleeding. For children whose stamina or cooperative ability is limited, the intraoral examination can be performed at the same time each dental area is scaled and polished. Frequent breaks may be best for the child with limited endurance. Planning to complete scaling over a series of appointments and more frequent preventive or treatment recalls may be a beneficial and appropriate modification of the typical dental protocol.

Sonic and ultrasonic scalers should be used with caution in children with dysphagia, cystic fibrosis, and moderate to severe asthma.

Plain unflavored prophylaxis paste is acceptable for use in the presence of ketogenic diet restrictions, but because of the presence of sweeteners, fluoride varnish is often avoided.

Considerations for Invasive Dental Procedures: Restorations, Extractions, and Subgingival Scaling

Huddle with your clinical staff, and be prepared to manage all emergencies in the dental office, and be ready to respond to an in-office crisis related to the child's condition. Discuss your plan to address known safety concerns for CMC (Table 3).

Each dental treatment plan will include the following for all children:

1. Level of treatment planned (examination under anesthesia, preventive sealants, interim therapeutic or caries control restorations, silver diamine fluoride, definitive care, no treatment)
2. Physical location where the child should be treated (community dental clinic, hospital dental clinic, hospital operating room, no treatment at all)
3. Under what conditions will the child be treated (awake +/− nitrous oxide, monitored, mild or moderate sedation, general anesthesia)

In addition to the above, the child with medical complexity will need additional planning:

4. Preoperative, intraoperative, and postoperative medication or device management (anticoagulation, blood products, prophylactic antibiotics, anesthetics, analgesics, vagus nerve stimulator or cardiac pacemaker adjustment, etc.)
5. Modification of the dental treatment protocol (hand vs. sonic or ultrasonic scaling, metal vs. non-metal restorations, tooth extraction vs. pulp therapy, etc.)

Table 3 Outpatient treatment modifications to consider for commonly encountered conditions

Pre-treatment preparation	Treatment modifications
Asthma [26, 27, 28]	
• Characterize severity and responsiveness to medication • Identify and avoid triggers such as fragrances (eugenol, surface cleansers) and stress • Patients should be directed to arrive with personal inhaler and spacer extension if applicable • Be prepared to stop treatment • Be prepared to manage asthma-related emergency	• Keep appointments short • Nitrous oxide is OK for anxiety-induced asthma, but avoid in patients with severe disease due to drying effects • Use NSAIDs with caution for severe asthmatics who are naïve to using them. Opiate drugs are contraindicated due to respiratory effect and histamine release. Acetaminophen is the analgesic of choice • Colophony-containing dental products such as some fluoride varnishes should be avoided for the severe asthmatic
Cardiac disease	
• After cardiac surgery, defer elective dental procedures for 6 months • Check with cardiologist regarding subacute bacterial endocarditis (SBE) recommendations. Follow AHA guidelines [29] • Facilitate the completion of all definitive dental care prior to cardiac surgery to avoid infection during the immediate post-surgery period • Oral anticoagulant (Coumadin): check INR • No need to alter aspirin therapy for dental procedures	• Confirm acceptability of plan to use nitrous oxide or local anesthesia with the cardiologist • Avoid epinephrine exposure in CMC with cardiac arrhythmia or transplanted heart. Mepivacaine plain is generally a good alternative • For patients at risk for infective endocarditis, consider extraction of primary teeth with deep caries over vital pulp therapy to avoid the consequence of the 5–20% which are at risk of failure
Congenital bleeding disorder (Hemophilia, von Willebrand's, platelet disorder) [30]	
• Procedures associated with bleeding: (extractions, scaling/root planning) work with hematologist to develop bleeding management plan—factor infusions (Advate), DDAVP (Stimate), posttreatment Amicar • Procedures not associated with bleeding: (routine restorative) infiltration, PDL, and intraosseous injections are safe • For severe bleeding disorders and extensive invasive dental treatment needs, refer for hospital-based general anesthesia	• Nerve blocks or injections in highly vascular regions such as the pterygoid plexus are contraindicated • Consider 4% articaine infiltration for restoring permanent molar teeth to avoid block anesthesia • Consider multi-surface restorations versus stainless crowns where possible to reduce tissue trauma and chronic gingival inflammation • Do not provide complete primary closure when suturing soft tissue wounds to avoid a dissecting hematoma • Avoid using optional monopolar electrosurgery in the patient with a severe bleeding disorder. Rebleeding may occur when resultant eschar sloughs

(continued)

Table 3 (continued)

Pre-treatment preparation	Treatment modifications
Acquired coagulopathy [31, 32]	
• Heparinized dialysis patients are best treated the day after dialysis. The half-life of unfractionated heparin is 4–6 hours • Low molecular weight heparin (LMWH) such enoxaparin (Lovenox) does not need to be discontinued for dental care if within therapeutic range • Oral anticoagulant Coumadin (warfarin). An INR of less than 3.5 is acceptable for clinic-based invasive procedures including extractions • Discontinue supplements affecting platelet function for 2 weeks if multiple extractions in single appointment are planned	• Minimum of 4 hours post-dialysis for emergency dental treatment • No modifications needed if pre-treatment preparation is complete • Avoid nerve blocks or injections in highly vascular regions such as the pterygoid plexus if INR >3.0. Consider 4% articaine infiltration instead
In situations where there is increased risk of bleeding, additional local measures such as placing resorbable sutures, absorbable gelatin, or hemostatic collagen are helpful. Postoperative protection of extraction sites with a surgical stent or administration of antifibrinolytics such as aminocaproic acid or tranexamic acid may be indicated	
Solid organ transplants	
Pretransplant • Ideally a dental screening clearance was undertaken prior to transplant, and all required dental procedures were completed • Check latest INR if severe liver disease • Check blood pressures on end-stage renal disease (ESRD) and renal transplant patients • ESRD on hemodialysis—best time to treat is the day following dialysis Posttransplant • Antibiotic prophylaxis is recommended for invasive dental procedures for 6 months after transplant. Follow AHA guidelines • Check with specialist regarding ongoing need for antibiotic prophylaxis beyond 6 months especially if history of transplanted organ rejection	• Timely completion of dental care pretransplant would ensure minimal need for an elective invasive dental procedure in the immediate posttransplant period • Children who are on a transplant list should be re-evaluated for dental concerns every 6 months if transplant has not yet occurred • Avoid NSAIDs in ESRD • Avoid acetaminophen for patients with liver disease Medication-induced gingival hyperplasia: • Cyclosporine immunosuppression—usually resolves after transition to tacrolimus • Calcium channel blocker antihypertensives such as amlodipine • Chronic gingival irritation caused by plaque and calculus buildup, and fixed orthodontic appliances exacerbate the hyperplastic response • Spontaneous resolution often occurs when the contributing factors are removed
Oncology [33]	
• Coordinate timing of care and antibiotic prophylaxis with the primary cancer team during any stage of chemotherapy and up to 6 months after completion • Check pre-treatment ANC and platelet count	• Antibiotic prophylaxis if ANC less than $500/mm^3$ • Minimum platelet count of 55,000/μl for local infiltration or 75,000/μl for nerve block local anesthesia

(continued)

Table 3 (continued)

Pre-treatment preparation	Treatment modifications
Hematopoietic stem cell transplant (HSCT)	
• Coordinate timing of invasive dental care and antibiotic prophylaxis with the HSCT team up to 12 months after transplant • Ongoing coordination may be required if immunosuppressed beyond 12 months or develops chronic graft-versus-host disease	• No elective invasive dental treatment including prophylaxis for 1 year (allogeneic) or 6 months (autologous) posttransplant until cleared by HSCT team • Remove fixed orthodontic appliances prior to transplant. Delay fixed orthodontics until 2 years posttransplant • Oral exams, including radiographs when indicated, and fluoride treatment important during first year posttransplant
Seizure history	
• Confirm compliance with therapy and continued absence of seizure events	• Patients with well-controlled seizure disorder are treated the same as typical patients

6. Anticipated postoperative course (bleeding, infection, delayed healing or self-injury risk; extended period of post-op observation; day surgery vs. admission for observation; socioeconomic factors influencing compliance; etc.)
7. Postoperative follow-up plan (timing, indications, etc.)

If procedural sedation is required for comprehensive dental treatment, most children with a complex medical condition will not qualify for sedation or GA in an outpatient setting. Risk is inherent in any sedated procedure, and multiple general anesthetics at a young age can affect neurocognitive development [25]. Therefore it is best practice to combine services under a single GA when possible. The benefit of delaying dental treatment to allow time to coordinate services must be weighed against the risk of the oral condition advancing toward pain, infection, and functional disability. Hearing tests (brainstem auditory evoked response (BAER)), sedated electroencephalography (EEG), otolaryngology procedures, and gynecologic procedures performed under GA are examples of procedures which may be possible to combine with dental treatment. When possible, it may be in the best interest of some CMC to schedule sedated dental care after permanent molar eruption to allow placement of preventive sealants. Caries control using interim therapeutic restorations and silver diamine fluoride can be valuable stabilizing alternatives if definitive dental treatment under GA must be delayed.

Bisphosphonates

Bisphosphonates are a group of drugs which act upon osteoclasts to reduce bone resorption. They are used in children with metabolic bone disease, avascular necrosis, osteoporosis, and hypercalcemia of malignancy [34]. High-dose corticosteroid therapy for asthma or immunosuppression can also lead to osteoporosis [35, 36]. Osteoporosis can also be a long-term problem, particularly in children who are not weight-bearing and are wheelchair/stroller dependent for mobility.

Although there is an absence of cases of bisphosphonate-related osteonecrosis of the jaws (BRONJ) in the pediatric literature, the evidence is lacking to rule out the risk of BRONJ altogether [37]. Until then, prudence would advise a conservative approach when treatment planning for elective extractions and oral surgical procedures as well as long-term monitoring for latent effects when a history of bisphosphonate use is revealed [38].

In contrast to the seemingly small risk of BRONJ, the side effects of bisphosphonate medications upon dental development are common, namely, prolonged primary tooth resorption and delayed permanent tooth eruption. Studies of orthodontic tooth movement in children exposed to bisphosphates are lacking. Adult orthodontic patients with a history of bisphosphonate use have been reported to have unpredictable orthodontic results and extended treatment times [39].

In addition to bisphosphonates, the dental provider should recognize that there are new therapies for the treatment of metabolic bone cancers. These treatments have short-term risks of jaw osteonecrosis. Denosumab is representative of this group of drugs used in children [40].

Case-Based Scenarios

Case 1: Seizure Disorder

Dillon, a 10-year-old boy with a seizure disorder, was referred to the dental clinic by the mother of a school classmate. On the health questionnaire, key responses were:

- Seizure disorder
- Mild intellectual disability
- Surgical history: vagus nerve stimulator (VNS) placed at age 5 years, most recent battery change 1 year ago
- Daily medications: valproic acid, lamotrigine, zonisamide, vitamin B6
- Allergies: none

Comment

A seizure disorder poses several challenges to quality of life. These may include restriction of activities, loss of independence, unease about telling others, prejudice and bullying, and side effects of medications. A matter of fact, calm, supportive dental team will be appreciated by these patients and their families. The dentist should obtain enough information about the seizure disorder to understand its presentation, management by the family, and impact on oral health. Periodic emergency drills by the dental team will ensure readiness to competently manage a seizure occurring in the dental office.

A phone interview with Dillon's mother in advance of the appointment is an efficient way to better understand his medical complexity. Questions to ask include, but are not limited to:

- Neurologist contact information
- Cause of seizures: unknown, epilepsy syndrome, trauma, brain tumor
- Age of first seizure
- Presentation of seizures: prodromal aura and form of aura, type and duration of seizures
- Frequency of seizures and date of most recent seizure
- Seizure triggers (time of day, emotional stress, sleep deprivation, flashing lights, illness, fever)
- Date of most recent emergency department visit or hospitalization related to seizures
- History of status epilepticus
- Seizure response plan: rescue medication/adjunct treatment for seizures (vagus nerve stimulator) and efficacy of rescue
- Typical postictal presentation
- Special diet
- History of dental trauma during a seizure
- History of prolonged bleeding following minor injuries

Additional Information from Phone Interview with Parent

Dillon has Dravet syndrome (SCN1A gene mutation). Febrile seizures started at 7 months of age and afebrile seizures at age 2 years. He has multiple seizure types: generalized tonic-clonic, myoclonic, and partial seizures with secondary generalization. A multifaceted approach to decrease seizures has included placement of a VNS, anti-seizure medications in various combinations, and the ketogenic diet. Current ketogenic diet ratio is 4:1 by weight of fat to combined protein and carbohydrate.

He has three or four seizures per month. His most frequent seizure type is a drop myoclonic seizure lasting between 2 and 4 min. Triggers include bright lights, flashing lights, and stress; most seizures occur between 6 and 9 A.M. Following a seizure, he sleeps soundly for up to 1 h. His parents have never needed to use rescue medication or activate the VNS device to stop a seizure. He has not suffered dental trauma during a seizure or required hospitalization for ongoing seizures. The family has never noticed prolonged bleeding following usual childhood accidents.

Dental Plan in Advance of the Dental Appointment

1. Review office emergency response to a seizure occurring anywhere in the dental office.
2. Look up details about Dillon's anti-epileptic medications, being aware that they may affect the gingiva, hemostasis, salivary flow, or salivary buffering.

3. Take steps to mitigate seizure triggers present in the dental environment
   (a) Most of Dillon's seizures occur in the morning—schedule an afternoon appointment.
   (b) Dim the room lighting as possible, and turn off or cover any items that flash or blink.
   (c) Invite him to wear his own dark glasses during the entire appointment.
4. Confirm that his parent will bring his seizure rescue medication and VNS activation magnet to the appointment.

During the Dental Appointment

1. Perform new patient examination, expose radiographs as indicated, provide preventive services as needed, and avoid flavored products such as prophylaxis paste and fluoride varnish.
2. Assess his risk for dental trauma during a seizure. Depending upon facial and occlusal relationships, protective measures to consider include no action, a helmet, sport mouth guard, thermal plastic retainer, or orthodontic treatment to decrease excessive overjet.
3. Due to very low carbohydrate allowed in the ketogenic diet, Dillon's diet is caries-protective. If his diet changes, his caries risk may change accordingly.
4. Be aware of carbohydrates in medications. In general, avoid liquids and chewable tablets because they can reverse the ketogenic state and decrease the seizure threshold.
5. If restorations are indicated, consider providing care under GA. Local anesthetics have an excitatory effect on the brain, lowering the seizure threshold.

Seizure Management

- Note the time seizure begins.
- Stay calm, and move onlookers away.
- Position patient to prevent injury: chair reclined and close to floor, nothing in the mouth, remove eyeglasses, and clear immediate area.
- Consider rescue medication (benzodiazepine).
- Activate emergency medical system if seizure lasts >5 minutes, a second seizure occurs with very little time between, first seizure ever for patient, and unable to awaken patient.
- Postictal patient support: place patient on his side if possible, with rolled towel under shoulders, suction airway, take vital signs, use pulse oximeter if available, and provide oxygen as needed.

Recommended Online Resources

- The Epilepsy Foundation
  - www.epilepsy.com

- National Institute of Neurological Disorders and Stroke
  - www.ninds.nih.gov/disorders/epilepsy/detail_epilepsy.htm
- National Library of Medicine
  - www.nlm.nih.gov/medlineplus/epilepsy.html
- International League Against Epilepsy
  - www.ilae.org
- Charlie Foundation (ketogenic diet)
  - https://charliefoundation.org
- Carbohydrate content of medications
  - http://ketomeds.com

Case 2: Congenital Heart Defect/Disease

Lisa, an 8-year-old girl, was referred to the dental clinic by her physician. Her family has relocated from another state. Important responses on the health questionnaire completed by her mother were:

- Congenital heart defect/disease.
- Surgical history:
  - Repair of aortic valve and pulmonary valve at age 2 months
  - Placement of mechanical aortic valve and mitral valve repair at age 7 months
  - Mitral valve replacement at age 3 years
  - Dental restorations under GA at age 4 years
- Hospitalizations: for heart surgeries as above. Dental surgery did not require an overnight stay.
- Daily medications: multivitamin, warfarin 4 mg daily.
- Allergies: none.

Comment

Lisa has severe congenital heart disease (CHD) as evidenced by multiple heart surgeries in early life. Presence of a mechanical aortic valve necessitates that she be maintained in an anticoagulated state. The highest risks for Lisa related to dental treatment are oral bleeding and bacteremia of oral origin causing infective endocarditis.

More specific information needed about Lisa's CHD is needed in advance of the dental appointment includes, but is not limited to:

- Cardiologist's contact information
- Date of most recent cardiology appointment and planned return interval
- Target value and monitoring method for international normalized ratio (INR)
- Restrictions on activities recommended by cardiologist

- Current cardiovascular symptoms such as shortness of breath, increased work of breathing, cyanosis, pallor, and fatigability
- Previous dentist's contact information
- Problems with oral bleeding
- Dental concerns and goals for dental care

Additional Information Obtained During Phone Interview with Parent

They have established local care with a cardiologist and with the PCP who referred Lisa to your dental practice. Lisa's most recent cardiology evaluation was 1 month ago. An echocardiogram done on that day showed her mechanical heart values were functioning well with no sign of ventricular hypertrophy. She is set to return to the cardiologist twice yearly. Target INR is between 2.5 and 3.5, monitored by home self-testing twice weekly. In recent weeks, the INR has varied between 2 and 5.4. Mom states that Lisa's health is good overall. She is growing and her energy level is excellent with no restriction on activities. When the INR is above 3.5, they notice bleeding around her mouth and bruising of her arms and legs. The cardiologist has advised antibiotics in advance of dental appointments for subacute bacterial endocarditis (SBE) prophylaxis. Lisa's parents express the hope to avoid the need for additional restorations as her permanent teeth come in.

Dental Plan in Advance of the Dental Appointment

1. Explain that the first dental appointment will be for acclimatizing Lisa to the dental team and office, performing examination, and taking any necessary radiographs. Pre-appointment antibiotics will not be prescribed because no invasive treatment is planned.
2. Contact her previous dentist to get radiographs, surgical operation report, and clinical notes.
3. Ask Lisa's mother to check INR level within 1 day prior to the appointment. Reschedule if INR is >3.5 due to high risk of oral bleeding with placement of radiography sensors.

During the Dental Appointment

1. Perform new patient clinical examination; expose radiographs as indicated.
2. Provide oral hygiene care coaching to Lisa and her parents. Meticulous daily oral care is essential for the health of her heart and her teeth. Maintenance of good oral health and hygiene may reduce the risk of oral bacteremia from daily activities.

3. Give anticipatory guidance appropriate for her age, developmental stage, and habits and as indicated by findings of clinical and radiographic examination.
4. Plan her next dental appointment.

Changes to Customary Dental Practice due to Patient Medical Complexity

1. Due to infection risk: Prescribe an antibiotic in advance of invasive treatment appointments including prophylaxis according to current AHA guidelines. Confirm that the medication was taken appropriately before beginning dental treatment. Manage oral infections definitively, and do not rely on host defense to clear an oral infection.
2. Due to bleeding risk: Lisa is at risk for oral bleeding during and after dental treatment. When the INR exceeds 3.0, persistent oral oozing from exfoliating primary teeth may result in anemia. Local anesthesia via nerve block in soft tissue spaces (posterior superior alveolar (PSA), inferior alveolar (IA)) is contraindicated due to the risk of trauma to adjacent blood vessels. Recognize that nonsteroidal anti-inflammatory medications cannot be given to this patient.
3. Consider GA with oral intubation (as opposed to nasotracheal intubation, which may cause bleeding from the nasal cavity) in a hospital setting for invasive dental treatment such as extractions, root canals, or restorations of teeth best anesthetized via IA or PSA nerve block.

Recommended Online Resource

- American Heart Association—Infective Endocarditis
  - http://www.heart.org

Conclusion

- The foundation of a dental home relies on a systematic approach to establishing family-oriented, comprehensive, coordinated, and safe delivery of dental care. However, locating professionally guided oral health services for children with medical complexities remains difficult for some individuals and their families.
- Current health-care trends expand outpatient management of complex medical conditions so that more children can experience a higher quality of life in the community. An adequate response to this trend from the dental community requires a commensurate expansion of community-based dental homes for CMC.
- After a thorough review of intake information, dentists can readily make an individualized assessment of the child's ability to tolerate proposed dental protocols and collaborate with the child's family and medical team to prevent oral problems treatment from negatively affecting health, well-being, or medical stability.

References

1. MacPherson M, Arango P, Fox H, et al. A new definition of children with special health care needs. Pediatrics. 1998;102(1 pt 1):137–40.
2. Cohen E, Kuo DZ, Agrawal R, Berry JG, Bhagat SKM, Simon T, Srivastava R. Children With medical complexity: an emerging population for clinical and research initiatives. Pediatrics. 2011;127(3):529–38.
3. Kuo DZ, Cohen E, Agrawal R, Berry JG, Casey PH. A national profile of caregiver challenges among more medically complex children with special health care needs. Arch Pediatr Adolesc Med. 2011;165(11):1020–6.
4. Bethell CD, Read D, Blumberg SJ, Newacheck PW. What is the prevalence of children with special health care needs? Toward an understanding of variations in findings and methods across three national surveys. Matern Child Health J. 2008;12(1):1–14.
5. Bramlett MD, Reda D, Bethell C, Blumberg SJ. Differentiating subgroups of children with special health care needs by health status and complexity of health care needs. Matern Child Health J. 2009;13(2):151–63.
6. Burns KH, Casey PH, Lyle RE, Mac Bird T, Fussell JJ, Robbins JM. Increasing prevalence of medically complex children in US hospitals. Pediatrics. 2010;126:638–46.
7. Feudtner C, Hays R, Haynes G, Geyer R, Neff J, Koepsell T. Deaths attributed to pediatric complex chronic conditions: national trends and implications of supportive care services. Pediatrics. 2001;107(6):E99.
8. Siffel C, Riehle-Colrausso T, Oster M, Correa A. Survival of children with hypoplastic left heart syndrome. Pediatrics. 2015;136(4):e864–70.
9. Klitzner TS, Rabbitt LA, Chang RK. Benefits of care coordination for children with complex disease: a pilot medical home project in a resident teaching clinic. J Pediatr. 2010;156(6):1006–10.
10. Scully C. Special care in dentistry: handbook of oral health care. Edinburgh: Churchill Livingstone; 2006.
11. Lockhart P. Dental care of the medically complex patient. Philadelphia: Elsevier Health Sciences; 2004.
12. Little JW, Falace DA. Dental management of the medically compromised patient. 4th ed. St Louis: Mosby; 1993.
13. Example of online medical topic update resource for medical professionals. https://www.uptodate.com/home/uptodate-subscription-options-clinicians
14. American Academy of Pediatric Dentistry. Pediatric medical history. Reference Manual Vol37/No6. 2016. Retrieved from http://www.aapd.org/media/Policies_Guidelines/RS_MedHistoryForm.pdf
15. Palisano R, Rosenbaum P, Walter S, Russell D, Wood E, Galuppi B. Development and validation of a gross motor function classification system for children with cerebral palsy. Dev Med Child Neurol. 1997;39:214–23.
16. Weiss A, Dym H. Review of antibiotics and indications for prophylaxis. Dent Clin N Am. 2012;56:235–44.
17. Lockhart PB, Loven B, Brennan MT, Baddour LM, Levinson M. The evidence base for the efficiency of antibiotic prophylaxis in dental practice. J Am Dent Assoc. 2007;138(4):458–74.
18. Fillmore WJ, Leavitt BD, Arce K. Dental extraction in the neutropenic patient. J Oral Maxillofac Surg. 2014;72(12):2386–93.
19. Behan J, Higgins S, Wysong A. Safety of cochlear implants in electrosurgery: a systematic review of the literature. Dermatol Surg. 2017;43(6):775–83.
20. Ogle OE, Mahjoubi G. Local anesthesia: agents, techniques, and complications. Dent Clin N Am. 2012;56:133–48.
21. Sanders RD, Weisman J, Maze MB. Biologic effects of nitrous oxide – a mechanistic and toxicologic review. Anesthesiology. 2008;109:707–22.
22. American Dental Association Council on Scientific Affairs and U.S. Food and Drug Administration. Dental radiographic examinations: recommendations for patient selection and limiting radiation exposure. 2012.

23. Stapleton MF, Sheller B, Williams BJ, Mancl L. Combining pediatric dental treatment in the OR with other procedures. Pediatr Dent. 2007;28:397–402.
24. Berry-Kravis E, Booth G, Taylor A, Valentino LA. Bruising and the ketogenic diet: evidence for diet-induced changes in platelet function. Ann Neurol. 2001;49(1):98–103.
25. Andropoulos DB, Greene MF. Anesthesia and developing brains – implications of the FDA warning. N Engl J Med. 2017;376:905–7.
26. Harrington N, Prado N, Barry S. Dental treatment in children with asthma – a review. Br Dent J. 2016;220(6):229–302.
27. Steinbacher DM, Glick M. The dental patient with asthma. An update and oral health considerations. J Am Dent Assoc. 2001;132:1229–39.
28. Rajan JP, Wineinger NE, Stevenson DD, White AA. Prevalence of aspirin-exacerbated respiratory disease among asthmatic patients: a meta-analysis of the literature. J Allergy Clin Immunol. 2015;135:676–81.
29. Wilson W, Taubert KA, Gewitz M, Lockhart PB, et al. Prevention of infective endocarditis: guidelines from the American heart Association (multiple councils). Circulation. 2007;116(1):1736–54.
30. Gupta A, Epstein JB, Cabay RJ. Bleeding disorders of importance in dental care and related patient management. JCDA. 2007;73(1):77–83.
31. Hepponstall M, Chanb A, Monaglea P. Anticoagulation therapy in neonates, children and adolescents. Blood Cell Mol Dis. 2017;67:41–7.
32. Beirne OR. Evidence to continue oral anticoagulant therapy for ambulatory oral surgery. J Oral Maxillofac Surg. 2005;63:540–5.
33. Zimmermann C, et al. Dental treatment in patients with leukemia. J Oncol 2015; 2015: 571739. 14 pages.
34. Ward LN, Petryk A, Gordon CM. Use of bisphosphonates in the treatment of pediatric osteoporosis. Int J Clin Rheumatol. 2009;4(6):657–72.
35. Chee C, Sellahewa L, Pappachan JM. Inhaled corticosteroids and bone health. Open Respir Med J. 2014;8:85–92.
36. Carpenter PA, Hoffmeister P, Chesnut CH, et al. Bisphosphonate therapy for reduced bone mineral density in children with chronic graft-versus-host disease. Biol Blood Marrow Transplant. 2007;13(6):683–90.
37. Kwot-Kit N, Bowe J, Goodger N. The risk of bisphosphonate-related osteonecrosis of the jaw in children. A case report and literature review. Dent Update. 2013;40:733–8.
38. Bhatt RN, Hibbert SA, Munns CF. The use of bisphosphonates in children: review of the literature and guidelines for dental management. Aust Dent J. 2014;59:9–19.
39. Krieger E, Jacobs C, Walter C, Wehrbein H. Current state of orthodontic patients under bisphosphonate therapy. Head Face Med. 2013;9:10–6.
40. Hernandez M, Phulpin B, Mansuy L, Droz D. Use of new targeted cancer therapies in children: effects on dental development and risk of jaw osteonecrosis: a review. J Oral Pathol Med. 2017;46:321–6.

Communication with Children with Special Healthcare Needs in Dental Practice

Kimberly M. Espinoza, Lisa J. Heaton, and Carolyn R. Baylor

Introduction

Children with special healthcare needs (CSHCN) are a diverse population with diverse communication needs. While there is no one-size fits all recommendation for communicating with CSHCN, by definition this population has a few things in common, which may all impact communication [1]:

- *CSHCN require more and/or different healthcare services*. CSHCN require more and/or different healthcare services than children without special healthcare needs. This may include the need for prescription medications, medical evaluations, tests, surgeries, occupational therapy, physical therapy, speech therapy, mental health services, or other types of healthcare services. Encounters with the broader healthcare system may affect how CSHCN view and/or respond to dental care. Dental care providers should be aware of the potential impact of these healthcare experiences and incorporate this knowledge when appropriate into maintaining respectful patient-provider communication.
- *CSHCN have chronic conditions*. The implications of treating a child with a chronic condition in dental practice include the need to understand (1) the potential impact of the chronic condition on dental care and oral health and (2) the

K. M. Espinoza (✉)
Department of Oral Medicine, University of Washington, Seattle, WA, USA
e-mail: kmespino@uw.edu

L. J. Heaton
Department of Oral Health Sciences, University of Washington, Seattle, WA, USA
e-mail: lheaton@uw.edu

C. R. Baylor
Department of Rehabilitation Medicine, University of Washington, Seattle, WA, USA

Department of Speech and Hearing Sciences, University of Washington, Seattle, WA, USA
e-mail: cbaylor@uw.edu

T. M. Nelson, J. R. Webb (eds.), *Dental Care for Children with Special Needs*,
https://doi.org/10.1007/978-3-030-10483-2_3

impact of the label itself. Dental providers should learn about facilitating communication with children whose chronic conditions impact communication. Additionally, dental providers should learn to communicate about patients' chronic conditions in culturally appropriate ways.
- *CSHCN are children.* CSHCN are, by definition, children. As with all children, there are several important considerations relevant to dental practice: (1) CSHCN develop throughout childhood. (2) CSHCN are not legally able to make their own healthcare decisions, unless emancipated. (3) CSHCN may have other people who help them with medical decision-making and access to healthcare. This may include giving informed consent, appointment scheduling, transportation to appointments, and financial responsibility for care received. While it is often the parents in these roles, other family members, court-appointed guardians, paid caregivers, nurses, or other types of caregivers may fill some of these roles. Dental providers should be familiar with triadic communication with children and their parents/caregivers and the complexity of medical decision-making for minors with special healthcare needs.

This chapter details how to address these diverse communication needs in dental practice.

Healthcare Experiences and Communication

The majority of CSHCN access healthcare services and/or have had experiences with the healthcare system that are more extensive or different than children without special healthcare needs. In some cases, CSHCN have extensive experience with the healthcare system, while in other cases, the experience is more limited [2]. The medically experienced child may have had a variety of healthcare encounters, positive, negative, and/or neutral, that affect her response to dental care. Children have various ways of coping with medical care. For some, the extensive experience of medical care may make the child an "expert patient." She may be courageous around medical providers, feel empowered to ask questions about her medical care, and/or be able to handle unpleasant medical procedures with ease. For others, medical care experiences may result in fear, development of negative coping skills, or overwhelm the child so much that even a small procedure feels insurmountable. Some CSHCN may feel their experiences with medical care have a limited impact on their receipt of dental care.

Recommendations for the dental provider:

- Understand that experience with the healthcare system varies among CSHCN.
- Understand that the emotional response to healthcare varies among CSHCN.
- Ask CSHCN, or their caregivers if appropriate, if they have any concerns about dental care.
- Avoid invasive questions about past medical experiences if not relevant to the dental encounter.

- Listen if CSHCN or their caregivers describe past negative healthcare experiences.
- Ask how you can alleviate concerns related to past negative experiences that have been disclosed.

Understanding Chronic Conditions

Dental providers should familiarize themselves with the chronic conditions of their patients with special healthcare needs. This will allow providers to ask relevant questions and understand specific concerns that the patient, parents, or other caregivers may bring up. Beyond this, it is prudent for the dental provider to become familiar with conditions that may impact communication, including communication disorders, autism, and intellectual disability.

Communication Disorders

Communication disorders are among the constellation of chronic conditions with which CSHCN may present. The purpose of this section is to review some of the main types and characteristics of pediatric communication disorders to familiarize the dental provider with the more common disorders they may see in patients. Much of this information can be found in introductory textbooks on communication disorders as well as on websites affiliated with the Centers for Disease Control (https://www.cdc.gov/ncbddd/actearly/index.html) and the American Speech-Language-Hearing Association (www.asha.org); thus these resources will not be referenced repeatedly throughout this section [3, 4]. This section will conclude with a framework that gives the dental provider some guidance as to how to interact with patients with communication disorders during the dental visit.

Speech and language disorders in children are often categorized as language disorders, speech sound disorders (SSDs), and social communication disorders. In all of these categories, communication disorders can be congenital or developmental, meaning the child does not have an initial period of typical function before the problems emerge. Examples include communication disorders associated with developmental delays or congenital conditions such as cleft palate or cerebral palsy. Communication disorders can also be acquired from an acute injury or trauma occurring in childhood. Whether congenital or acquired, an important issue to consider in pediatric patients is that the communication disorder occurs in the context of ongoing speech, language, and cognitive development. While trajectories are highly individualized, many children with communication disorders will continue to develop communication skills throughout childhood, but that developmental trajectory may be slower (delayed) or different (disordered) than typical development. To further contribute to the unique presentation of each child, any of these types of communication disorders can occur by themselves but often are found in combination either with other types of communication disorders, or with other health conditions. Each of these categories is described below, followed by a summary of another important type of communication disorder—hearing loss.

Language Disorders

A discussion of speech and language disorders must begin by drawing the distinction between speech and language. Language is essentially a code used by humans to transmit meaning to each other. Languages are systems of symbols that are used in a rule-based manner to both encode and decode meaning between communication partners. Language symbols come in many forms. In spoken language, the symbols are the speech sounds that speakers of a language combine into meaningful words and sentences. In written language, the symbols are the letters combined to form words and sentences according to the rules of the language. Likewise, in sign languages such as American Sign Language, the symbols are the gestural movements that create shared meaning for sign language users. The term "speech" is reserved for the physical act of talking—that of producing spoken language.

Language can be characterized by three aspects—form, content, and use. *Language form* refers to the symbols in the language and the rules for combining the symbols to create meaning. Rules for language form can be broken down further into rules regarding phonology, morphology, and syntax (grammar).

- *Phonology* refers to the rules governing how sounds are combined for spoken language—what sounds carry meaning in a language, as well as which sound combinations are "allowed" in the language and which are not. The difference between the "r" sound and the "l" sound does not inherently carry any meaning. In English, however, the difference in those two sounds does convey meaning because there are words that differ only in those two sounds that mean different things, for example, "rate" versus "late."
- *Morphology* refers to the smallest unit in the grammar of a language that carries meaning. For example, in English, the "-ed" is the past tense morpheme. When it is added to the end of regular verbs, it changes the meaning of the verb to past tense: "pick" changes to "picked."
- *Syntax* specifies the correct sequence of words to make sense in the language. For example, in English, adjectives typically come before the noun they are describing ("white dog"), whereas in Spanish, the adjectives typically come after the noun ("perro blanco").

While there are many rules governing language form, language content and language use are also important aspects of a language. *Language content* refers to the meaning or semantics of language units. For example, English speakers recognize the combination of letters or sounds in the word "dog" to mean a four-legged animal that barks and is happy to see you come through the door at the end of the day. Alternatively, they understand that the word "cat" describes an animal that meows and might not deign to greet you when you arrive home from work. *Language use* refers to knowing the rules of how we implement language to accomplish various tasks. For example, we learn that using the word "please" is a polite way to request something, and that "hello" and "good-bye" are appropriate terms to use when meeting and departing from people, respectively.

Early childhood is a period of very rapid language development. Most typical language development happens automatically from the natural exposure children receive in their environments, assuming their early childhood environments are "language-rich" with frequent and ongoing interactions with people around them. Around the first birthday, typically developing children will produce their first spoken words, although they have likely understood spoken language long before they say their first words. The toddler and preschool years are periods of explosive vocabulary growth and advancing sophistication of understanding and using the rules of language. At the time children enter elementary school, many of the foundational aspects of language are established, although children continue to develop more abstract and complex language constructs throughout their childhood years. The critical developments occurring in the school years focus around developing literacy skills.

When children experience language delays or disorders, the problems can arise in any aspect of language including form, content, or use. Most often, children will have difficulties with both expressive and receptive language, although perhaps not to the same degree. Language impairments may also impact all modalities of language, including spoken language, reading, and writing, although not necessarily to the same degree. Language problems can be categorized as either language delays or disorders. In a *language delay*, the child may be progressing through the typical stages of language development but at a slower than expected pace. Children typically develop language at varying paces so judicious use of developmental guidelines is recommended in judging if a child might have a language delay. *Language disorders* typically refer to situations in which a child is not progressing in language development even at a delayed pace, or if delayed language is following an atypical pattern of development.

Dental providers should be alert that children presenting with complex neurological conditions affecting cognitive function are likely to also present with language delays and disorders. However, language impairments can also occur without any other coexisting cognitive or other condition. The term "specific language impairment (SLI)" is the diagnoses used to refer to situations in which a child's language is impaired, but there are no other accompanying cognitive, emotional, or other disorders or delays that might explain the language disorder. SLI is an isolated disorder of language only.

From this introduction to language and language disorders, the dental provider can likely imagine that language delays and disorders present in a myriad of ways. Severity may range from very mild to profound, and the different combinations of receptive and expressive difficulties with form, content, and use can create many different profiles of language disorders and delays. Furthermore, different communities may choose to use different terms for concepts such as SLI and other language delays and disorders.

Recommendations for the dental provider:

- Ask caregivers for information about the characteristics of each child's language abilities.
- Get specific examples of what level of language input the child understands and how the child typically expresses herself using language.

With school-aged children, consider inquiring about the child's literacy skills. This provides information regarding the extent to which a child might be able to take responsibility for following written instructions.

Speech Sound Disorders

As mentioned above, speech refers to the physical ability to produce sounds to talk. Speech sound disorders can arise from underlying problems with neurologic control of the speech mechanism, from structural impairments to the speech mechanism (e.g., cleft palate), or from developmental delays and disorders for which a cause might not be apparent. Speech sound disorders (SSDs) are often sorted into three categories: articulation disorders, phonologic disorders, and motor speech disorders.

- *Articulation disorders.* The term "articulation disorder" is usually reserved for those situations in which a child presents with difficulties producing one or two specific speech sounds beyond the age of expected mastery, with all other sounds in the child's speech inventory produced correctly. Common examples of articulation disorders include problems producing the "r," "s," or "th" sounds. Different speech sounds are typically mastered at different ages. For example, early developing sounds such as "p," "m," and "b" are mastered by most typically developing children by the age of 3 years old, whereas more complex sounds such as "s," "z," or "th" might not be fully mastered by typically developing children until the age of 7 or 8 years old. Again, developmental norms are used judiciously due to considerable variability in typically developing children. Because these types of articulation disorders usually impact only one or two sounds, these children will likely be mostly intelligible, but their speech may sound "young" for their age, particularly if these speech errors persist beyond early elementary school. Many children with these errors will enter speech therapy in the early elementary school years, and these isolated articulation errors are typically very responsive to therapy.
- *Phonologic disorders.* Phonologic disorders are speech production disorders in which multiple speech sounds are impaired, and the errors occur in patterns according to underlying rules of phonology in spoken language. Many of these error patterns are normal in typically developing children, but as children develop, the phonologic error patterns, or processes, will resolve at different ages. For example, one phonologic error pattern is referred to as fronting. In fronting, sounds that are usually produced in the back of the mouth such as "k"

and "g" are produced in the front of the mouth; hence "cat" is pronounced as "tat" and "gum" is pronounced as "dum." In typically developing children, fronting resolves naturally between the ages of 3–4 years old. Another phonological process is called "cluster reduction" and occurs when a group of consonants normally "cluster" together, such as the "sp" in "spy" and the "bl" in "blow." In cluster reduction, the more complex speech sound is dropped from the cluster so that there is only one consonant left—hence "spy" is pronounced "pie," and "blow" is pronounced "bow." Typically developing children will stop using cluster reduction around the ages of 4–5 years old, with different stages of resolution depending on the speech sounds involved. When phonologic processes do not resolve by the expected age, phonologic process disorders are suspected. Depending on the number of phonologic processes involved, children's speech intelligibility can be highly variable, but at times can be significantly impaired. One strategy that can help with understanding a child with phonologic processes errors is to remember that the errors occur in patterns. If the listener can learn the pattern the child is using, the listener may find it easier to decipher the speech and understand the child's message. Caregivers are often very familiar with a child's speech patterns and can often help a new listener learn to understand the child's speech.

- *Motor speech disorders*. The term "motor speech disorders" refers to speech disorders of neurologic origin and can be related to problems with either programing the movements for speech (apraxia) or executing speech movements (dysarthria).
  - *Apraxia of speech* is a condition in which the brain has difficulties programming the movements for speech. Common speech errors observed in apraxia of speech include substitutions or distortions of speech sounds, slower rate, and distortions in the prosody or intonation of speech. Errors typically get worse as utterances become more lengthy, novel, and complex. Individuals with apraxia often visibly struggle or "grope" to form speech sounds. The term "apraxia of speech" was traditionally used to refer to an acquired disorder caused by damage to the speech motor programming area of the brain. However, speech error patterns that are characteristic of apraxia are also observed as a developmental condition in children with no known acute onset of neurologic trauma. In this latter situation, where apraxic speech appears to be developmental in children, the term "childhood apraxia of speech" is now used to differentiate the condition from the traditional acquired apraxia of speech occurring after neurologic injury later in life.
  - The term *dysarthria* refers to a collection of neuromotor speech disorders that are the result of damage to any location along the neuromuscular pathway for executing speech movements including the primary motor cortex, the upper and lower motor neurons, the neuromuscular junction, and the muscle fibers. The characteristics of dysarthria can vary widely depending on the site of neurologic damage. For example, damage to upper motor neurons will cause symptoms of spasticity in muscles (spastic dysarthria), whereas damage to the lower motor neurons will cause flaccidity in muscles (flaccid dysarthria), and

damage to the cerebellum will lead to discoordination (ataxic dysarthria). Problems can involve all aspects of speech production including having sufficient respiratory support for speech, voice quality, articulation accuracy, and resonance (e.g., hypernasal or hyponasal voice). While the specific speech characteristics can vary across different types of dysarthria, the common problem is reduced speech intelligibility as well as reduced naturalness. Speech errors will be fairly consistent in dysarthria as opposed to the more variable errors in apraxia. One of the most common childhood diagnoses associated with dysarthria is cerebral palsy.

- *Fluency disorders*, commonly referred to as *stuttering*, can take several forms including repetitions of words and sounds, prolongations of sounds, and prolonged silent blocks. Stuttering typically emerges in the preschool years. While the exact cause of stuttering is unknown, there are some distinct patterns: it tends to run in families, it is more common in boys than girls, and there is some evidence of neurologic differences that may relate to problems with timing and coordination of speech. Environmental and social stressors such as fast-paced and demanding communication environments that are not sensitive to the child's communication level and pace, as well as emotional stressors in the environment, might also contribute to speech difficulties. Some people who stutter often experience a cycle where speech fluency contributes to feelings of fear or anxiety about a speaking situation, and that anxiety can then contribute to increased dysfluency in that situation in the future. The primary characteristics of stuttering are repetitions, prolongations, and blocks. Many people also develop secondary behaviors that they adopt, sometimes unintentionally, in an effort to push through the dysfluency. These may include facial grimaces, gestures, or other body movements. Some of the key communication strategies to use with children who stutter are to allow them ample time to talk without putting any pressure on them to rush and to respond to the content of what they say without drawing any attention to their dysfluency.

Disorders in Social Use of Communication

Disorders in the social use of communication include difficulties using communication in the "right" ways for the "right" purposes according to the context a child is in at a particular moment. This is closely related to the concept of language use or pragmatics described above in the section on language disorders. However, this category of social use of communication is intended to highlight that the child is able to use pragmatic skills flexibly and adaptively to match or fit each situation. A child may learn rules of pragmatics such as what we typically say or do when meeting someone for the first time, when requesting something that we want, or when we have hurt or inconvenienced someone and need to apologize. Although there may be certain underlying "rules" about what we do in each of those situations, most people will implement those rules differently depending the situation and communication partners involved. For example, we would use a more formal greeting with someone in a professional setting than we would with a friend or family member. Children with disorders in the social use of communication might learn that there is a rule, but they might not be able to adapt and apply that rule flexibly to different situations. They might memorize that they should say "How do you do" when meeting someone. However, they might not realize this formal greeting is appropriate when meeting an adult but makes them stand out as unusual if used with peers at school. This type of challenge is common in children with autism.

Hearing Loss

Hearing loss in children is of paramount concern because of the importance of hearing to developing speech and language, as well as maintaining general connection to the environment. Hearing loss is generally described as either conductive or sensorineural. Conductive hearing loss is due to damage in the outer ear or the middle ear. A typical example is the hearing loss associated with middle ear infections which are common in childhood. Sensorineural hearing loss is associated with damage to the inner ear (the cochlea) and associated neural pathways. While sensorineural loss can certainly occur in children, it is most often associated with aging and noise-induced hearing loss. Children with suspected hearing loss need to be followed closely by their pediatrician and an audiologist to ensure that protracted periods of hearing loss are addressed with the appropriate medical or audiologic services, including hearing aids if needed. When working with a child with hearing loss, the dental provider should be sure the child can see the provider at all times when the provider is talking. This includes removing a mask so the child can see the provider's entire face. The child may use cues from the providers' facial expressions and body language to help them understand what the provider is saying. Also, if a child wears hearing aids, be sure the aids are in place and working before addressing the child.

The term "deaf" refers to situations when hearing loss is profound or complete, and thus an individual has no usable residual hearing. Some families may choose to use sign language as the primary mode of communication, particularly if the family has multiple members who are deaf. A cochlear implant is a series of electrodes surgically implanted into the inner ear and connected to a sound processor worn externally much like a hearing aid. When turned on, the implant allows the child to perceive sound. Children who receive cochlear implants early in their speech and language development years can become very proficient with spoken language.

Dental providers working with families with deaf children should be aware of and sensitive to the issue that the choice about communication methods can have strong ties to culture and identity for some families. The Deaf culture is a very rich culture with strong roots in sign language and close community identity. Many people who are deaf and who associate strongly with Deaf culture will not regard deafness as an impairment or disorder that in any way needs remediation, whereas people who associate strongly with hearing cultures will likely seek to remediate hearing loss through hearing aids or cochlear implants. This is another example of cultural diversity that warrants the full respect of the dental provider. Children who use sign language for communication should be provided with a sign language interpreter for dental visits much as a medical interpreter might be present when a dental provider works with someone who speaks a different language than the provider.

Augmentative and Alternative Communication

Augmentative and Alternative Communication (AAC) methods are useful for individuals who are not able to communicate through verbal messages alone and can be used for a wide variety for communication disorders. A literature review by Millar and colleagues found that 89% of individuals with developmental disabilities demonstrated gains in speech through use of AAC technologies [5]. The use of AAC in dental practice has also been shown to improve communication outcomes [6]. The primary categories of AAC are *unaided*, *low-technology*, and *high-technology* communication strategies [7].

- *Unaided AAC*. Unaided AAC strategies refer to nonverbal communication techniques. These may include informal sign language (personalized hand signals) and formal sign language, pointing, blinking, or squeezing another's hand to indicate "yes" or "no."
- *Low-technology AAC*. This type of AAC involves techniques such as communication boards, books, drawing, writing, or picture exchange systems (Fig. 1). Communication boards and books can either be handmade or purchased. For individuals who are able to spell, an alphabet board is a commonly used type of communication board. Individuals can also point, gesture, or use eye-gazing techniques to select symbols, words, or phrases on a communication board. Symbols, words, phrases, and photographs can be organized into personalized communication books for individuals to use.
- *High-technology AAC*. Electronic devices used to aid communication fall into the category of high-technology AAC techniques. These devices may include electronic communication boards, e-mail, or voice amplification (Fig. 2). Individuals may use speech-generating devices to digitize their speech when they select or spell words, phrases, symbols, or pictures using touch-based or eye-tracking systems. In addition to devices specifically designed as AAC tools, individuals may use tablets or laptop computers that contain communication software or personal photographs.

Dental providers should be sure to be aware of nonverbal cues from their patients using AAC methods. Dental staff may consult with parents and/or caregivers regarding the pediatric patients' individual strategies and preferences in their use of AAC methodologies. Referrals to a speech-language pathologist are warranted for all children along any point of the spectrum of severity of speech and/or language disorders. Because of the critical role that communication plays in a child's social, emotional, and academic development, every effort should be made to maximize the

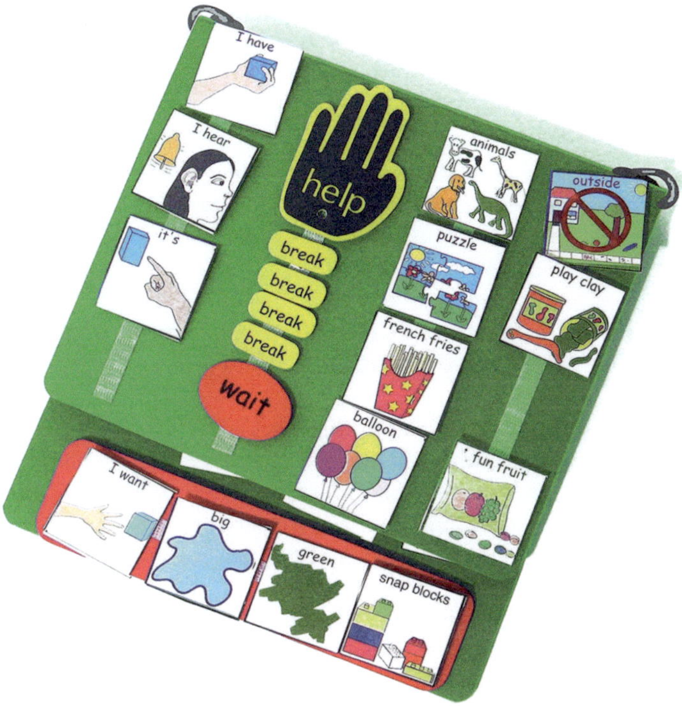

Fig. 1 An example of a low-tech AAC device (Picture Exchange Communication System by Pyramid Educational Consultants)

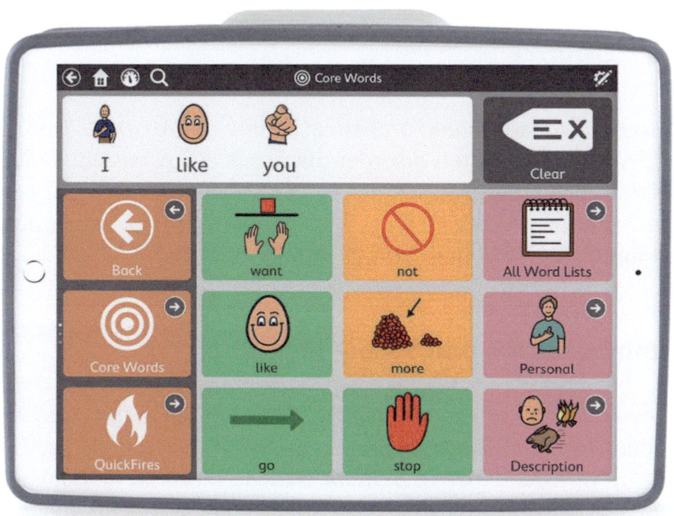

Fig. 2 An example of high-tech AAC device (Tobii Dynavox Speech Case with iPad)

child's access to communication regardless of the nature or severity of the impairment. Children with mild-moderate impairments may benefit from intervention to help them maximize their communication abilities and to perhaps progress toward speech and language function that is typical for their age. Children with more severe impairments, including nonverbal children, are particularly in need of speech-language pathology services to assist them and their families in establishing the least restrictive means of communication possible, including possible use of high-tech or low-tech augmentative communication systems.

Accommodating the Needs of Children with Communication Disorders: The FRAME Mnemonic

Many individuals with communication disorders are able to communicate more productively when people in their environments provide communication supports. Much as a ramp can provide someone in a wheelchair with access to a physical environment, communication supports can give people with communication disorders access to participating in the communication that is happening in their environments [8]. The kinds of communication supports that people need can vary widely with different types of communication disorders, as well as across varying situations that pose unique communication demands and barriers. However, a mnemonic referred to as FRAME can help healthcare providers prepare for, or frame, their interactions with people with communication disorders for a more respectful and productive healthcare encounter [9, 10, 11]. The FRAME model was initially developed for use with adults with communication disorders but is adapted for use with children in Table 1:

Autism

According to the *Diagnostic and Statistical Manual of Mental Disorders, 5th edition* (DSM-5), autism spectrum disorder manifests as "persistent deficits in social communication and social interaction" and "restrictive and repetitive patterns of behavior, interests or activities" [12]. A review of how these manifestations can impact communication in dental settings is detailed below.

Social Communication and Social Interaction

Autism is considered a "spectrum disorder." People with autism may have varying levels of deficits in social communication and social interaction. The DSM-5 notes three categories of these types of deficits: deficits in social-emotional reciprocity, deficits in nonverbal communicative behaviors, and deficits involved in developing, maintaining, and understanding relationships.

Table 1 The FRAME framework for communicating with children with communication disorders

	General strategy	Examples of how to apply to children with communication disorders
F	*Familiarize* Familiarize yourself with how the patient communicates before the medical or dental session. This helps to avoid communication breakdowns by setting the "ground rules" for communication before the conversation starts	• If the child is old enough and able to respond, ask her how she would like to communicate and if there is anything she would like you to do to help with communication • Ask caregivers how they communicate with the child. Ask them to show you how to communicate with the child • Review chart notes, particularly for information from speech-language pathologists and audiologists, pediatricians, or other healthcare providers • If a child uses any communication device or materials, ask them to demonstrate it, and learn how you should interact with them before starting the appointment • Do not reinvent the wheel if the child has existing communication strategies that work for her
R	*Reduce rate* Reduce your rate of speech. The pace of most communication is too fast for most people with communication disorders	• Be sensitive to the pace of communication that is comfortable for the child and maintain that pace • Slow your speech down a bit, but keep the tone natural. Pause frequently and use shorter sentences to help children with comprehension problems understand you • Be very patient and allow children time to express themselves. Do *not* rush a child to talk or to respond
A	*Assist with communication* Directly assist and participate in the communication process. Be willing to "step forward" to help with communication—do not wait for the child to solve a communication breakdown. If existing communication strategies are not working, try a new one	• Try asking questions in different ways—open ended, multiple choice, yes/no. Different types of questions might work better at different times or for different purposes • Verify that you and the child understand each other. Frequently repeat or summarize what the child says and check that the child understands you, without making her feel that she is being quizzed • Do *not* pretend to understand the child when you do not. Acknowledge when you are not understanding each other—but do so in a kind and supportive manner—and keep working to find a strategy to communicate

(continued)

Table 1 (continued)

	General strategy	Examples of how to apply to children with communication disorders
M	*Mix communication modalities* Do not rely on speaking/listening only. Supplement conversations with additional ways to communicate—either to help the child understand you or to help the child express herself	• Use body language and facial expression to add actions to words to help convey meaning • Encourage a child who has difficulty talking to *show* you if she cannot tell you. Can she point, gesture, or otherwise demonstrate what she wants to say? • Keep communication materials on-hand, such as picture boards that contain pictures of things the child will see and do in the dental visit. These can be used to aid your explanation of what is happening; and help the child express herself • Both of you can write or draw on whiteboards or pads of paper to convey information • If a child uses eye gaze to communicate, try using the eyes to point (e.g., pointing to choices held in your hands or responses pictured on page held in front of child) instead of using blinking which can be confusing • If a child uses an augmentative device, learn how the device works and how you should interact with the child in the context of the device
E	*Engage* Engage the patient first	• Respect the child's autonomy to a degree that is appropriate for her age and developmental level • Include the child in communication about the dental visit as you would any child—requesting preferences when appropriate, informing her about what will happen, etc. • Show interest in the child as a person by building rapport as you would with any child: by asking about hobbies, family, school, etc. • Position yourself at eye level with the child so you are not looking down at her • To the extent possible and appropriate for developmental level, caregivers should help you communicate *with* the child but should not communicate *for* the child

Adapted from Burns MI, Baylor CR, Morris MA, McNalley TW, Yorkston KM. Training health-care providers in patient-provider communication: what speech language pathology and medical education can learn from one another. Aphasiology. 2012;26(5):673–688

- *Deficits in social-emotional reciprocity*. Reciprocity is the "mutual and symmetrical exchange between individuals while talking, working or playing together, including finely timed turn taking and a steadily increasing dynamics as the interaction unfolds" [13]. While the DSM-5 does not define social-emotional reciprocity, the manual lists the following as examples of deficits in this area:
  - Abnormal social approach
  - Failure of normal back-and-forth conversation
  - Reduced sharing of interests, emotions, or affect
  - Failure to initiate or respond to social interactions

Children develop skills in social-emotional reciprocity over time as they age. Deficits in social-emotional reciprocity may make it more difficult for children with autism to respond to communication cues from a dental provider, to maintain turn taking in communication with the dental provider, and to engage in conversations in ways that are sensitive to social cues. As reciprocity is a two-way street, reciprocity may be increased when dental providers are attentive to the child's interests, engage with her, match her pace, and adapt to the child's communication styles [14].

- *Deficits in nonverbal communicative behaviors used for social interaction*. Nonverbal communication is a cornerstone of communication. Individuals with autism have varying levels of deficits in nonverbal communicative behaviors. The DSM-5 gives the following examples of deficits in this area:
  - Poorly integrated verbal and nonverbal communication
  - Abnormalities in eye contact and body language
  - Deficits in understanding and use of gestures
  - Total lack of facial expressions and nonverbal communication

Discomfort with eye contact is often present among individuals with autism. Children with autism may have selective deficits in recognizing facial expressions, being more comfortable with familiar faces and less comfortable with new faces. The reasons for this are still being researched. The eye avoidance hypothesis is that eye contact is avoided due to being perceived as socially threatening and that this eye avoidance makes it harder to recognize facial expressions [15]. Eye contact is often used in dental practice, especially with children who might experience procedural anxiety. It may help the provider to become familiar with the patient's preferences and comfort level regarding eye contact.

In addition to deficits in nonverbal and social-emotional communication, individuals with autism may have language and speech deficits as well. Techniques for facilitating communication with patients with communication disorders, including language and speech disorders, were presented earlier in this chapter (FRAME framework).

- *Deficits in developing, maintaining, and understanding relationships*. Individuals with autism may have difficulty in developing, maintaining and understanding

relationships. This can include relationships with healthcare providers. Examples from the DSM-5 of how these deficits can manifest are listed below:
- Difficulties adjusting behavior to suit various social contexts
- Difficulties in sharing imaginative play or in making friends
- Absence of interest in peers

Patterns of Behavior, Interests, or Activities

In addition to the social-emotional communication deficits discussed above, individuals with autism exhibit "restrictive, repetitive patterns of behavior, interests or activities." Examples from the DSM-5 are listed below:

- Stereotyped or repetitive motor movements, use of objects, or speech (e.g., simple motor stereotypies, lining up toys or flipping objects, echolalia, idiosyncratic phrases)
- Insistence on sameness, inflexible adherence to routines, or ritualized patterns of verbal or nonverbal behavior (e.g., extreme distress at small changes, difficulties with transitions, rigid thinking patterns, greeting rituals, need to take same route or eat same food every day)
- Highly restricted, fixated interests that are abnormal in intensity or focus (e.g., strong attachment to or preoccupation with unusual objects, excessively circumscribed or perseverative interests)
- Hyper- or hyporeactivity to sensory input or unusual interest in sensory aspects of the environment (e.g., apparent indifference to pain/temperature, adverse response to specific sounds or textures, excessive smelling or touching of objects, visual fascination with lights or movement)

Familiarization with these potential manifestations of autism can help the dental provider facilitate care and communication with patients who have an autism spectrum disorder diagnosis. For example, stererotypies, such as echolalia (repeating another's words), hand flapping, rocking, lip smacking, chewing, or humming may occur. Historically, these behaviors were considered nonfunctional. There are some hypotheses that these behaviors may serve a function, such as maintaining focus and mediating sensory input [16]. Other manifestations of autism may include hypersensitivity to light, sound, and touch. For some children with autism, maintaining a quiet and low light environment may help them engage in communication in the dental visit.

Intellectual Disability

Children with intellectual disability (ID) have wide variation in communication abilities, even among the same severity categories. They may have impairments in both expressive and receptive communication. *Expressive communication* is communication to convey messages to others. This includes communicating preferences, decisions, and emotions via verbal and nonverbal means. Impairments in this area can vary widely among children with ID and may be due to the intellectual impairment itself, a co-occurring developmental disorder, and/or another communication disorder. Some children with ID will have minimal to no expressive communication impairments. Some may communicate with 1–2 word phrases or sentences in addition to nonverbal methods. Others may rely on nonverbal methods exclusively, such as pointing, facial expressions, reaching gestures, vocalizations, and/or eye gaze [17, 18].

Receptive communication involves understanding messages from others. Similar to expressive communication, there is wide variation in receptive communication abilities in children with ID. Causes of receptive communication impairment among individuals with ID include impairments in memory and attention span, as well as processing verbal and nonverbal messages. Receptive communication abilities also vary by context [19]. An unfamiliar context, such as a new dental office, can make understanding messages more difficult. Individuals with ID typically have stronger receptive communication abilities than expressive communication abilities [20].

Recommendations for the dental provider:

- Familiarize yourself with manifestations of communication disorders, autism, and intellectual disability to gain awareness of the communication needs that may be present in children with these conditions.
- Utilize the FRAME framework with children who have communication disorders and other conditions which may impact communication.

Culturally Appropriate Communication

There are many cultural influences on health and healthcare. Many of the most important of these are included in Pamela Hay's ADDRESSING Framework of Cultural Influences [21]. These include:

- Age and generation
- Developmental and other disabilities
- Religion
- Ethnicity/race
- Socioeconomic status
- Sex
- Indigenous status
- Nationality
- Gender and gender identity

These influences act in intersecting ways and have varying levels of personal importance to individual people, including CSHCN. For those who have developmental and other disabilities, there are many considerations that factor into culturally appropriate patient-provider communication. Chapter 1 details cultural factors specific to developmental and other disabilities, including ableism, the social model of disability, and structural barriers to accessing healthcare. Disability is one aspect of a person's identity or life circumstances that may overlap with many other cultural identities. Fifty percent of CSHCN come from homes with low socioeconomic status and/or a minority ethnic/racial group [22]. Additionally, many CSHCN come from families with limited English proficiency [23]. Language barriers and variations in health literacy can increase the risk of communication vulnerabilities in practice, especially if providers are not responsive to addressing these barriers. Sensitivity to the cultural identities and needs of CSHCN will help facilitate communication in practice.

Recommendations for the dental provider:

- Become familiar with cultural factors specific to disabilities, including ableism and the social model of disability.
- Commit to lifelong learning in the development of cultural humility.

Triadic Communication

Triadic communication in pediatric dental care involves communication between three individuals, the dental provider, the patient, and the caregiver (often a parent). There are three sets of communication dyads in triadic communication (Fig. 3) [24, 25]. These are:

- The dental provider and child
- The child and parent
- The parent and dental provider

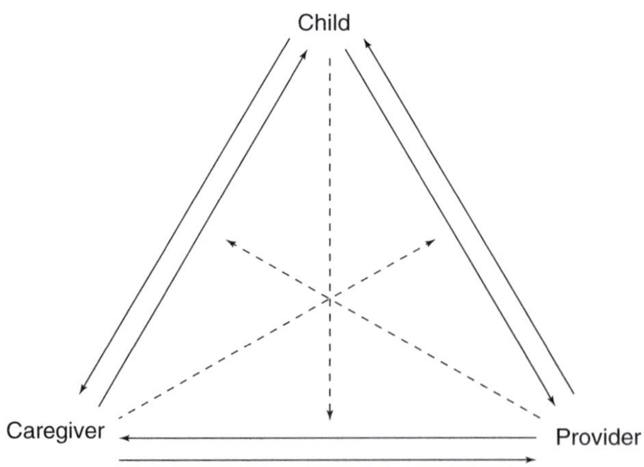

Fig. 3 Communication triad. Contains three communication dyads: child-provider, child-caregiver, provider-caregiver. Each individual in the triad may influence communication in any of the dyads

Each of these communication dyads may involve communication along the same theme or may involve communication along different themes.

- *Communication between the dental provider and child.* Healthcare outcomes improve when children are involved in communication with their healthcare provider. However, studies show that children are often overlooked in communication triads in medical settings [25, 26]. The authority of adults, both parent and provider, influences this communication. Children are generally able to make meaningful contributions to communication regarding treatment decisions as young as 5 years old [27]. By 7 years old, children are often better at communicating their own health information to providers than their parents [25]. Children are more likely to be overlooked in communication processes if they have cognitive delays or communication disorders or a frequently stigmatized chronic condition. Dental providers should involve children in discussions on decision-making to the extent possible. This may include verbal and nonverbal communication and the use of AAC.
- *Communication between the child and parent.* The relationship between parents and CSHCN is complex, as is any parent-child relationship. During dental appointments, some children may look to their parents to reduce their anxiety, answer questions for them, or help them make decisions. Other children may be more independent in a dental setting. Parents often advocate for their CSHCN in dental practice. Child-parent communication may focus on alleviating patient anxieties or advocating for the child to be more involved in communication herself. If a CSHCN has a behavioral or medical condition that necessitates the parent's attention, the parent may attend to the needs of the child while simultaneously trying to communicate with the provider. It was historically assumed that when a child received a diagnosis of a disability, parents experienced primarily sorrow and negative emotions. Newer theories recognize the complex role a disability diagnosis can have on both the parent and child. Parents experience various feelings reflective of the joys and difficulties of parenthood, whether or not a child has a disability or SHCN [28, 29, 30, 31].
- *Communication between the parent and dental provider.* The provider-parent interaction may focus on parental concerns about the child's oral health, her ability to tolerate dental care, the length of the appointment, the treatment recommended, obtaining consents for procedures, and/or the cost of care. For many CSHCN, the parent's role as advocate plays a big part in parent-provider communication, especially when a communication disorder or other communication barrier is at play. Generally, when a child is unable to verbally communicate her concerns, parents can give the dental provider excellent insight into her concerns and what she can tolerate. Sometimes parents may not accurately assess what their child can tolerate in the dental chair, including overestimating or underestimating her ability to tolerate and follow instructions for dental care. Listening to their concerns and keeping an open mind about the patient's abilities can help address the needs of both the patient and parent.

Discussing Sensitive Topics

One barrier to communication with parents of CSHCN is the stigma that sometimes accompanies a child's disability. As an example, mothers of children who have been diagnosed with fetal alcohol spectrum disorder (FASD) may feel stigmatized and judged negatively due to their alcohol consumption during pregnancy. The National Organization on Fetal Alcohol Syndrome (NOFAS) has adopted a "Stamp Out Stigma" campaign to help lessen the stigma in parents, particularly biological/birth mothers of children with FASD [32]. When discussing a child's health history that may be associated with stigma with parents (e.g., alcohol consumption during pregnancy), it is critical to use language that is nonjudgmental. For example, NOFAS suggests defining FASD as "The range of effects that occur when a baby is prenatally exposed to alcohol," rather than saying to a parent that "FASD is what happens when a mother drinks alcohol while she's pregnant." Using noncritical, nonjudgmental language increases the likelihood that a parent will report a child's symptoms accurately and can significantly improve communication between parents and healthcare providers. Other scenarios where disclosure of disability may be a sensitive topic include disability from accidental drowning, a motor-vehicle accident, or a congenitally acquired infection. The same principles of using nonjudgmental language apply.

Complexity of Decision-Making

Parents typically give consent for medical care for their children. In some cases children will have another family member who serves the role of legal guardian for the child. It is generally preferred to have assent from the child as well. In some cases this not possible, such as might occur with an infant or someone who is not able to communicate her preferences for care. Once the child turns 18, she has reached legal adulthood and is able to give consent herself. This process becomes complicated if the person has a condition that impacts her ability to make healthcare decisions. *Capacity* to consent is defined as the cognitive ability to make medical decisions, including the ability to understand the treatment proposed, the risks and benefits of treatment or refusal, and the alternatives to treatment [33]. *Competency* is a legal definition that an individual is able to give her own consent. Once a minor becomes an adult, she becomes legally competent to consent unless a court has declared otherwise. When a court has decided that an individual does not have the capacity to consent, she is considered not competent to consent and is appointed a guardian to make medical decisions. When it appears that an adolescent with special healthcare needs may not have medical decision-making capacity, it becomes important to address this issue prior to adulthood to avoid delays in care. In cases where the capacity to consent is questionable, it may help to involve the patient's primary care physician or psychiatrist to determine capacity [34]. In some cases, a person may lack the capacity to consent, regardless of legal status. In these cases, a caregiver or parent may need to pursue medical guardianship in order to proceed with care.

It is often helpful to have children participate in the decision-making processes. Children in general may be very susceptible to the influence of others, including in how they communicate decision-making. For example, some children may have a tendency to respond "yes" to every question asked, as a learned adaptation to avoid "getting into trouble." This is called acquiescence or *yea-saying* and can occur in all children, but especially among children with intellectual disabilities [35, 36]. Children may also respond this way in the dental setting when they do not understand what the dentist or dental staff is asking. A related concept is *nay-saying*. In this case a child learns to respond "no" to all questions as an adaptive technique to avoid unwanted or unpleasant situations. If the dental staff suspect that the child is using this communication method, they may change how they ask questions so that she is encouraged to choose between one of two options. Both options, however, arrive at the same outcome. For example, the dental provider may ask a child, "Would you like to get in the chair by yourself, or would you like me to help you get into the chair?" In both instances, the outcome is that the child is seated in the dental chair. When given a list of choices, some children may tend to choose the option they heard most recently, regardless of what they truly want to do. This type of response is known as *recency*. Dental staff can alternate the order in which they present the choices in order to avoid this type of response bias.

Case-Based Scenario

Part 1

An 18-month-old female with severe oral aversion, avoidant/restrictive food intake disorder (ARFID), and a heart murmur presents for a new patient evaluation with her parents. The parents' chief dental concerns are chipped teeth and how dental treatment might impact feeding issues. The other major concern is tolerance of an oral exam given her sensory issues and extreme fear of strangers.

The provider listened to the parents discuss their concerns regarding oral aversion, feeding issues, and sensory concerns for approximately 20 minutes prior to initiating the exam. The mother held the child on her lap during the exam, and the child tolerated the exam well. After the examination the dentist told the parents that some teeth needed to be extracted and other teeth needed restorations. The dentist attempted to schedule the patient for dental surgery. The parents left the appointment "horrified and in tears."

What Went Wrong?

The mother reported that "the dentist gave us no explanation of why she needed her teeth out or how it would affect her it. It seemed like he had not listened to a single thing I said." The provider did not address one of the major chief complaints, which is how dental care might impact a special healthcare need (ARFID).

Part 2

The parents took the child to another dentist for a second opinion. The appointment proceeded as described above, with a 20 minutes discussion prior to the exam, an exam that was well tolerated, and recommendations for extractions and restorations. The dentist followed the exam with a discussion of the dental problems the child was experiencing, the risks and benefits of treatment, the risks and benefits of no treatment, the relationship between feeding issues and dental problems, and what to expect once treatment was completed. The patient received dental care under general anesthesia followed by routine care in the dental office.

By 2.5 years of age the patient had been diagnosed with autism. She was able to sit in the dental chair independently, although still was fearful of dental care. The dental hygienist was able to clean her teeth using tell-show-do, positive reinforcement, and breaks, to which the child responded very well. The mother described the most recent dental hygiene visit as "amazing."

What Went Right?

The family's chief concerns were addressed, and they felt heard. The provider used patient/family centered interviewing principles to "iteratively explain diagnostic and/or prognostic information and incorporate [the patient/family's] informational needs" [37]. The family felt confident in proceeding with care.

On recall, the mother reports that the dental hygienist "explained everything she was going to do beforehand. She let her feel each instrument on her hand and showed her each time what she would do with it, how it would feel, and what noise it would make and asked her if the noise was okay. She took several breaks to make sure she was okay and gave her time to reset. I think this is a big thing because the sensory stuff plus the anxiety can overload her."

Lessons Learned

- Having a dental exam or procedure go well in the eyes of the provider does not necessarily mean the appointment went well from the perspective of the parent.
- Addressing patient/family concerns, including those related to the special healthcare need, is a critical aspect of communication in dental practice.
- Listening to a patient or family member does not mean that they will feel heard. Principles of patient/family-centered interviewing can facilitate effective healthcare communication.
- Behavioral facilitation techniques make up a critical part of communication between providers and many patients with special healthcare needs.

Conclusion

Communication in healthcare settings is complex. Communication needs of CSHCN are not universal; they are affected by individual history with the medical care system, personal and cultural needs and preferences, and health conditions that affect communication. Commitment to lifelong learning to address complex communication needs can help providers better serve CSHCN.

Take-Home Points

- CSCHN have diverse communication needs in dental settings that will vary with their experiences in the healthcare system and communication preferences.
- Communication disorders can occur in isolation or co-occur with other special healthcare needs.
- Individuals with autism spectrum disorder may have varying levels of deficits in social communication and social interaction, including discomfort with eye contact and nonverbal communicative behaviors.
- When treating patients with intellectual disability, there will be significant variation in both expressive and receptive communication abilities.
- Dental providers should take time to familiarize themselves with the child's experiences in the healthcare system, her preferences for communication methods, the nature of any communication disorders she may have, and her ability to participate in the decision-making process about her dental care.
- The FRAME mnemonic (*F*amiliarize, *R*educe Rate, *A*ssist with Communication, *M*ix Communication Modalities, and *E*ngage) is a valuable tool in helping dental providers frame their interactions with patients with communication disorders.
- Dental providers should engage with both the child and her parents or caregivers in developing effective communication strategies for the dental setting (triadic communication).
- Excellent communication with CSHCN requires dental providers to practice cultural humility.

Acknowledgments Julie Dunlap, MS, CCC-SLP
University of Washington, Department of Speech and Hearing Sciences
For the conceptual organization of section on communication disorders

References

1. McPherson M, Arango P, Fox H, Lauver C, McManus M, Newacheck PW, Perrin JM, Shonkoff JP, Strickland B. A new definition of children with special health care needs. Pediatrics. 1998;102(1):102–37.
2. Kuo DZ, Melguizo-Castro M, Goudie A, Nick TG, Robbins JM, Casey PH. Variation in child health care utilization by medical complexity. Matern Child Health J. 2015;19(1):40–8.
3. Anderson N, Shames G, editors. Human communication disorders: an introduction. 8th ed. Upper Saddle River, NJ: Pearson; 2011.
4. Paul R, Norbury C, Gosse C. Language disorders from infancy through adolescence: listening, speaking, reading, writing, and communicating. 5th ed. Maryland Heights, MO: Mosby; 2017.
5. Millar DC, Light JC, Schlosser RW. The impact of augmentative and alternative communication intervention on the speech production of individuals with developmental disabilities: a research review. J Speech Lang Hear Res. 2006;49(2):248–64.
6. Grewal N, Sethi T, Grewal S. Widening horizons through alternative and augmentative communication systems for managing children with special health care needs in a pediatric dental setup. Spec Care Dentist. 2015;35(3):114–9.

7. Beukelman DR, Garrett KL, Yorkston KM. Augmentative communication strategies for adults with acute or chronic medical conditions. Baltimore, MD: Paul H Brookes Publishing; 2007.
8. Kagan A. Supported conversation for adults with aphasia: methods and resources for training conversation partners. Aphasiology. 1998;12:816–30.
9. Burns MI, Baylor CR, Morris MA, McNalley TW, Yorkston KM. Training healthcare providers in patient-provider communication: what speech language pathology and medical education can learn from one another. Aphasiology. 2012;26(5):673–88.
10. Burns M, Baylor C, Dudgeon BJ, Starks H, Yorkston K. Health care provider accommodations for patients with communication disorders. Top Lang Disord. 2017;37(4):311–33.
11. Yorkston K, Baylor C, Burns M, Morris M, McNalley T. Medical education: preparing professionals to enhance communication access in healthcare settings. In: Blackstone S, Beukelman D, Yorkston K, editors. Patient provider communication: roles of speech-language pathologists and other health care professionals. San Diego, CA: Plural Publishing; 2015. p. 37–72.
12. American Psychological Association. Autism spectrum disorder. In: Diagnostic and statistical manual of mental disorders. 5th ed. Arlington, VA: American Psychological Association, 2013. Print; p. 50–59.
13. van Ommeren TB, Begeer S, Scheeren AM, Koot HM. Measuring reciprocity in high functioning children and adolescents with autism spectrum disorders. J Autism Dev Disord. 2012;42:1001–10.
14. Gernsbacher MA. Toward a behavior of reciprocity. J Dev Process. 2006;1(1):139–52.
15. Tanaka JW, Sung A. The "eye avoidance" hypothesis of autism face processing. J Autism Dev Disord. 2016;46(5):1538–52.
16. Barry S, Baird H, Lascelles K, Bunton P, Hedderly T. Neurodevelopmental movement disorders – an update on childhood motor stereotypies. Dev Med Child Neurol. 2011;53:979–85.
17. Schalick WO, Westbrook C, Young B. Communication with individuals with intellectual disabilities and psychiatric disabilities: a summary of the literature. Ann Arbor, MI: University of Michigan Retirement Research Center; 2012.
18. Cascella PW. Expressive communication strengths of adults with severe to profound intellectual disabilities as reported by group home staff. Commun Disord Q. 2005;26(3):156–63.
19. Purcell M, Morris I, McConkey R. Staff perceptions of the communicative competence of adult persons with intellectual disabilities. Br J Dev Disabil. 1999;45(1):16–25.
20. Belva BC, Matson JL, Sipes M, Bamburg JW. An examination of specific communication deficits in adults with profound intellectual disabilities. Res Dev Disabil. 2012;33:525–9.
21. Hays PA. The new reality: diversity and complexity. In: Addressing cultural complexities in practice. 3rd ed. Washington, DC: American Psychological Association; 2016. p. 3–18.
22. van Dyck PC, Kogan MD, McPherson MG, Weissman GR, Newacheck PW. Prevalence and characteristics of children with special health care needs. Arch Pediatr Adolesc Med. 2004;158(9):884–90.
23. Eneriz-Wiemer M, Sanders LM, Barr DA, Mendoza FS. Parental limited English proficiency and health outcomes for children with special health care needs: a systematic review. Acad Pediatr. 2013;14(2):128–36.
24. Solomon O, Angell AM, Yin L, Lawlor MC. "You can turn off the light if you'd like": pediatric health care visits for children with autism spectrum disorder as an interactional achievement. Med Anthropol Q. 2015;29(4):531–55.
25. Greene MG, Adelman RD. Beyond the dyad: communication in triadic (and more) medical encounters. In: Martin LR, DiMatteo MR, editors. The Oxford handbook of health communication, behavior change, and treatment adherence. 2013. http://www.oxfordhandbooks.com/view/10.1093/oxfordhb/9780199795833.001.0001/oxfordhb-9780199795833-e-003. Accessed 22 Feb 2018.
26. Carnevale FA, Teachman G, Bogossian A. A relational ethics framework for advancing practice with children with complex health care needs and their parents. Compr Child Adolesc Nurs. 2017;40(4):268–84.

27. Cahill P, Papageorgiou A. Triadic communication in the primary care paediatric consultation. Br J Gen Pract. 2007;57:904–11.
28. Green SE. “We’re tired, not sad”: benefits and burdens of mothering a child with a disability. Soc Sci Med. 2007;64:150–63.
29. Lalvani P, Polvere L. Historical perspectives on studying families of children with disabilities: a case for critical research. Disabil Stud Q. 2013;33. https://doi.org/10.18061/dsq.v33i3.3209.
30. Kandel I, Merrick J. The child with a disability: parental acceptance, management and coping. Sci World J. 2007;7:1799–809.
31. Neely-Barnes SL, Graff JC, Roberts RJ, Hall HR, Hankins JS. “It’s our job”: a qualitative study of family responses to ableism. Intellect Dev Disabil. 2010;48(4):245–58.
32. NOFAS. National Organization on Fetal Alcohol Syndrome. NOFAS Statement on the Stigma of Fetal Alcohol Syndrome. 2018. https://www.nofas.org/2015/08/24/nofas-statement-on-the-stigma-of-fasd/. Accessed 5 Mar 2018.
33. Leo RJ. Competency and the capacity to make treatment decisions: a primer for primary care physicians. Prim Care Companion J Clin Psychiatry. 1999;1(5):131–41.
34. Applebaum PS. Assessment of patients’ competence to consent to treatment. N Engl J Med. 2007;357:1834–40.
35. Finlay WM, Lyons E. Acquiescence in interviews with people who have mental retardation. Ment Retard. 2002;40(1):14–29.
36. Heal LW, Sigelman CK. Response biases in interviews of individuals with limited mental ability. J Intellect Disabil Res. 1995;39(Pt 4):331–40.
37. Fortin AH, Dwamena FC, Frankel RM, Smith RC, editors. Smith’s patient-centered interviewing: an evidence-based method. 3rd ed. New York, NY: The McGraw-Hill Companies, Inc.; 2012.

Adapting Oral Care Protocols to Support Children with Sensory Sensitivities: Occupational Therapy and Dentistry

Leah I. Stein Duker

Introduction

Difficulties processing sensory information can occur in typically developing children but are even more prevalent in clinical populations. Specifically, sensory sensitivities can negatively impact how children experience and interact with the world around them. It is essential to take sensory sensitivities into account when providing oral care to children with special health care needs (CSHCNs) in order to improve both the oral care experience and the success of the encounter for children and their caregivers. With a little knowledge and a willingness to be flexible and try different strategies, great potential exists to provide a holistic and comprehensive approach to improve care.

An Overview of Occupational Therapy

Occupational therapy (OT) is a widely utilized and recognized health profession. It is client-centered and focused on helping:

> "people across the lifespan to do the things they want and need to do through the therapeutic use of daily activities (occupations). Occupational therapy practitioners enable people of all ages to live life to its fullest by helping them promote health and prevent—or live better with—injury, illness, or disability" [1].

OT provides a unique holistic perspective to patient challenges and works to either remediate issues or adapt the task and/or environment to enable participation. These principles guide all of occupational therapy practice, but OT may look very different depending on the setting (e.g., home, school, clinic, hospital, community) and the

L. I. Stein Duker (✉)
Chan Division of Occupational Science and Occupational Therapy, University of Southern California, Los Angeles, CA, USA
e-mail: lstein@chan.usc.edu

T. M. Nelson, J. R. Webb (eds.), *Dental Care for Children with Special Needs*,
https://doi.org/10.1007/978-3-030-10483-2_4

population (e.g., individuals with developmental disabilities, autism, physical disabilities, spinal cord injuries, stroke survivors, mental health diagnoses, etc.).

Occupational therapists (OTs) can assist children in developing the foundational sensory and motor skills that support good oral care. Specifically, OTs may work with children on fine motor skills, feeding difficulties, postural stability/positioning, and sensory processing challenges. Adequate fine motor skills are essential for maintaining good oral hygiene in the home with toothbrushing and flossing activities. When there are delays in fine motor skills, OTs can address motor coordination and control difficulties through development of skills and/or adaptation of equipment (i.e., "building up" of toothbrush handles). Good oral hygiene can also be impacted by feeding difficulties, especially in children who have atypical tongue or lip function, which may lead to challenges with swallowing and/or chewing. Some chewing problems result in nutritional management that includes the use of the bottle for prolonged periods of time and/or the use of soft and easy-to-chew diets that are often rich in carbohydrates and easily become stuck between the teeth. OTs work with children who have feeding difficulties and can improve the foundational skills necessary for improved oral care. Additionally, some children have postural instability due to muscle weakness, paralysis, or spasticity and may require positioning techniques to facilitate home and professional oral care that can be provided by OTs. Lastly, sensory processing difficulties, the emphasis of this chapter, may lead to cariogenic food repertoires and can significantly negatively impact adequate oral care both in the home and dental office.

Sensory Processing

Sensory processing refers to the way in which our nervous system organizes incoming sensory information so that we can successfully interact with the world around us. Through modulation of sensory input from all seven of our sensory systems, facilitation and inhibition in the central nervous system (CNS) allow us to respond to relevant information, ignore that which is not, and generate appropriate behavioral responses [2, 3]. Sensory processing abilities are typically measured and diagnosed by OTs in a variety of ways including standardized, norm-referenced tests, caregiver-/teacher-completed questionnaires, and clinical observations. However, many disciplines commonly utilize parental questionnaires or interviews, such as the Short Sensory Profile 2 [4], Sensory Profile 2 [4], or the Sensory Processing Measure [5].

Parents and/or dental professionals may suspect the presence of sensory processing difficulties, specifically over-responsivity to sensory stimuli (sensory sensitivities), if a child exhibits behaviors such as:

- Visual: covering eyes or complaining about bright lights that do not bother others
- Auditory: covering ears or responding negatively to noises that do not bother others
- Tactile: avoiding being touched and/or grooming activities, wearing only clothes that fit the body loosely

- Gustatory/olfactory: exhibiting picky eating behaviors and/or avoiding certain smells or foods that children of a similar age often eat/enjoy
- Vestibular (movement): displaying distress behaviors when feet leave the ground, difficulty moving head upside down or backwards in space (e.g., leaning head back to wash hair in bathtub)

These difficulties may occur throughout all sensory modalities or present themselves only when a child is exposed to certain types of sensory stimuli.

Sensory Processing Difficulties

Sensory processing difficulties occur when sensory information is processed and perceived by the brain atypically, such that responses to differing types of sensory stimuli are not graded appropriately, either leading to over- or under-reactions to stimulation or problems with sensorimotor control [6]. According to Dunn's model of sensory processing, people's responses to sensory input vary based on differing neurological thresholds (how reactive they are to stimuli), which exist along a continuum [7]. Those with low neurological thresholds require less intense or less frequent sensory stimulation to excite the nervous system and elicit a behavioral response, while people with high thresholds require stronger and more intense input to elicit a behavioral response [7]. It is important, however, to note that neurological threshold can vary within an individual based on internal and external conditions as well as the type of sensory input [7]. These sensory processing challenges may be pervasive across the lifespan and have been reported to exist through adulthood in populations with autism spectrum disorder (ASD) and attention deficit hyperactivity disorder (ADHD) [8, 9].

Sensory processing difficulties include a wide array of responses, including sensory over-responsiveness (defensiveness) and sensory under-responsiveness, and can occur across all sensory domains (e.g., tactile, auditory, visual, olfactory, vestibular) [6]. Difficulties modulating sensory information can lead to inappropriate reactions to sensory stimuli, which can be detected both behaviorally and physiologically [10, 11].

People with low neurological thresholds are said to have an *over-responsive* nervous system, causing them to notice stimuli present in daily life more so than others [7]. This leads to an exaggerated and often aversive response to stimuli that others would consider non-noxious, often resulting in *fight, fright, or flight* reactions, including physical withdrawal, vocal outbursts, aggressive behaviors, tantrums, or attempts to block the stimuli [12].

Populations Experiencing Sensory Processing Difficulties

Sensory processing difficulties have been reported in a number of clinical populations including individuals with ASD [13, 14], ADHD [15, 16], developmental delay [13, 14], Fragile X syndrome [17], and fetal alcohol spectrum disorder [18] and children who have experienced prolonged institutional care [19]. Although clearly more frequent in clinical populations, reports of sensory processing abnormalities also exist in typically developing populations. Research indicates that, based on parent perception, approximately 5–33% of typically developing children experience difficulty with sensory processing [8, 20].

The patients with sensory processing difficulties that dental practitioners will most likely encounter are children with ASD, as 1 in 59 children is diagnosed with ASD [21] and research indicates that up to 95% of children with ASD exhibit some form of sensory processing difficulties [22]. In fact, sensory differences (specifically hyper- or hyporeactivity to sensory input) are now included in the new DSM-5 (Diagnostic and Statistical Manual of Mental Disorders) diagnostic criteria as an example of the restricted, repetitive patterns of behavior, interests, or activities that may be exhibited by individuals with ASD [23].

The remainder of this chapter will focus on sensory sensitivities (also termed sensory over-responsivity). Due to the frequency of sensory-related concerns experienced by children with ASD, the majority of current research examining the impact of sensory sensitivities on dental care has been conducted on individuals with ASD.

Impact of Sensory Sensitivities

Challenges with sensory processing difficulties, particularly sensory over-responsivity, have been found to be positively correlated with anxiety [24]. Feelings of anxiety may result in adherence to strict daily routines [7] and have both psychological and physiological effects that can adversely interfere with optimal patient outcomes and overall well-being during healthcare encounters [25]. These difficulties have the ability to impede participation in a variety of activities, decrease quality of life [26], and have been shown to be negatively correlated with a patient's ability to function on a day-to-day basis [27]. Additionally, it has been reported that that children with ASD with greater differences in taste/smell sensitivity or auditory/visual sensitivity exhibit decreased receptive and expressive language skills [28]. These diminished language skills have the potential to negatively impact traditional dental behavior guidance techniques such as tell-show-do. Therefore, it is no surprise that sensory sensitivities have the potential to negatively impact oral health and dental treatment [29–31].

Negative Impact on Diet

Limited diet/food repertoire. Children with sensory sensitivities may experience hyper-sensitivities to taste, texture, or smells. This can potentially lead to avoidance and restriction of foods, resulting in limited and/or "picky" diets [32]. For example, high sensitivities to taste, smell, and/or tactile sensory stimuli in children have been found to be associated with lower fruit and vegetable preference and consumption [33].

Children with ASD who have greater sensory impairment also experience more feeding and mealtime problems [34]. For example, the presence of sensory over-responsivity in different domains (e.g., overall, taste/smell sensitivity, oral sensory sensitivity) has been linked to higher food selectivity, food refusal, and disruptive feeding and mealtime behaviors [35, 36]. Overall, children with ASD are reported to refuse foods based on texture and prefer soft, sweet, or sticky foods [37, 38]. These limited food repertoires and modified dietary habits and preferences in children with sensory sensitivities have the potential to negatively impact oral health and increase caries risk.

Use of food as reward. Using food as a reward for desired behaviors in children has the potential to adversely affect nutrition and oral health [39]. Parents who frequently provided food rewards reported that their children consumed more total fat and carbohydrates daily as compared to those who did not use food rewards [39]. In children with ASD, parents reported that almost half were currently or had a history of receiving food rewards and 46% of those were sweet rewards [38]. Of these children, 41% exhibited new caries activity, and 60% had a history of caries [38]. Frequent consumption of sugar-containing food rewards may be a detriment to children's oral health, especially as consumption of foods that easily adhere to the tooth surface (e.g., fruit roll-ups, candy, gummy bears) increases the risk for dental caries.

Packing/pouching food. Packing or pouching food in the oral cavity without swallowing is a problematic feeding behavior which can place a child at risk for aspiration, decreased caloric intake [40], as well as caries development due to the prolonged exposure of food to the child's teeth. Pouching of food is one of the feeding challenges commonly reported for children with ASD [41], and this type of behavior has been associated with higher-textured foods [40]. Although this type of mealtime behavior has not yet been explicitly linked to sensory sensitivities, it is possible that pouching may occur as a result of higher-textured foods which are perceived as noxious due to intraoral tactile sensory sensitivities, thereby placing children at increased caries risk.

Challenges with Oral Care in the Home

Oral care in the home has been reported to be significantly more challenging for children with ASD and sensory over-responsivity, as compared to children with ASD without sensory over-responsivity. These challenges included toothbrushing, dislike of the taste or texture of toothpaste, as well as the presence of gagging during toothbrushing [30, 42]. Parents have explicated that anything touching the mouth can exacerbate oral sensitivities, with toothbrushing being particularly challenging [43].

Challenges with Oral Care in the Dental Office

Not surprisingly, sensory-related challenges in the home have been significantly associated with professional oral care difficulties in the dental office. These have included challenges obtaining a dental cleaning as well as the presence of behavioral difficulties that interfered with professional dental care [42]. For example, children with ASD and sensory over-responsivity, compared to children with ASD and no sensory over-responsivity, were reported to experience more difficulty with dental prophylaxis and a negative last experience at the dental office [30]. Parents believe their children's sensory sensitivities make dental appointments more challenging and that their children are afraid of, complain, or dislike some or all of the sensory features of the dental office [30, 43].

Differences in sensory processing have been correlated with both physiological distress (sympathetic nervous system activation) and behavioral distress in children with ASD undergoing routine dental prophylaxis [44, 45]. In children with ASD with sensory over-responsivity, uncooperative behaviors were reported to increase at the dental office significantly more than in children with ASD without sensory over-responsivity. These behavioral difficulties made dental appointments more challenging for all involved—the child, caregiver, and dental practitioner [30]. Subsequently, the use of protective stabilization or pharmacological method adjuncts for routine oral exam and prophylaxis were reported more often by parents of children with ASD and sensory over-responsivity as compared to children with ASD with no sensory over-responsivity [30].

Due to the relationship between sensory sensitivities and uncooperative behaviors exhibited in the dental clinic, sensory stimuli present in the dental environment are of extreme importance. Many sensory stimuli in the everyday environment may be experienced as aggravating or noxious by a child with sensory sensitivities, but these can become even more problematic in the dental office. Of the many sensory systems that may be affected by sensory sensitivities, tactile, gustatory, visual, and olfactory sensitivities require special attention in the dental setting [31].

Tactile sensitivities may be exacerbated when the dental practitioner touches around and inside the child's mouth during treatment. The mouth and face are extremely sensitive areas, and standard procedures such as examination, prophylaxis, and fluoride application may be perceived by the patient as noxious stimuli. In one study investigating barriers to dental care, 35% of parents reported that their child with autism, developmental delay, or Down syndrome didn't like to have anything done to his/her mouth [46]. The texture, taste, and smell of products used in the dental office may aggravate *gustatory and olfactory sensitivities*; likewise, scented perfumes or soaps and even medical gloves worn by dental staff may be perceived as noxious to children with olfactory sensitivities. The overhead lighting in dental offices is very bright, often using fluorescent lights that commonly flicker and may make quiet humming or buzzing noises, intensifying *visual and/or auditory sensitivities*. Additionally, loud, unfamiliar noises will surround the child, especially during prophylaxis or if a dental handpiece is used; likewise, the suction equipment produces a loud noise, also emitting an audible sound even when not in use. Lastly, the dental chair itself may be especially noxious to children with *vestibular (movement) sensitivities* during the slow backward reclining of the dental chair.

Due to the relationship between sensory sensitivities and uncooperative behaviors, a child with sensory sensitivities may exhibit fight, flight, or fright reactions to these stimuli. He or she may try to cover his or her eyes or ears in response to bright lights or unfamiliar machinery noise, avoid looking at or be bothered by decorations that may be pleasing to others, flinch or move away from being touched by instruments or people on the dental team, and/or exhibit fear responses to noises and reclining movements of the dental chair. These responses may escalate into physical reaction as the child tries to escape from the noxious stimuli [12, 47].

Sensory-Related Strategies to Improve Oral Care

When a child experiences severe sensory sensitivities that impact his functional abilities, especially everyday oral care, he should receive an evaluation by an occupational therapist who has training in sensory integration. When available, an occupational therapist can assist the dental practitioner and families in finding the right sensory strategies to improve oral care. It is important to note that finding the right strategy for children is often a process of trial and error, so there must be patience and creativity involved [47–49]. Ultimately, utilizing strategies that are individualized based on a specific child's strengths and challenges, practicing flexibility, employing new techniques, and valuing parental input are crucial to achieving positive results. The following strategies may help facilitate successful and positive oral care experiences in the home and dental office settings.

Strategies to Improve Oral Care in the Home

Visual Supports

It can be helpful for children to have a firm end time and/or understanding of duration when experiencing something noxious. Verbal preparation and using visual cues can help make oral care more predictable (visual schedule) and finite (visual clock) [12, 47]. Visual schedules, which are visual representations of a task or activity, break down tasks like toothbrushing into discrete step-by-step tasks, which can be checked off once completed. These can be made in the home by caregivers with support from professionals like OTs and dental practitioners or even found online. Box 1 provides links to examples of visual supports.

Routine and Continuity

Routine and continuity are also essential for children with sensory sensitivities. As stated earlier, over-responsivity to sensory stimuli has been linked to anxiety and may be related to adherence to strict daily routines. Emphasize to parents that oral care routines should be undertaken at the same time each day and carried out with the same sequence of tasks (e.g., first brush bottom teeth, second brush top teeth, third floss, fourth done). Visual schedules, as mentioned above, have the potential to make oral care more predictable and decrease anxiety around home oral care activities.

Sensory-Based Strategies

Visual and/or auditory sensitivities may make the location of toothbrushing in the home important. *Location of brushing* traditionally occurs in a bathroom. What individuals without sensory sensitivities often forget is how bright and loud bathrooms can be. They are often equipped with bright fluorescent light bulbs that may flicker and/or give off a slight but audible hum. These rooms can also be very loud as they echo noises, especially the toilet flushing. For typical individuals, a bathroom is just a bathroom, but for a child with sensory sensitivities, it may be a loud, bright, scary room which can activate the sympathetic "fight or flight" nervous system. For children with toileting challenges, the bathroom is a place of additional stress. For these reasons, taking toothbrushing out of the bathroom can sometimes yield success for children with visual and/or auditory sensitivities.

Tactile sensitivities. To lessen the child's dislike of the feeling of the toothbrush in the mouth, parents can attempt the following strategies: start with an oral massage or vibration to the face/mouth area. Deep pressure sensations have been linked to decreased tactile sensitivity and may help prepare the patient for brushing [12]. Clinicians may also suggest wiping teeth with a washcloth before a toothbrush, using a toothbrush with very soft bristles if oversensitive, allowing the child to brush his face and lips with the brush, and/or try using an electric toothbrush. If parents are interested in trying an electric toothbrush, advise them to purchase an inexpensive brush prior to investing in a more expensive electric toothbrush in order to ensure the child will tolerate the vibration. While a child who is sensory seeking may prefer a hard bristle toothbrush, families should be cautioned against this due to the negative effects on the gingiva.

Gustatory and olfactory sensitivities. In the home, parents can experiment with different toothpastes to identify the least noxious to their child with a mild taste/smell and preferred texture. Anecdotally, mild toothpaste tastes such as strawberry and bubble gum flavors may be better tolerated than stronger flavors such as mint.

Strategies to Improve Oral Care in the Dental Office

Preparation is key to promoting successful dental office visits for children with sensory sensitivities. This preparation can occur in the home or the dental office and may be facilitated by the parent/caregiver or professionals such as dentists or occupational therapists. However, success is most likely to be achieved if a collaboration is undertaken by the parent/caregiver, dental professional, and other healthcare provider(s) or therapist(s) working with the child.

Practice

Practicing in the home supports positive dental treatment in the office. In the home environment, this may include toothbrushing, positioning, and exposure to practice examination kits. In the dental office, this could include desensitization visits.

Positioning may be important for children with sensory sensitivities that have difficulties lying back in a dental chair. For children that will not sit in a dental chair or respond negatively to the reclining feature of the chair (vestibular input), toothbrushing in the home can be completed with the child lying supine (with a pillow below the head to elevate it) on a bed or reclining chair. This can help to acclimate the child to oral care in a reclined position which may help to facilitate care in the dental office. Utilizing a *practice exam kit* to practice oral care in the home can help familiarize a child with the sensations provided by the use of gloves, a mask, and/or a disposable dental mirror. In a recent study, one dentist participant even reported sending bitewing radiograph tabs home with a therapist to practice using with a child with ASD [49]. See chapter "Desensitization and Therapeutic Behavioral Approaches to Dental Care" for more details regarding practice exam kits.

Lastly, *desensitization visits* to address difficulties experiencing new situations and change are utilized frequently by oral health providers working with CSHCN [50, 51]. These visits diminish aversion to the dental clinic through gradual exposure to the myriad of sensory stimuli present in that environment. Providers may allow or encourage children to stop by the dental office to merely come into the clinic, sit in the dental chair, and/or experience the clinic without an exam or treatment performed [49].

Visual Supports

Visual supports may also facilitate successful dental care encounters. As mentioned above, aids may include visual cues such as *visual schedules* and/or *visual clocks*. Tools such as these provide information to the child regarding the structure and length of the visit, increasing predictability and feelings of control and thereby reducing fear and/or anxiety [52, 53]. Visual schedules that break dental treatment into discrete tasks have been implemented in the home and/or with professionals to improve cooperation in children with ASD, yielding some success [54, 55]. These visual schedules can likewise be utilized during dental treatment, with tasks removed or checked off once completed.

Social Stories™ are another type of visual support, originally developed as an intervention strategy to help children with ASD address difficulties in social skills, behaviors, functional skills, and/or academic settings by providing important information about an upcoming event [56]. These stories allow individuals to anticipate and predict what experiences will occur and what sensory stimuli will be encountered, thereby diminishing anxiety [53]. In order to ensure that the story facilitates understanding, the following rules should be followed when writing a social story [56]:

- Written from the perspective of the child.
- Written at the child's comprehension level.
- Behavioral responses should be stated in positive terms (e.g., "I will lay still" vs. "I will not wiggle").
- Directive statements identifying appropriate responses to guide behavior should occur at a 1:2+ ratio to other sentence types (e.g., descriptive, perspective, cooperative, affirmative). For example, "I will keep my mouth open wide. The dentist will clean my teeth with a moving toothbrush. The toothbrush might tickle." Here, the first sentence is directive (guides child's behavior), while the following two sentences are descriptive (describing situation and people involved), perspective (describing reactions or feelings), and cooperative (what other people will do).

Social Stories™ do no not require the use of illustrations; however, photos and drawings are often included to enhance the child's understanding. Research suggests that stories written with illustrations are associated with higher effectiveness compared to stories without illustrations [57]. Illustrations may include sketches, cartoon characters, photographs, or even photographs of the individual who will be reading the book and of the actual dental office in which he will be receiving care.

A child's caregiver or occupational therapist should develop the social story with detailed feedback and input from the dental provider. This enables the story to accurately reflect the dental encounter. As with visual schedules, these stories should be read in the home to prepare for dental visits and may be utilized during dental treatment itself. The language utilized by the dental professionals during care should reflect the language choices of the story that was read in the home. Although most frequently used for children with ASD, Social Stories™ have also been examined for children with ADHD, Fragile X syndrome, language delays, and Down syndrome [57]. Research suggests that Social Stories™ decrease disruptive behaviors in children with ASD; however, fewer studies have examined effects on children with other disabilities [58].

See Box 1 for links to examples of visual supports and Fig. 4 of Chap. 5 (Desensitization and Therapeutic Behavioral Approaches to Dental Care) for an example dental Social Story™.

Box 1: Visual Support Resources

A variety of resources are available to clinicians, parents, and children to improve dental treatment utilizing visual supports, including:

- Visual Supports and Autism Spectrum Disorders (Autism Speaks™): https://www.autismspeaks.org/docs/sciencedocs/atn/visual_supports.pdf
- Community Connections Dental Guide—see Visual Schedule example (Autism Speaks™): https://www.autismspeaks.org/sites/default/files/documents/dentalguide.pdf
- Healthy Smiles for Autism (National Museum of Dentistry): http://vkc.mc.vanderbilt.edu/assets/files/resources/healthy-smiles-for-autism.pdf
  - Brushing and Flossing Visual Sequencing Cards
  - I Can Brush My Teeth Social Story
  - Visiting the Dentist Visual Sequencing Cards
  - My Visit to the Dentist Social Story
- My Visit to the Dentist: Social Story (Center for Pediatric Dentistry, University of Washington & Seattle Children's Hospital; see also [52]): http://www.thecenterforpediatricdentistry.com/intranet/ss/socialstory.pdf
- Visiting the Dentist Social Story (Children's Village): https://www.yakimachildrensvillage.org/pdf/social-story.pdf
- My Visit to the Dentist: Social Story (Western Health and Social Care Trust): http://www.westerntrust.hscni.net/pdf/Social_Story_-_Omagh_(3).pdf
- Social Narrative: Visit to Dentist's Office (Hands in Autism; Indiana University School of Medicine): https://handsinautism.iupui.edu/pdf/StrategyAtWork_VisitToDentistSocialStory.pdf
- "My Trip To The Dentist" [29]

Pre-visit Questionnaire/Interview

Obtaining additional information about a child from caregivers can facilitate positive dental care encounters. One effective way to do this is with a pre-visit questionnaire. A discussion of this topic and an example questionnaire are provided in Chap. 5 (Desensitization and Therapeutic Behavioral Approaches to Dental Care). In these questionnaires it is important that several sensory-related questions are answered by caregivers, especially if the caregiver reports that his child exhibits sensory sensitivities. Caregivers can provide important insight into their child's responses to sensory stimuli as well as previously successful or unsuccessful strategies implemented in response to these stimuli. Caregivers "know best" and should be involved in the care process. Clinicians can leverage caregiver knowledge by seeking their advice regarding the best approach for the child's care [48, 49]. Box 2 provides examples of sensory-related questions to ask prior to the dental visit.

Box 2: Sensory-Related Questions to Ask Prior to the Dental Visit

1. Is your child over-responsive, or does he/she respond differently to any of the following sensory stimuli (circle all that apply)?

Visual (sight)	Auditory (sound)	Gustatory (taste)	Olfactory (smell)	Tactile (touch)	Vestibular (movement)

Home-Related Follow-Up Questions:

- *If yes*, does your child experience challenges with toothbrushing/flossing in the home due to his/her sensory sensitivities?
  Examples: doesn't like the feeling of the toothbrush in mouth, the taste/texture of toothpaste, gags during toothbrushing
- *If yes*, does your child experience dislike or refuse certain foods based on taste/texture/etc.? Are the foods/drinks your child most frequently eats sugar- and/or carbohydrate-rich (e.g., chicken nuggets, crackers, juice)?

Dentist-Related Follow-Up Questions:

- *If yes*, describe how your child responds to these sensory sensations? Is this how he/she responds in the dental office?
  Examples: runs away/tries to escape, becomes aggressive, cries
- *If yes*, what would help make the dental visit easier for your child based on his/her sensory sensitivities?
  Examples: Does your child prefer a dimly lit room? Does your child prefer quiet or music (which kind)? Do certain tastes bother your child? Will your child tolerate wearing a hat/headphones/sunglasses? Does your child like/dislike smells (candle or aromatherapy scents)?
- *If distress behaviors occur in the dental clinic*, what strategies might be successful to reduce or stop them?

2. Does your child use visual schedules or social stories to complete multiple-step procedures or tasks?
   - *If yes*, does your child already have one for treatment in the dental clinic? For toothbrushing/flossing in the home?

3. Do you or other adults use food items as rewards for your child (e.g., in school or home environments)?
   - *If yes*, what food items are used?

4. Does your child currently receive therapy services (e.g., occupational therapy) to help address challenges with sensory processing?

5. Is there anything else we should know prior to the visit that may help us better prepare for a successful visit?

Routine and Continuity

In addition to their importance during home oral care practices, routine and continuity are often critical during professional dental treatment. In the dental office environment, care should be taken to establish a routine and document it so that same routine can be followed during subsequent visits. If possible, the dental team should utilize the same exam sequence, dental provider and assistant, and room and schedule the appointment at the same time of day. If visual supports are used, the same language should be repeated.

Environmental Adaptations in the Dental Office

A holistic and comprehensive approach to care considers the myriad of potential sensory and environmental barriers that individuals with sensory sensitivities may encounter during a dental visit. Occupational therapists have in-depth knowledge of sensory integration and universal design principles and can assist dental providers in identifying possible challenges and developing a plan to alleviate them.

The *waiting room* is often the first experience an individual encounters at a dental visit. This can either support or hinder a positive dental encounter for children with sensory sensitivities. Often waiting rooms are large, noisy, visually stimulating areas that may exacerbate anxiety and sensory sensitivities [59]. It is possible to adapt the visual, auditory, tactile, olfactory, and vestibular sensory stimuli of the waiting room to enhance relaxation and diminish noxious responses to sensory stimuli. Modifications can include, but are not limited to, replacing fluorescent lighting with softer or natural lighting, dimming lighting, and/or placing an aquarium or projecting nature scenes in the waiting room (visual), playing classical music or providing noise-cancelling headphones to patients (auditory), offering bean bag chair seating and/or weighted blankets/lap pads (tactile), using mild aromatherapy scents (olfactory), and providing rocking chairs as a seating alternative (vestibular). Additionally, utilizing strategic scheduling (e.g., first appointment in the morning,

Table 1 Examples of sensory-related modifications for the waiting room to reduce anxiety

Visual modifications	– Paint walls with neutral, cool colors – Replace fluorescent lighting with soft, warm, or dimmed lights – Use natural sunlight (windows, skylights) – Hang nature artwork – Project slow-moving images on walls – Place an aquarium, plants, or bubble tube in the corners of the room – Remove unnecessary flyers from walls
Auditory modifications	– Play calming classical or nature sounds – Have noise-cancelling headphones available – Soundproof doors leading to treatment areas – Provide a quiet room separate from the waiting room – Have a patient privacy talking area
Tactile modifications	– Provide various seating options (e.g., bean bag chairs, different fabrics, different sizes) – Offer a basket of fidget toys or objects – Supply weighted blankets, lap pads, or weighted stuffed animals
Olfactory modifications	– Use aromatherapy scents (e.g., lavender) *Note.* Some people may be bothered by aromatherapy scents
Vestibular modifications	– Offer rocking chairs as a seating alternative

Note. Adapted from "Occupational Therapists' Distinct Value in Creating a Sensory-Friendly Waiting Room," by E.Y. Hong, S.A. Cermak, & L.I. Stein Duker, 2018 [59]. Originally published in the *Special Interest Section Quarterly Practice Connections, 3,* p. 11–13. Copyright (c) 2018 by the American Occupational Therapy Association. Reprinted with permission.

last appointment in the evening) to ensure shorter wait times and decrease the stimulation in the waiting room may be successful [49].

Table 1 offers a list of potential sensory-based modifications that may be used in the waiting room.

Stimuli encountered during *dental treatment* also have the potential to exacerbate sensory sensitivities. Environmental modifications can be implemented to adapt the dental cleaning experience as well as the room itself. First, if possible, utilizing a private or semi-private room instead of large open bays may facilitate a positive encounter. This decreases the amount of stimulation encountered and shelters the child from other children exhibiting uncooperative or anxious behaviors. During the dental examination and cleaning, adaptations may be made to many other sensory stimuli. For example, dimming lights or suggesting the child to wear sunglasses may counteract *visual sensitivities*. *Auditory stimuli* encountered during care may be diminished by wearing headphones or earmuffs and/or playing calming music. *Tactile sensitivities* may be reduced by the application of deep pressure sensations which provide "hugging" pressure designed to facilitate a calming effect [60, 61]. In the dental office, use of a weighted blanket or the X-ray vest laid across the child could provide this input. Perceived control and predictability may help to diminish patient anxiety [53]; therefore, allowing children, when able, to choose the prophylaxis paste or fluoride flavor may facilitate cooperation when encountering *gustatory sensitivities*; use of unflavored pumice instead of prophylaxis paste may also be helpful if the child is able to tolerate the texture. Instructing dental staff to not use scented perfumes or soaps may help to avoid exacerbating *olfactory sensitivities*; likewise, the application of certain aromatherapy scents has been reported to decrease patient anxiety [62]. Nasal hoods to provide nitrous oxide sedation can be purchased either unscented or with various scents, which the child can choose from during care. Lastly, as mentioned previously if a child is sensitive to *vestibular (movement) stimuli*, it may be helpful to practice in the home to acclimatize a child to receiving dental care in a supine position. It can also benefit the patient to have the dental chair pre-reclined when the child enters the dental room. Dental staff should also provide instructions using the same language the patient has practiced in the home (e.g., "climb into the chair like a bed").

It is important to reiterate that these strategies are not one-size-fits-all and that finding the best techniques will take time and require some trial and error. For example, donning sunglasses and knitted hat/earmuffs to attenuate visual and auditory stimuli may be successful strategies for some children. Others may find the experience of wearing these items as noxious as the originally offending stimuli.

Table 2 offers a list of potential sensory-based modifications for use during dental treatment.

Table 2 Examples of sensory-related modifications during dental prophylaxis

Visual modifications[a]	– Paint walls with neutral, cool colors – Turn off overhead lights, and utilize the dental unit light or headlamp carefully directing light into child's mouth and not eyes – Replace fluorescent lighting with soft lighting and provide sunglasses for the child to wear – Project slow-moving images on ceiling above chair
Auditory modifications[a]	– Have noise-cancelling headphones available – Instruct child to don knitted hat or earmuffs – Play calming classical or nature sounds – Soundproof doors of treatment areas
Tactile modifications	– Utilize weighted blankets, lap pads, weighted stuffed animals, or an X-ray vest to provide deep pressure calming sensations. Some families may already own deep pressure sensory or compression vests or shirts
Gustatory modifications	– Allow child to choose prophylaxis paste flavor when possible – Use mild-tasting or "no taste" cleaning products (e.g., pumice)
Olfactory modifications[a]	– Instruct staff to forgo scented perfumes and/or soaps – Use aromatherapy scents (e.g., lavender, orange) *Note.* Some people may be bothered by aromatherapy scents
Vestibular modifications	– Pre-recline dental chair before child enters exam room, or, if child is willing and able, recline chair very slowly after a verbal warning

[a]*Note.* Some children may be equally bothered by visual/auditory stimuli present during dental care and modifications (e.g., wearing sunglasses, hat, headphones); for these children, other adaptations should be chosen. Additionally, some people may be bothered by aromatherapy scents. Information about potential successes of these strategies may be obtained via use of the pre-visit questionnaire completed by the parent/caregiver.

The Sensory Adapted Dental Environment

A specific combination of these sensory adaptations, the *Sensory Adapted Dental Environment*, has recently been studied in children with developmental disabilities, children with autism spectrum disorders, and typically developing children [45, 63, 64]. Both studies utilized visual, auditory, and tactile deep pressure modifications; see Table 3 and Fig. 1. Results from these pilot studies are promising, suggesting that dental cleanings provided in a sensory adapted dental environment, as compared to a regular dental environment, cause less overt behavioral distress as well as physiological stress and anxiety (sympathetic nervous system activation as measured by electrodermal activity) in children with developmental disabilities and autism spectrum disorders. In these studies, equipment costs were minimal, no permanent renovations were made, and the equipment was portable, able to be cleaned between participants, and relatively simple to set-up and remove. This approach recognizes that it is often difficult to manage maladaptive behaviors and the challenges they create [65], and reducing problem-causing stimuli in the environment may limit negative patient responses.

Table 3 The sensory adapted dental environment for children with developmental disabilities and children with autism spectrum disorder

	Children with developmental disabilities ($n = 16$ DD; $n = 19$ TD) [63, 64]	Children with autism spectrum disorder ($n = 22$ ASD; $n = 22$ TD) [45]
Visual modifications	• All direct overhead fluorescent lighting and dental overhead lamp turned off • Adapted lighting included dimmed upward fluorescent lighting • Dental practitioner used head-mounted lamp to see in child's mouth • Slow-moving visual color effects (Snoezelen) projected on ceiling	• All direct overhead fluorescent lighting and dental overhead lamp turned off • Darkening curtains placed on windows • Dental practitioner used head-mounted lamp to see in child's mouth • Slow-moving visual color effects (Snoezelen) projected on ceiling
Auditory modifications	• Rhythmic nature and piano music projected through portable speakers	• Rhythmic nature and piano music projected through portable speakers
Tactile modifications	• Wings of a specially designed "butterfly" wrapped around child to provide deep pressure "hugging" sensations (DD group); X-ray vest only (TD group) • Bass vibrator connected to dental chair to provide vibration sensations	• Wings of a specially designed "butterfly" wrapped around child to provide deep pressure "hugging" sensations • X-ray vest placed over child's chest under the butterfly wrap
Vestibular modifications	• Dental chair was pre-reclined before child entered room	• Dental chair was pre-reclined before child entered room

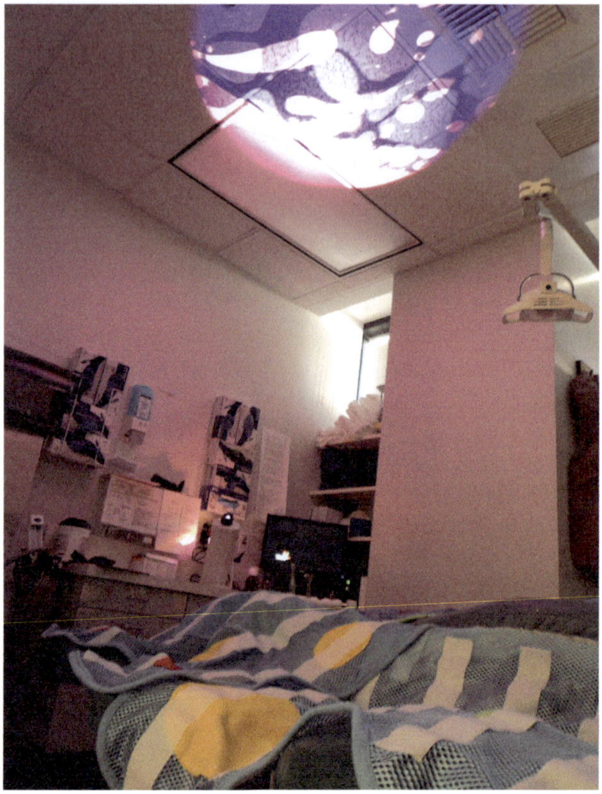

Fig. 1 Side view of butterfly wings and visual ceiling projections in sensory adapted dental environment [45]. Picture provided by L.I. Stein Duker

Collaborating with Other Professionals

Both parents and dental professionals report that collaborating and coordinating with other professionals (e.g., behavioral and/or occupational therapists) has the potential to help achieve desired outcomes during dental care [49]. These professionals may be able to assist the oral health provider with many of the strategies/techniques discussed in this chapter, including:

- Creation and implementation of visual supports (visual schedules and/or Social Stories™)
- Development of pre-visit questionnaires/interviews
- Providing parents with strategies to assist with oral care in the home
- Providing parents and the dental team with strategies to assist with oral care in the dental office
- Identification and implementation of strategies to assist dental practitioners with oral care in the dental office, including the design and implementation of sensory-friendly and/or sensory adapted environments in the dental office
- Training of dental office staff and practitioners regarding sensory sensitivities and their relationship to oral care

There are three broad options for obtaining an occupational therapy consultation for children with sensory sensitivities. First, speak with a child's caregiver to determine if the child is already receiving OT services. If he is, the dental practitioner would likely be able to obtain OT contact information from the caregiver. Contacting an OT who is already familiar with and treating that child will provide the oral health provider with additional insights and support to develop and possibly even implement strategies to address oral care in the home and/or dental environments. Second, funding for pediatric occupational therapy services is covered by the Individuals with Disabilities Education Act (IDEA), which includes services both for children 0–3 years of age (early intervention) and for school-aged children. Under IDEA, any approved referring entity (e.g., physician, medical insurance, childcare worker) is able to refer a child for an OT evaluation which will determine eligibility for OT services. The sole presence of sensory sensitivities alone, however, will not qualify a child to receive OT services. But, as stated above, these difficulties are often comorbid with a number of qualifying diagnoses. Therefore, if sensory sensitivities are present, OT services would appropriately address these sensory difficulties as a goal in treatment. Third, a dental clinic and/or caregiver could hire an OT per diem or fee-for-service consultation work. Although more expensive, the financial outlay may be worth the cost for clinics that work with a number of children who might benefit from this type of dental/OT collaboration.

Case-Based Scenario

Bobby is a 9-year-old boy diagnosed with autism spectrum disorder (ASD) referred to your dental practice by another parent of a child with special healthcare needs. When Bobby's mother called to schedule the appointment, she explained to your intake personnel that no successful dental examination or cleaning had occurred in over 2 years but that she does not believe there are any immediate dental needs. As part of your regular practices, your personnel sent Bobby's parent an introductory letter and a pre-visit questionnaire with specific questions to assess possible sensory sensitivities because those are commonly observed in individuals with ASD.

Prior to Bobby's visit, you reviewed his parent-completed questionnaire, which indicated that he attends elementary school in a general education class with the assistance of a one-on-one aide and that he receives speech therapy, occupational therapy, and resource specialist support in the school setting. Based on the parent responses, it appears that Bobby has challenges with sensory over-responsivity, fine motor skills, social skills, and attention. Specific to the dental office, Bobby is over-responsive to visual, tactile, auditory, and vestibular (movement) stimuli, becomes easily overwhelmed in waiting rooms, and is most calm during the morning hours of the day. He uses social stories in the school and home environments but does not have one to specifically assist with his oral care. Bobby's mother reported that he has only been to the dentist a total of four times and that each of those visits was a struggle, often with no successful dental procedures completed. Bobby's mother specifically described that she hated when "they strapped him to a board" to keep him still during the dental procedures. During one of the four visits, Bobby underwent dental treatment with general anesthesia to complete a dental cleaning and X-rays and to treat multiple cavities.

In order to minimize overstimulation in the waiting room and take advantage of his preferred time of day, you directed your staff to schedule Bobby for the first appointment of the day. On the day of Bobby's dental visit, Bobby and his mother were taken to a private dental room immediately following check-in. During the visit, Bobby sat on the dental chair with no difficulty while you discussed the questionnaire with his mother, including Bobby in the discussion when possible. Bobby's mother stated that she doubted he would allow an exam or cleaning but acknowledged she would be thrilled if those were possible. Encouraged by Bobby's behavior during the interview, you told Bobby that you were going to recline the dental chair. As you did, Bobby quickly leapt out of the chair and started screaming that he was "going to fall and get hurt" and that the room was "too bright!" His mother quickly helped calm him down by sitting him on her lap and hugging him tightly, and then she convinced him to open his mouth so you could visually inspect his teeth. However, Bobby did not allow you to conduct a thorough oral examination, prophylaxis, or even brush his teeth with a toothbrush. At the end of the visit, you spoke with Bobby's mother about developing a social story for the next dental visit and inquired if you could ask Bobby's occupational therapist (OT) for assistance. Bobby's mother agreed and provided you with the contact information for Bobby's OT. For the follow-up, you instructed your receptionist to schedule another dental visit for Bobby, allowing enough time for you to contact his OT to develop strategies to support his success before the next visit.

During your subsequent phone meeting with Bobby's OT, you began by recounting your experiences with Bobby during his dental visit. The OT asked about your typical procedures during a dental exam and cleaning to aid understanding (e.g., sit in chair, chair reclines, dental examination, dental prophylaxis, fluoride application, visit over) and asked you to send pictures of your waiting room, private dental room, and equipment. When you described the specific meltdown Bobby experienced when you reclined the chair, the OT suggested that you fully recline the chair before he enters the room so he can simply "lie on it like a bed" as this may reduce his aversive response to the movement of the chair. The OT also suggested that you instruct Bobby's mom to practice toothbrushing while he is lying supine in bed or on a couch in his home so that he can get used to oral care occurring in that position. The OT suggested placing the X-ray vest over Bobby's chest while he is supine to help keep him calm during his next visit. The X-ray vest provides the deep pressure sensations that help him stay calm, similar to those provided by his mother's tight hug during the previous visit. Lastly, the OT encouraged you to turn off any overhead lights that are not necessary to complete his dental care.

Bobby and his OT developed and fabricated the social story during therapy time, and a copy was sent home with instructions to read it once a day for at least a week before a dental visit. At his next dental visit, Bobby entered the private operatory, laid down on the pre-reclined chair with verbal prompting to "lie on it like a bed," and opened his mouth for the dentist to "count" his teeth. The dentist laid an X-ray bib over his chest, and Bobby commented that it "felt good." Bobby allowed the prophylaxis brush to spin on his finger but would not let in his mouth; he did allow the dentist to brush his teeth with a toothbrush and apply a tasteless fluoride varnish. Both you and Bobby's mother were happy with the progress and discussed next steps, such as using an electric toothbrush at home and including additional pages about prophylaxis ("the spinning toothbrush" and the "water sucker") in his social story prior to his next visit.

Conclusion

- Children with sensory sensitivities may experience greater challenges tolerating oral care in the home and dental office.
- There is a need for a holistic and comprehensive approach to the myriad of potential sensory-related barriers that individuals with sensory sensitivities may encounter.
- To address challenges with oral care in the home, strategies may include the use of visual supports and sensory-based strategies, alongside a focus on routine and continuity.
- To address challenges with oral care in the dental office, strategies may include preparation and practice prior to the visit (e.g., positioning, use of an exam practice kit, desensitization visits, visual supports, pre-visit questionnaire), as well as sensory-based strategies including adaptations to the waiting room, clinic environment, and dental treatment itself.
- Multidisciplinary collaboration with other professionals, such as occupational therapists, may help to facilitate positive dental encounters for children with sensory sensitivities.

References

1. American Occupational Therapy Association. What is occupational therapy? Available at: https://www.aota.org/Conference-Events/OTMonth/what-is-OT.aspx. Accessed 25 Feb 2018.
2. Ayres AJ. The nervous system within: understanding how the brain works and the importance of sensation. Sensory integration and the child: understanding hidden challenges. Los Angeles, CA: Western Psychological Services; 2005.
3. Lane SJ. Sensory modulation. In: Bundy AC, Fisher K, editors. Sensory integration: theory and practice. 2nd ed. Philadelphia, PA: FA Davis Company; 2002. p. 101–22.
4. Dunn W. Sensory profile 2 user's manual. San Antonio, TX: Psychological Corporation; 2014.
5. Parham L, Ecker C, Miller-Kuhaneck H, Henry D, Glennon T. Sensory processing measure. Los Angeles, CA: Western Psychological Services; 2007.
6. Tomchek SD. Sensory processing in individuals with an autism spectrum disorder. In: Miller-Kuhaneck H, Watling R, editors. Autism: a comprehensive occupational therapy approach. 3rd ed. Bethesda, MD: AOTA Press; 2010. p. 135–62.
7. Dunn W. The sensations of everyday life: empirical, theoretical, and pragmatic considerations. Am J Occup Ther. 2001;55:608–20.

8. Leekam SR, Nieto C, Libby SJ, Wing L, Gould J. Describing the sensory abnormalities of children and adults with autism. J Autism Dev Disord. 2007;37:894–910.
9. Bijlenga D, Tjon-Ka-Jie JYM, Schuijers F, Kooij JJS. Atypical sensory profiles as core features of adult ADHD, irrespective of autistic symptoms. Eur Psychiatry. 2007;43:51–7.
10. Gavin WJ, Dotseth A, Roush KK, Smith CA, Spain HD, Davies PL. Electroencephalography in children with and without sensory processing disorders during auditory perception. Am J Occup Ther. 2011;65:370–7.
11. Reynolds S, Lane SJ. Diagnostic validity of sensor over-responsivity: a review of the literature and case reports. J Autism Dev Disord. 2008;38:516–29.
12. Miller-Kuhaneck H. Going to the dentist. Available from: https://www.spdstar.org/basic/going-to-dentist. Accessed 25 Feb 2018.
13. Baranek GT, David FJ, Poe MD, Stone WL, Watson LR. Sensory experiences questionnaire: discriminating sensory features in young children with autism, developmental delays, and typical development. J Child Psychol Psychiatry. 2006;47:591–601.
14. Baranek GT, Boyd BA, Poe MD, David FJ, Watson LR. Hyperresponsive sensory patterns in young children with autism, developmental delay, and typical development. Am J Ment Retard. 2007;112:233–45.
15. Ghanizadeh A. Sensory processing problems in children with ADHD: a systematic review. Psychiatry Investig. 2011;8:89–94.
16. Panagiotidi M, Overton PG, Stafford T. The relationship between ADHD traits and sensory sensitivity in the general population. Compr Psychiatry. 2018;80:179–85.
17. Baranek GT, Roberts JE, David FJ, et al. Developmental trajectories and correlates of sensory processing in young boys with Fragile X Syndrome. Phys Occup Ther Pediatr. 2008;28:79–98.
18. Wengel T, Hanlon-Dearman AC, Fjeldsted B. Sleep and sensory characteristics in young children with Fetal Alcohol Spectrum Disorder. J Dev Behav Pediatr. 2011;32:384–92.
19. Wilbarger J, Gunnar M, Schneider M, Pollak S. Sensory processing in internationally adopted, post-institutionalized children. J Child Psychol Psychiatry. 2010;41:1105–14.
20. Ahn RR, Miller LJ, Milberger S, McIntosh DN. Prevalence of parents' perceptions of sensory processing disorders among kindergarten children. Am J Occup Ther. 2004;58:287–93.
21. Centers for Disease Control and Prevention. Autism spectrum disorders: data and statistics. Available at: http://www.cdc.gov/ncbddd/autism/data.html. Accessed 13 Aug 2018.
22. Tomchek SD, Dunn W. Sensory processing in children with and without autism: a comparative study using the short sensory profile. Am J Occup Ther. 2007;61:190–200.
23. American Psychiatric Association. Diagnostic and statistical manual of mental disorders: text revision. 5th ed. Arlington, VA: American Psychiatric Publishing; 2013.
24. Pfeiffer B, Kinnealey M, Reed C, Herzberg G. Sensory modulation and affective disorders in children and adolescents with Asperger's disorder. Am J Occup Ther. 2005;59:335–45.
25. Biddiss E, Knibbe TJ, McPherson A. The effectiveness of interventions aimed at reducing anxiety in health care waiting spaces: a systematic review of randomized and nonrandomized trials. Anesth Analg. 2014;119:433–48.
26. Koenig KP, Rudney SG. Performance challenges for children and adolescents with difficulty processing and integrating sensory information: a systematic review. Am J Occup Ther. 2010;64:430–42.
27. Baker AEZ, Lane A, Angley MT, Young RL. The relationship between sensory processing patterns and behavioural responsiveness in autistic disorder: a pilot study. J Autism Dev Disord. 2008;38:867–75.
28. Tomchek SD, Little LM, Dunn W. Sensory pattern contributions to developmental performance in children with autism spectrum disorder. Am J Occup Ther. 2015;69:6905185040:1-10.
29. Charles JM. Dental care in children with developmental disabilities: attention deficit disorder, intellectual disabilities, and autism. J Dent Child. 2010;77:84–91.
30. Stein LI, Polido JC, Cermak SA. Oral care and sensory over-responsivity in children with autism spectrum disorders. Pediatr Dent. 2013;35:230–5.
31. National Institute of Dental and Craniofacial Research. Practical oral care for people with autism. Available at: http://www.nidcr.nih.gov/OralHealth/Topics/DevelopmentalDisabilities/PracticalOralCarePeopleAutism.htm. Accessed 10 Feb 2018.

32. Cermak SA, Curtin C, Bandini LG. Food selectivity and sensory sensitivity in children with autism spectrum disorders. J Am Diet Assoc. 2010;110:238–46.
33. Coulthard CR, Blissett J. Fruit and vegetable consumption in children and their mothers: moderating effects of child sensory sensitivity. Appetite. 2009;52:410–5.
34. Johnson CR, Turner K, Stewart PA, et al. Relationships between feeding problems, behavioral characteristics and nutritional quality in children with ASD. J Autism Dev Disord. 2014;44:2175–84.
35. Chistol LT, Bandini LG, Must A, et al. Sensory sensitivity and food selectivity in children with autism spectrum disorder. J Autism Dev Disord. 2018;48:583–91.
36. Lane AE, Geraghy ME, Young GS, Rostorfer JL. Problem eating behaviors in autism spectrum disorder are associated with suboptimal nutrient intake and taste/smell sensitivity. Infant Child Adolesc Nutr. 2014;6:172–80.
37. Hubbard KL, Anderson SE, Curtin C, Must A, Bandini LG. A comparison of food refusal related to characteristics of food in children with autism spectrum disorder and typically developing children. J Acad Nutr Diet. 2014;114:1981–7.
38. Marshall J, Sheller B, Mancl L. Caries-risk assessment and caries status of children with autism. Pediatr Dent. 2010;32:69–75.
39. Lu J, Xiong S, Arora N, Dubé L. Using food as reinforcer to shape children's noon-food behavior: the adverse nutritional effect doubly moderated by reward sensitivity and gender. Eat Behav. 2015;19:94–7.
40. Patel MR, Piazza CC, Layer SA, et al. A systematic evaluation of food textures to decrease packing and increase oral intake in children with pediatric feeding disorders. J Appl Behav Anal. 2005;38:89–100.
41. Levin D, Volkert VM, Piazza CC. A multi-component treatment to reduce packing in children with feeding and autism spectrum disorders. Behav Modif. 2014;38:940–63.
42. Stein LI, Polido JC, Mailloux Z, Coleman GG, Cermak SA. Oral care and sensory sensitivities in children with autism spectrum disorder. Spec Care Dentist. 2011;31:102–10.
43. Stein Duker LI, Henwood BF, Bluthenthal RN, et al. Parents' perceptions of dental care challenges in male children with autism spectrum disorder: an initial qualitative exploration. Res Autism Spectr Disord. 2017;39:63–72.
44. Stein LI, Lane CJ, Williams ME, et al. Physiological and behavioral stress and anxiety in children with autism spectrum disorders during routine oral care. Biomed Res Int. 2014;694876:1–10.
45. Cermak SA, Stein Duker LI, Williams ME, et al. Sensory adapted dental environments to enhance oral care for children with autism spectrum disorders: a randomized controlled pilot study. J Autism Dev Disord. 2015;45:2876–88.
46. Nelson LP, Getzin A, Graham D, et al. Unmet dental needs and barriers to care for children with significant special health care needs. Pediatr Dent. 2011;33:29–36.
47. Miller-Kuhaneck H, Chisolm EC. Improving dental visits for individuals with autism spectrum disorders through an understanding of sensory processing. Spec Care Dentist. 2012;32:229–33.
48. Lewis C, Vigo L, Novak L, Klein EJ. Listening to parents: a qualitative look at the dental and oral care experiences of children with autism spectrum disorder. Pediatr Dent. 2015;37:e98–104.
49. Stein Duker LI, Floríndez LI, Henwood BF, et al. Strategies for success: A qualitative study of caregiver and dentist approaches to improving oral care for children with autism. Pediatr Dent. In press.
50. Weil TN, Bagramian RA, Inglehart MR. Treating patients with autism spectrum disorder – SCDA members' attitudes and behavior. Spec Care Dentist. 2011;31:8–17.
51. Nelson TM, Sheller B, Friedman CS, Bernier R. Educational and therapeutic behavioral approaches to providing dental care for patients with autism spectrum disorder. Spec Care Dentist. 2015;35:105–13.
52. Marion IW, Nelson TM, Sheller B, et al. Dental stories for children with autism. Spec Care Dentist. 2016;36:181–6.
53. Pfeiffer B, Stein Duker LI. The impact of the sensory environment on patient care for individuals with autism spectrum disorders. In: Giarelli E, Fisher K, editors. Integrated health care for people with autism spectrum disorder: interdisciplinary planning and delivery of care. Springfield, IL: Charles C. Thomas Publishers; 2016. p. 69–92.

54. Backman B, Pilebro C. Visual pedagogy in dentistry for children with autism. ASDC J Dent Child. 1999;66:325–31.
55. Cagetti MG, Mastroberardino S, Campus G, et al. Dental care protocol based on visual supports for children with autism spectrum disorders. Med Oral Patol Oral Cir Bucal. 2015;20:e598–604.
56. Gray C. The new social story™ book. 10th ed. Arlington, TX: Future Horizons; 2010.
57. Reynhout G, Carter M. Social Stories™ for children with disabilities. J Autism Dev Disord. 2006;36:445–69.
58. Rhodes C. Do social stories help to decrease disruptive behavior in children with autistic spectrum disorders: a review of the published literature. J Intellect Disabil. 2014;18:35–50.
59. Hong EY, Cermak SA, Stein Duker LI. Occupational therapists' distinct value in creating a sensory-friendly waiting room. Am J Occup Ther SIS Quarterly Practice Connections. 2018;3:11–3.
60. Edelson SM, Edelson MG, Kerr DCR, Grandin T. Behavioral and physiological effects of deep pressure on children with autism: a pilot study evaluating the efficacy of Grandin's hug machine. Am J Occup Ther. 1999;53:145–52.
61. Grandin T. Thinking in pictures: my life with autism. New York: Vintage Books; 2006.
62. Jafarzadeh M, Arman S, Farahbakhsh Pour F. Effect of aromatherapy with orange essential oil on salivary cortisol and pulse rate in children during dental treatment: a randomized controlled clinical trial. Adv Biomed Res. 2013;2(1):10.
63. Shapiro M, Sgan-Cohen HD, Parush S, Melmed RN. Influence of adapted environment on the anxiety of medically treated children with developmental disability. J Pediatr. 2009;154:546–50.
64. Shapiro M, Melmed RN, Sgan-Cohen HD, Parush S. Effect of sensory adaptation on anxiety of children with developmental disabilities: a new approach. Pediatr Dent. 2009;31:222–8.
65. Green D, Flanagan D. Understanding the autistic dental patient. Gen Dent. 2008;56:167–71.

Desensitization and Therapeutic Behavioral Approaches to Dental Care

Travis M. Nelson

Introduction

Our tendency as clinicians is often to focus on a patient's immediate dental condition: calculus buildup, a retained primary tooth, or an unsealed permanent molar. Unfortunately, many children with special healthcare needs (CSHCN) will not readily tolerate the dental procedures that address these issues. Pressuring the child to receive treatment can overwhelm her, resulting in a negative dental experience. Our duty as pediatric providers is twofold: treat the patient's immediate needs and position her for optimum health in adulthood. Behavior modification techniques can be used to teach patients dental skills needed to achieve both short- and long-term oral health goals. This process requires patience and dedication, but the results make the effort worthwhile. Ultimately, the greatest gift we can give a child with special needs is graduating from pediatric care with the ability to receive dental services as an adult.

Education and Behavioral Therapy in the Medical Environment

Educational and behavioral therapies are an integral part of daily life for CSHCN. For example, nearly all CSHCN have an Individualized Educational Plan (IEP) developed and implemented at their school. These plans are customized to help the child reach educational goals for each calendar year. Other examples include applied

T. M. Nelson (✉)
Department of Pediatric Dentistry, University of Washington, Seattle, WA, USA
e-mail: tmnelson@uw.edu

T. M. Nelson, J. R. Webb (eds.), *Dental Care for Children with Special Needs*,
https://doi.org/10.1007/978-3-030-10483-2_5

behavior analysis (ABA) therapy (the mainstay of treatment for children with autism), feeding therapy for children with nutritional challenges, and a wide variety of other physical and occupational therapies. These programs identify areas for improvement, develop the child's skills in that area, and provide positive reinforcement for target behaviors [1]. Members of the child's care team work together to optimize the child's potential. The interdisciplinary team that participates in a child's care may include:

- Parents
- Social worker
- Primary care provider (PCP)
- Developmental pediatrician
- Psychologist or psychiatrist
- Neurologist
- Nutritionist
- Behavioral therapist
- Physical therapist
- Occupational therapist
- Speech and language pathologist
- Teacher and teacher's aid
- Other medical subspecialists (e.g., nephrologist, rheumatologist, pulmonologist, endocrinologist, cardiologist)

The care team works with the child in multiple settings: the home, school, and in medical offices. Recognizing that children and families are accustomed to receiving these types of services, we can adopt a similar approach to help children cope with unfamiliar dental settings and develop dental skills. Giving children the opportunity to prepare and learn at their own pace frequently facilitates cooperation for dental care. This often requires only minor modification of behavioral techniques that clinicians are accustomed to using with typically developing patients.

Behavior Management Versus Behavior Modification

Behavior management (also known as behavior guidance) is a mainstay of pediatric dental practice. It is comprised of a wide variety of techniques used to facilitate cooperation for dental care. Behavior modification, on the other hand, is focused on changing problem or avoidance behaviors to facilitate dental treatment. The basic tenet of behavior modification is that the patient's behavior is learned and that the principles of learning can be applied to develop or change behavior [2].

Behavior modification programs recognize that patient behavior is dependent upon the environment. By adapting the patient's environment, we can alter behavior [3–5]. Systematic desensitization is a common example of a behavior modification technique that has been used to facilitate dental care for fearful children. It was developed by Joseph Wolpe in the 1950s for the treatment of neurosis and has been used in dentistry with patients who have developmental disabilities since at least the 1970s [2, 6–12]. Avoidance increases anxiety, but controlled exposure to stimuli can reduce it. Through "successive approaches" the child is gradually exposed to anxiety-provoking stimuli while being reinforced with pleasant experiences. Ultimately the fearful patient no longer experiences a stress response, allowing her to relax during dental procedures. Behavior modification programs reduce the patient's negative responses through gradual exposure to a triggering stimulus. For example, a patient may fear dental equipment such as the panoramic radiograph machine, making it impossible to obtain a diagnostic image. However, after repeatedly watching a video that shows how the machine is used, being allowed to touch the equipment, and practicing standing with the mouthpiece between her teeth, the patient can learn to have a panoramic radiograph taken.

Terminology

The following key terms are commonly used to describe procedures in the behavior conditioning process:

- *Reinforcement* is provided when the child is given a reward for performing a desired behavior. It is most effective when given immediately after a behavior [9].
- *Shaping* is the process of gradually modifying behavior toward a target or goal. It is initiated by engaging the patient in activities that are minimally stressful and gradually proceeding to more stressful procedures. For example, mouth opening may be shaped by initially providing reinforcement for narrow opening. Over time only wider opening is reinforced, and opening time is increased from short durations (5 s) to greater intervals.
- *Cueing and Prompting* are clear physical or verbal indications that signal for the patient to perform a behavior. This could involve tactile sensation such as a light touch to the child's lip when requesting that she open her mouth. A toothbrush is a familiar item that can be used very effectively to prompt the child to open for an examination.
- *Fading* occurs when a cue or prompt is gradually withdrawn until the need for it fades away. For example, the patient no longer needs a prompt to sit in the chair—she simply sits in it once she enters the room. Fading can also refer to gradual introduction of a new stimulus, while a desired behavior is occurring (e.g., a mouth open response is maintained, while a dental handpiece is introduced; a tongue depressor is first replaced by a mirror, then by a probe) [2].
- *Escape extinction* occurs when a child learns to tolerate a procedure or stimulus without escape behavior, aggression, or protest.

- *Modeling* is a process of learning by observation [13]. Live or video models of peers can be used to demonstrate dental behaviors. Narration or verbal instructions are typically used during modeling. This process allows the patient to anticipate and become familiar with procedures and instruments without actually having to experience them herself. The behavior management technique of tell-show-do utilizes basic principles of modeling.
- *Distraction* takes the patient's focus away from noxious dental stimuli and refocuses it on something more pleasant. Music and videos are common forms of distraction used in dental offices. Contingent distraction can be very powerful. This technique gives a child access to a preferred distraction as long as she is cooperative ("You can watch your show while we clean your teeth as long as you stay wide open").

Effectiveness

Dental behavior modification has existed in dentistry for some time, but protocols have varied considerably. This makes it challenging to determine effectiveness. The population of CSHCN is also very diverse, and generalization from one patient to another is difficult. Still, evidence suggests that these techniques can be effective. While sample sizes are typically small, many reports suggest that behavior modification programs improve behavior in a significant number of patients [2, 3, 5, 14–16].

Children with autism spectrum disorder (ASD) have been a major focus in the behavior modification research. The population of patients with ASD is very heterogeneous, yet common features such as a preference for consistency and familiarity make desensitization well suited to these individuals. In general the literature suggests that 30–50% of children on the autism spectrum can learn to receive needed services through dental desensitization [17–20]. One study showed that within five desensitization visits, >85% of children in the sample were able to have an oral examination while seated in a dental chair. Three-quarters of the children in that study achieved the exam in 1–2 visits [21].

Every patient is unique, so it is impossible to accurately predict how well an individual will do in a behavioral program. Most caregivers hope for their child to receive dental care like typically developing peers, but that is not always realistic. Therefore, it is important for clinicians to have a frank discussion with families about factors that promote success. Inquire into what other life skills the patient has learned at home and in occupational therapy programs. This provides insight into the patient's aptitude for learning dental skills. Also consider how involved the patient's caretakers are likely to be in the education process. Patients with more profound disability have greater challenges learning to receive dental care. For these children, practicing skills outside the dental office is critically important. Repeated exposure and habituation may be the difference between success and failure. While the clinician's expectations are based upon scientific data and clinical experience, the parent's expectations are based on knowledge of their own child. Therefore, they may measure success differently. Sometimes accomplishments that seem minor to the dental team may be perceived as significant victories for the family. Similarly, some families have expectations that are overly optimistic.

Patient Selection

Ideally patients would arrive to their first dental appointment without fear or avoidance behaviors they have learned through aversive dental or medical visits. In reality, many CSHCN may have been "sensitized" to difficult dental procedures and present to the dental office with preconceptions that must be overcome. On the first visit, many patients may not willingly sit in the dental chair for an exam. The question then arises:

> Is it best to force the exam and determine if the child has urgent dental needs or is it preferable to postpone examination and use behavioral modification techniques to teach dental skills?

Most families and clinicians prefer to avoid forcing an exam on the child, but it is not always appropriate to rely solely on behavioral modification techniques. Some children are just not good candidates for this approach. Similarly, we should avoid engaging in "supervised neglect" of pressing dental issues. While success has been reported in over 50% of patients, outcomes vary widely depending upon which patients are included in the program and the treatment goals [16, 21]. For example, most studies have evaluated a child's ability to learn skills associated with dental examination, not operative dentistry [9]. It is important to consider these factors, focusing resources on patients who do not have urgent dental needs and those that are most likely to benefit.

Patients with severe intellectual disability, low baseline cooperation, few social and communication skills, and those who are prone to aggressive behavior may not be good candidates for behavioral modification [3, 22]. In one study children with high levels of challenging home behavior were more than ten times less likely to cooperate for an oral health screening [22]. Table 1 shows factors that the clinical team should consider when making this decision [20, 21, 23].

Providing dental care in the least restrictive method is a major focus of this text. However, as indicated above, clinicians who care for CSHCN will invariably encounter children who have dental needs that cannot be addressed using behavioral methods. Therefore, it is important to have access to protective stabilization and sedation/general anesthesia services when caring for this patient population. Being able to provide surgical and restorative services in an atraumatic fashion will help preserve the child's ability to cooperate for routine diagnostic and preventive services.

Table 1 Factors to consider before implementing behavioral strategies

	Factors that encourage behavior modification	Factors that encourage obtaining initial exam, even if child is unwilling
Dental disease	Has received dental care elsewhere and has no history of dental disease Caregiver and/or child are able to perform good oral hygiene Minimally cariogenic diet (e.g., g-tube fed, ketogenic diet, limited snacking or sugared beverages)	Caregiver is aware of an urgent dental condition (decay, pain, infection, etc.) Poor oral hygiene: child unable to cooperate for home hygiene measures Highly cariogenic diet
Age	Older patient, able to participate in the exam process	Pre-cooperative age (expect behavior similar to typically developing peers)
Intellectual disability	Mild intellectual disability (ID)	Severe intellectual disability (ID)
Cooperation in other settings	Tolerates medical exams Has a history of learning social skills	Not cooperative for other medical visits Generally has extreme difficulty learning social skills
Communication	Patient is able to communicate with caregiver and dental team (expressive and receptive language skills)	Patient has extreme difficulty communicating with caregiver and dental team
Caregiver desires	Caregiver engaged and interested in pursuing behavioral techniques in home and dental office	Caregiver uninterested in pursuing behavioral techniques Limited time to practice in home
Self-care	Child able to perform self-care (dressing, bathing, toileting, oral hygiene, hair brushing)	Child cannot independently perform self-care

Clinical Strategies

The following clinical strategies are presented as a multicomponent package. In practice, a dental office might choose to incorporate some or all of these strategies into a hybrid program of its own. A successful behavior modification program incorporates simple, repeatable techniques based upon principles that are known to work. Caregiver engagement is critical, and providing a variety of options for the child's dental care facilitates a positive therapeutic relationship. Each patient's behavioral plan must be individualized, allowing families to select treatment options that support the child's ability to receive care. The dental team must remain flexible and open to input from families. While provider experience and skill are important in caring for CSHCN, emotional intelligence and positive energy are the key attributes needed for success.

The First Impression

The patient relationship begins before the family has even stepped foot through the door of the dental practice. Preparing patients and caregivers for what to expect on the first visit relieves anxiety and sets the stage for a positive experience. This is true

Dear Parent,

As you know, children with special health care needs often have a difficult time receiving dental care. We recognize that each child has unique strengths and challenges and must be treated as an individual. To more effectively care for our patients, we have adopted a specific care approach.

- New patients are asked to complete the *Pre-Visit Questionnaire* included in this packet. Please complete the form to the best of your ability and return it to our clinic. Once received, our team will review the information and call to schedule your child's first visit.
- During the first visit you and your child will have the opportunity to see the clinic, meet the staff, and discuss treatment strategies with the dentist. The first visit is an opportunity for us to learn more about your child's unique strengths, determine any special accommodations required, and develop an individualized plan for his/her care. We don't want you to feel pressure to have any treatment completed at this visit. Some children allow a dental exam on the first trip to our clinic, but for others it may take a few more appointments.
- Subsequent visits to our clinic will focus on 1) completing dental care 2) obtaining a set of skills which will enable your child to maintain optimal oral health for a lifetime. These visits are typically scheduled for 30 minutes, but will vary depending on your child's needs.
- We have placed a dental story, Pictures of our dentists, and a YouTube introduction to the clinic on our website. Please make use of these resources before your visit if you think they would help your child:

  http:// practicewebsite

We understand that this approach requires a considerable amount of your time, and we thank you for your participation. If this approach does not seem appropriate for your child, please call our office at: **---/---/----**to speak with our team. It is always possible to make alternate arrangements for care.

We look forward to meeting you soon,

Sincerely

Name of Dental Practice

Fig. 1 Introductory letter

for all patients, but it is even more critical for CSHCN. It is helpful to greet new patients with an introductory letter or email (Fig. 1). The introductory letter provides an opportunity to:

1. Inform the family that the office is accustomed to caring for CSHCN.
2. Explain rationale for and deliver pre-visit intake forms.
3. Introduce caregivers to resources that may be available on the practice website (pictures of the dental team, dental stories, videos, etc.).
4. Set expectations for the first visit.

Information Gathering

Gathering patient information is a critical first step in behavior modification. This can be accomplished by conducting an in-person interview or by having the caregiver complete a pre-visit questionnaire. Standard medical and dental histories effectively capture important clinical information, yet they often fail to provide a complete picture of the patient. When engaging with children and families at this level, it is important to ask questions that reveal a wide variety of details about the individual. An in-person interview is very effective, but it can be time intensive. When gathering information in-person is not practical, a pre-visit questionnaire provides an effective way to learn important details about the patient. Knowing more about the child enables the dental team to make supportive treatment accommodations, facilitates effective communication, and perhaps most importantly helps build rapport with families. A thorough questionnaire may include (Fig. 2):

Pre-Visit Parent Questionnaire for CSHCN

Date____________

Child's First and Last Name____________________________ Age ____________

Address____________________________ Phone #____________

Medical Diagnosis____________________________

Medications____________________________

Allergies____________________________

You may include a separate written list of medications and allergies if there are a large number of items

Who referred you to us?____________________________

Your Child's Primary Care Doctor____________________________

PLEASE CHECK OR CIRCLE All THE RESPONSES THAT ARE APPROPRIATE FOR YOUR CHILD

Your child's educational support system

☐ Has an educational assistant or behavioral therapist

☐ Has an personalized school program in place (IEP)

☐ Classroom type (Circle one) Integrated class Special Education

☐ Other____________________________

How would you describe your child's developmental/intellectual disability?

Mild Moderate Severe Don't Know

How does your child communicate?

Language Understanding	Limited	Some	Most
Speech	Non-verbal	Limited verbal	Highly Verbal
Reading	Non-reader	Some reading	Fluent reader
Complies with simple instructions	Rarely	Sometimes	Usually

What tools does your child use to communicate?

Social Stories Visual Schedules iPad Pictures

Other____________________________

Fig. 2 Pre-visit parent questionnaire for CSHCN

Which activities can your child do on their own?

Toileting Toothbrushing Bathing Hair brushing Dressing

What are your child's strengths?

What are your child's interests?

Is your child sensitive to any of the following?

Loud Noises Bright Lights Unfamiliar Smells Unfamiliar Tastes

Other____

What are the best rewards for your child?

iPad/tablet time Prize/trinket from dentist Special food/meal Special outing

Other____

What kind of treatment would you like our team to provide?

Routine Exam Cleaning Filling/Crown Extractions A lot of work Orthodontics

What would be your preferred way to accomplish your child's care?

☐ Desensitization/Behavioral Approach

☐ Sedation/General Anesthesia

☐ Restraint/Protective stabilization

☐ Other, Describe

How did your child's last dental visit go? What could have made it easier?

Is there anything else that you would like us to know about your child?

Thank you for completing this form. The information will be used to help your child with dental treatment

Fig. 2 (continued)

- Medical diagnoses, medications, and allergies
  - A baseline for providing safe dental care.
  - Number and complexity of medical conditions offer clues to ID severity.
- Child's educational support system
  - Gives insight into degree that child and family are participating in other therapeutic and behavioral services.

  - Some strategies may be adapted to the dental environment.
  - Members of the child's care team (e.g., behavioral therapists) may accompany the patient to dental visits and/or work on skills outside the dental office.
  - The child may have an IEP that describes goals and accommodations for the child at school. It is often possible to have oral care added to the patient's IEP (e.g., toothbrushing is completed by an aid daily at school).
- Communication
  - Enables provider to engage with patient in her own communication "currency."
  - Parents can often be used as "interpreters" for the patient.
  - If the patient is accustomed to using visual schedules or Social Stories (discussed at length below), dental stories or sequence cards can be offered to the family at or before the initial visit.
- Ability to perform specific self-care
  - Greater number and complexity of self-care skills may indicate increased ability to participate in dental behavior modification.
- Child's strengths and abilities
  - Leveraging current strengths is a good starting point for development of new skills.
  - The practitioner gains trust and encourages engagement by learning about the patient's interests and discussing topics she cares about.
- Sensitivities that "trigger" avoidance or escape behaviors
  - Avoiding items that trigger negative behaviors facilitates a calm learning environment.
- Preferred rewards
  - Many patients enjoy standard rewards such as stickers or tokens, but it is common for items that are not typically thought of as reinforcers to be highly motivating to the patient.
- Sensory responsiveness
  - Patients may be hyper- or hypo-responders, indicating that they avoid or seek stimulation during visits.
  - Accordingly, the team should encourage or avoid sensory input (e.g., smells, tastes, etc.).
- Questions about dental history
  - Provides insight into what has worked or failed previously.
  - Some patients may have preconceived notions of dental care based upon negative past experiences.
- Parent expectations
  - The people who live with the patient understand her best and will be responsible to prepare her for appointments.
  - Caregiver satisfaction and treatment success hinge upon mutually agreed upon goals.

The Initial Office Visit

After the office has received the pre-visit questionnaire, it is time to schedule the first visit. When reception staff call to make arrangements, they should inform the family that the team has reviewed the informational packet that the family took the time to complete. This shows caregivers that the office is prepared to make the first visit a positive experience. If possible, staff should offer appointments at select times of the day. Many children do best in the morning when they are well-rested, but some may benefit from later appointment times that occur after school or therapy sessions. If possible, CSHCN should be scheduled in a private operatory for the initial visit. This reduces stimuli that may distract or distress the patient. For some patients who are fearful of dental and medical offices, it may be better to arrange for an initial visit in a consultation room or other nonclinical area. This provides an opportunity for the family to become acquainted with the office, so that at the subsequent visit, the child is familiar with the setting.

Once the date of the appointment has been set, ask caregivers to consider bringing comfort objects that keep the patient calm and comfortable during the dental visit. These items could include a favorite toy or stuffed animal, blanket, sound-elimination ear muffs, fidget toys, tablet computers, and other communication devices. When the patient arrives for the initial evaluation, wait times should be kept short to minimize patient anxiety. It may help to schedule particularly sensitive patients for the first or last appointment of the day. If it is not possible to seat the child right away, ask the family if they would prefer to wait in their vehicle or take a walk outside. While the patient is waiting in the exam room, conceal instruments so they don't become a source of worry. Having a variety of toys, games, and movies is also a good strategy for keeping patients relaxed before the dentist arrives.

The first in-person conversation with the family is an opportunity to flesh out information obtained in advance of the visit. Clinicians should confirm responses on the medical history or pre-visit questionnaire (e.g., "I see here that you use pictures to prepare for dental and medical visits. Can you show me an example?") and ask additional questions to learn more about the patient. This is also a good time to discuss caregiver expectations and set goals. Success requires a partnership between the patient, family, and provider. Therefore, it is critical that the family provide input on the treatment approach and assist in developing treatment protocols. Caregivers possess a wealth of information, and frequently provide tips and techniques that have worked to facilitate cooperation in other settings.

An Example Behavior Modification Protocol

Some CSHCN readily adapt to the dental environment with only a few supportive accommodations. For these children, simple behavior guidance techniques may be enough to facilitate a good exam. For others, a more involved behavior modification protocol may be appropriate. The first step is setting immediate and long-term goals. Examples include having the patient sit in a dental chair for a thorough examination, allowing radiographs, or having a restorative procedure. Once the goal is mutually agreed upon, the next step is to establish a plan for achieving it. Principles of behavior modification suggest engaging the patient at a minimally stressful level and shaping behavior from that point. Therefore, it is helpful to break down the dental visit into discrete skills and focus on obtaining success at each point before proceeding to the next (Fig. 3). Skills can be broken into multiple small steps to facilitate working with the patient at a pace that is appropriate to her developmental level. Patients who participate in therapy programs such as applied behavior analysis will be very familiar with this approach [24].

Steps in the oral exam sequence:

1. Patient sits in the dental chair.
2. Parent brushes teeth.
3. Dentist brushes teeth.
4. Dentist touches teeth with gloved finger.
5. Introduce dental mirror.
6. Introduce probe/explorer.
7. Perform dental examination.

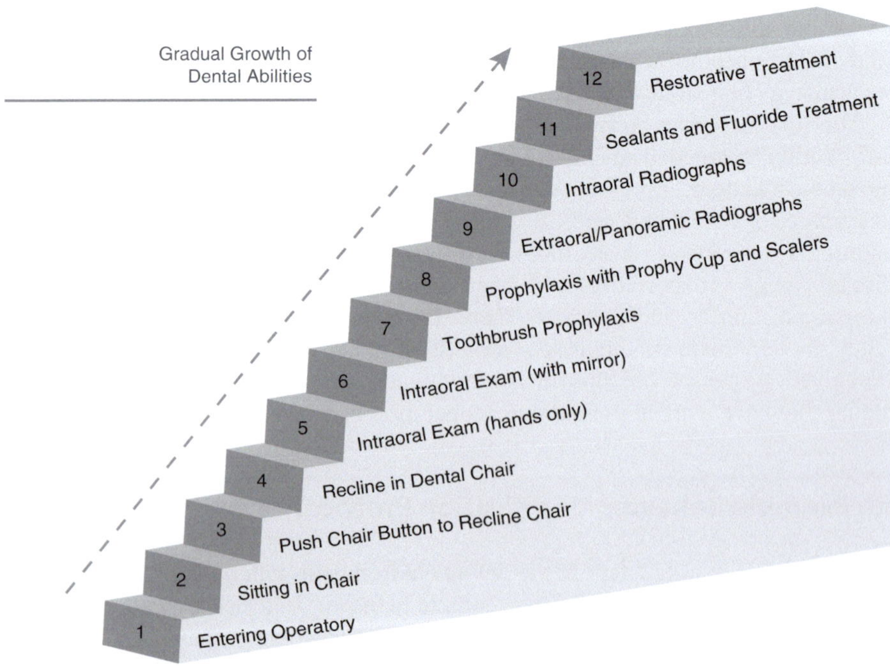

Fig. 3 Building on simple skills to learn more complex dental treatment

At the beginning of each visit, review the session goal with the caregiver to ensure that team and family expectations are congruent. Then, proceed with the visit, taking time to reward and reinforce the patient when the goal is achieved. In many cases it is possible to proceed past the goal, stopping at a point that is mutually agreed upon. At the conclusion of the visit, the dentist and caregiver should discuss the goals and preparation plan for the subsequent appointment. This should be based upon the accomplishments of the visit. New skills should only be added after the initial goals have been achieved and reinforced. Procedures that involve increased physical proximity, intensity, or touch are gradually introduced into the behavioral program [4].

There is no consensus on how frequently behavior modification patients should be appointed for follow-up. Some practices initially appoint patients for very frequent visits (e.g., weekly) until the treatment goal has been achieved. Others may schedule longer intervals to accommodate the family's preferences and allow for increased home practice. There is no magic time interval, but generally patients who are learning dental skills should be seen more frequently than other patients in the dental practice. It may be helpful to suggest an initial follow-up of 2–4 weeks, subsequent visits at 1–2 months, and recall visits at 3–4 months until the child is quite comfortable with procedural goals. Caregivers have good insight into what will work for the child, so they should provide input regarding the appointment intervals. Patients also vary considerably in how rapidly they acquire new skills, so flexibility is important. Remember that children who are learning other life skills through behavioral therapy may have the opportunity to practice the skills daily or weekly. In contrast, dental visits occur much less frequently. Therefore it may not be realistic for many patients to acquire new dental skills through standard biannual visits. Behavioral programs in dentistry have reported that some CSHCN are able to achieve an oral examination in as little as one to two visits, but others require five, ten, or even more visits before an exam is possible [3, 7, 9, 21].

Strategies to Increase Success

Modeling

Modeling involves having the patient watch a typically developing "model" receive dental services. It has been used historically to assist children in decreasing fears and displaying less negative behavior for dental treatment [25]. It is also an effective way to modify behavior and teach CSHCN dental skills. The model may be a parent, sibling, or other peer that can perform the specified tasks without displaying anxiety. When the patient views the model successfully accomplishing these tasks, she sees how they are performed and that the procedures do not cause harm. This allows the patient to learn by observation, without actually having to practice the procedures. Typically modeling is most effective with patients who do not already have experience with the procedure (e.g., the patient has not yet received a dental restoration). It is highly effective to show the model receiving praise or another reward for correctly completing the requested action. Once the patient is ready to practice the skill, it may be helpful to use a hand mirror so that she can see what is occurring in her mouth. Video modeling can also be a good way to prepare CSHCN for procedures. The advantage of video modeling is that the patient can mentally rehearse procedures as many times as she likes within the comfort of her own home. Dental offices can produce short videos of common procedures and post them to practice websites as a convenient resource for families. Having caregivers record video of the child using a smart phone or tablet while she performs skills is also a very effective strategy. Many children love to watch videos of the dental visit once they return home. This provides powerful reinforcement and a pleasant souvenir of the appointment.

Dental Stories

Many CSHCN are visual learners. Dental stories leverage this by displaying a series of photographs with captions showing a sequence of actions required to complete a task. Also known as Social Stories or Visual Pedagogy, these short learning tools are used in many areas of the child's life to reduce fear of the unknown and help prepare for unfamiliar tasks or procedures [26]. Dental stories may be incorporated into the visit in a number of ways, but commonly caregivers read the story to the patient multiple times before an upcoming appointment. Individual photos in the story can also be used as prompts during the exam. Caregivers sometimes deconstruct photos to make flip books, visual sequence charts, and other aids (Fig. 4). These strategies reflect the fact that many CSHCN use augmentative and alternative communication (AAC) techniques like communication boards and electronic devices rather than speech to express thoughts, needs, wants, and ideas [27].

During treatment, the child can be shown cards that demonstrate specific actions. Once an action is performed, it can be removed from the chart so that the child understands that aspect of the visit has been accomplished. It can help to show the child how the number of photos/cards decreases after each task. Research indicates that dental stories are well received by families and can be effective in teaching skills and reducing anxiety. It is not clear however which patients benefit most from dental stories [28]. Some may not find them useful or may even be more anxious when viewing them. This information can often be elicited during an initial interview or on a pre-visit questionnaire.

It is also important to note that dental stories vary considerably. Some show actual photos of children visiting the dentist. Others are cartoon depictions of patients receiving dental procedures. Stories may be printed or displayed on a tablet computer. Patients have a wide variety of preferences, so it is generally best to simply make parents aware that the dental stories are an option for their child. Not all children will find them useful, but making the resource available shows families that the team is accustomed to caring for CSHCN and is invested in each patient's success. If caregivers are presented with stories in a number of formats, they will likely adapt and use them in ways that are appropriate for their child.

Practice Exam Kit

Many CSHCN participate in occupational and physical therapy, so they are accustomed to in-office therapies. While this is common in the medical community, most dental offices are not equipped to provide that level of support. Generally the practice provides standard dental care for the majority of patients, with a behavioral modification program targeted toward specific individuals. Therefore, time devoted to desensitization and dental training programs may be limited. Practice exam kits are one way to extend and amplify the affect of office-based training. A practice kit typically would include a disposable dental mirror, exam gloves, and a mask (Fig. 5). These items are inexpensive and can easily be given to caregivers. This

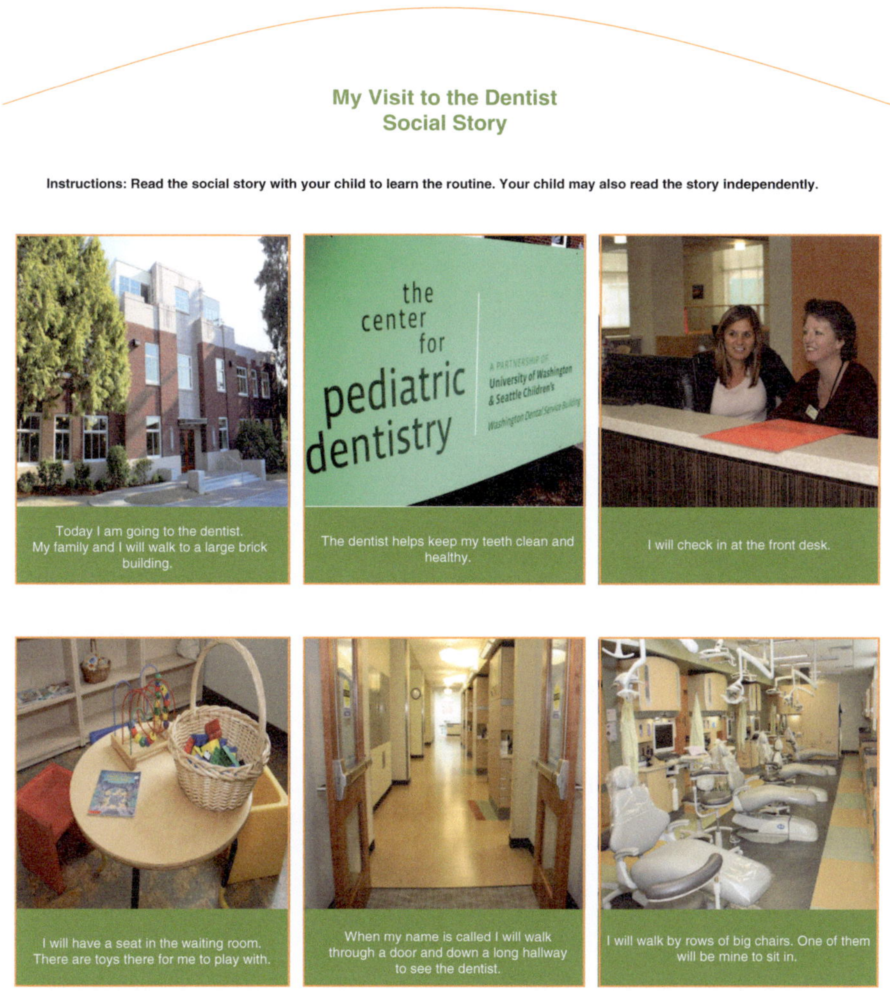

Fig. 4 A dental story that can be used to teach patients about aspects of the dental visit

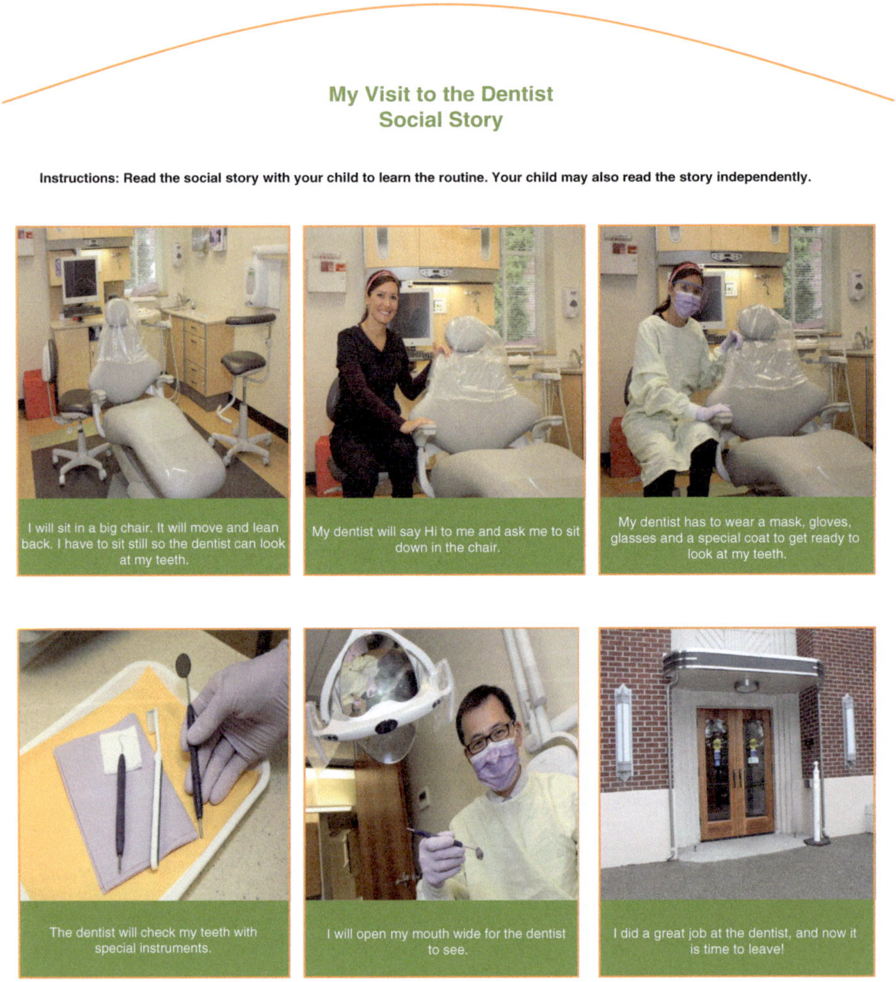

Fig. 4 (continued)

offers the family an opportunity to rehearse dental procedures at home. One effective strategy is to use the kit daily when toothbrushing. The caregiver wears the mask and/or gloves and begins by initiating a toothbrushing sequence that the child is familiar with. At the conclusion of the routine, the caregiver examines the child's mouth using the disposable mirror. Caregivers can be instructed to perform a specific examination sequence:

- Touch the patient's lips with the mirror (count to 5).
- Touch the right cheek mucosa (count to 5).
- Touch the left cheek mucosa (count to 5).
- Touch the tongue (count to 5).

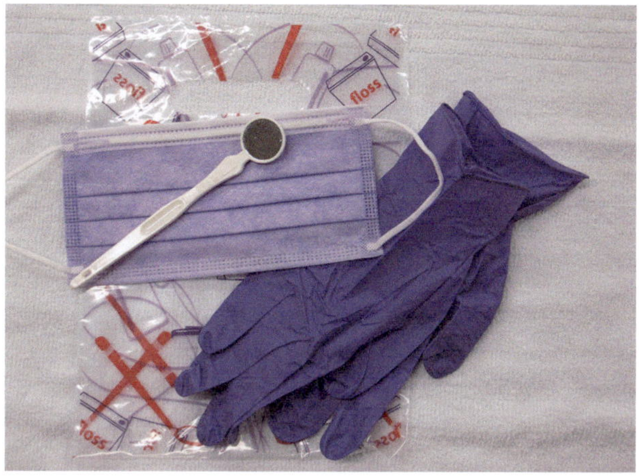

Fig. 5 A practice dental examination kit for home use

- Have the patient open wide with the mirror above the tongue (count to 5 four times, once for each quadrant).

Practicing this at home familiarizes the patient with the procedure. The next step is transferring the skill to the dental office. Once the patient is seated, the caregiver can initiate the oral hygiene routine, followed by the examination. A disposable mirror can be used if necessary because the patient will already be comfortable with it. The dentist should watch how the caregiver and child interact during toothbrushing and the examination. After they conclude, the dentist can say "my turn" and take over from the caregiver replicating the same exam sequence. With experience, the time periods that the child is accustomed to can be extended to facilitate thorough examination. Other adjuncts such as gauze sponges and the air/water syringe may also be added. This practice kit is an incredibly powerful tool that can be expanded to teach the patient other dental skills. For example, the patient can be sent home with impression trays or sample bitewing radiograph tabs for practice before attempting procedures in the dental office.

Individualized Reinforcement

Nearly all behavior modification programs are based on the principle of exposure to new experiences, repeating learned skills, and reinforcing desired behaviors. Providing the patient with rewards is perhaps the most basic and fundamental aspect of successful programs. Behavioral experts recognize that rewards should be highly individualized and offered as close as possible to the time the patient successfully completes a requested task [2, 6, 8, 9]. The pre-visit questionnaire is an effective way to obtain information about rewards that are motivating to the patient, but it is also important to ask caregivers to provide details about the best reinforcers during the initial visit. Items that are used in outside behavior therapy sessions can be very powerful motivators. Asking about items that motivate the child is also an opportunity to determine if she receives food as a reward during therapy sessions. Food is considered a primary reinforcer because it satisfies visceral cravings [9]. These types of reinforcers can be highly effective for patients who require that level of reinforcement. This is particularly true in the initial stages of therapy. While effective, providing cariogenic rewards puts the patient at risk for decay. Families may be unaware of this and should be counseled to consider sugar-free or nonfood alternatives.

Social reinforcement, recreation, prizes, and money are considered secondary reinforcement [9]. Secondary reinforcers that are well suited to the patient can also be highly motivating. During the treatment visit, it is common to provide continuous social reinforcement. Praising the patient for small accomplishments builds confidence and keeps the visit on track (e.g., "you are doing a great job of sitting still"). For minor accomplishments during the visit, it may be helpful to provide the child with access to "preferred items" such as a tablet or a favored toy (e.g., "we are going to brush your teeth for 10 s, and then you will be able to watch a short clip of your show"). Many patients can be encouraged to proceed with requested tasks by reminding them of an agreed upon reward throughout the visit (e.g., "remember, if you finish everything today we will go and get an ice cream afterward"). In practice, it is usually best to find a way to end the visit on a high note. Even if it is clear that the child is not going to accomplish the stated goal, she can usually be encouraged to achieve something minor. Once she has done that, the parent and dentist should congratulate her on a job well done. This leaves a positive impression of the visit and sets the stage for future successes. Initially a patient may need relatively large rewards as an incentive for learning simple dental skills. As the patient gains confidence in these areas, the rewards should gradually be thinned or tapered. Larger rewards can be then reserved for accomplishing new skills. This places the patient on an upward treatment trajectory.

Other Clinical Strategies

Success in behavior modification is contingent upon building rapport, good planning, and consistency. Table 2 provides a number of clinical pearls that can be used to help achieve care goals.

Cost

It is important to consider how the clinic will be reimbursed for the dental behavior modification program. In the USA most dental insurance programs do not cover the cost of behavioral therapy, so the family is generally responsible to pay for these services. Clinics that employ behavioral strategies for only a few patients may choose not to charge for initial consultation and brief training visits. Other clinics that routinely work with CSHCN may provide these services frequently, so it

Table 2 Tips to facilitate clinical care

Communication	• Use speech that is calm, clear, concrete, simple, slow, and repetitive • Provide one instruction at a time • Use terminology consistently • Address the patient directly, not through the caregiver • Use the caregiver to interpret patient communication
Office setup	• Avoid bright lights and stimulating office design in areas intended for CSHCN • Avoid using strong flavors and odors in fluoride, prophy paste, and other dental products • Keep instruments covered
Appointment design	• Schedule short appointments (15–20 min) • Divide procedures into discrete parts • Attempt to schedule patient with the same provider, assistant, room • Establish a routine, document it, and adhere to it
Exam technique	• Have parent demonstrate a skill they practiced at home, and take over when skill is demonstrated • Provide patient with control, "are you ready?" • Proceed slowly when moving the dental chair; fully reclined is a vulnerable position for patients • For patients who have difficulty with chair motion, consider reclining before the patient is seated • Be willing to change your own posture to facilitate exam • Don't force a patient to perform a task, but be persistent in asking • Consider patient sensory profile: e.g., scalers may be easier to tolerate than rubber cup prophylaxis • Having parents massage limbs may calm sensory seeking children • Counting to an established number during procedures lets children know how long they must cooperate for
Props and tools	• Keep fidget toys, bubble wrap, and other objects that patient enjoys at office • X-ray vests, compression clothing, and weighted blankets calm some patients • Have multiple sizes of sunglasses available for light-sensitive patients • Headphones for television programs or sound-cancelling earmuffs may calm sensitive patients • Movies and tablet apps are an effective reward that can be used as a contingent distraction [29] • Large digital timers can be used with children who like numbers • Let the child play music she likes during the appointment

becomes important to develop a fee schedule that provides appropriate compensation for time spent teaching dental skills. Ultimately the decision is up to the clinic, but the author has found that most families are accustomed to paying for out-of-pocket behavioral services. Many parents are happy to be provided with the option of paying a small fee to visit the dental clinic for educational sessions. A good starting point can be to charge a fee that is in line with that of other brief clinical visits (e.g., a limited evaluation, fluoride and hygiene instructions for high-risk patients, etc.). One very rewarding part of behavior modification programs is that over time, many children no longer need frequent training visits. They become familiar with dental procedures and can "graduate" to a standard recall interval, receiving services like examination, dental prophylaxis, and fluoride that are paid for by insurance plans.

Office Forms

In addition to the introductory letter and the pre-visit questionnaire, practices that incorporate behavior modification programs may find it useful to have specific office forms. The developers of the D-Termined program of Familiarization and Sequential Tasking have created forms to assist in obtaining consent for behavioral techniques, identifying the correct approach for each patient, and charting patient progress. These are available online and can be used as is or adapted to meet the specific needs of individual offices [16, 30]. A sample care plan and progress chart are included with this chapter to assist practices as they develop their own programs (Fig. 6).

Case-Based Scenario

Jonathan, an 8-year-old boy with Down syndrome, was referred to the dental clinic by his pediatrician. The referral stated that the patient had no obvious signs of decay or dental infection and he was being referred to establish a dental home. After receiving the referral, reception staff called the patient's family to inquire if they were interested in participating in the clinic's desensitization program. The patient's parents informed the front office staff that they were not aware of any acute dental needs and they would be open to that approach. Reception staff sent out an introductory letter and a pre-visit questionnaire.

Two weeks later the office received Jonathan's questionnaire in the mail. Upon receipt the dentist reviewed the questionnaire noting that Jonathan is in an integrated classroom at school and has an IEP in place and that he receives speech therapy outside the home. The questionnaire also described the patient as a nonreader with limited verbal ability. It stated that he was able to comply with simple instructions and could do some dressing and toileting by himself. According to his caregivers, Jonathan was accustomed to using pictures for communication, and he was very interested in "anything with wheels." Caregivers also noted that the patient was sensitive to loud noises and had a hard time around new people. The questionnaire stated that visiting a local fast-food restaurant would be an effective reward for the patient. When asked "What would be your preferred way to accomplish your child's care (e.g., desensitization, protective stabilization, sedation, general anesthesia)?", the family checked all the responses and stated "we are willing to try anything." At the end of the form, a write-in section showed: "The last time we went to the dentist was when Jonathan was 5 years old. He wouldn't let the dentist look in his mouth, so we had to hold his hands and legs to check his teeth."

Jonathan was accompanied to the first dental visit by both mother and father. He was scheduled at 1:00 PM, right after the lunch break to avoid being seated late. After check-in the family was escorted to a private operatory by a dental assistant. The assistant verified medical history, medications, and allergies. The dentist

Care Plan/Progress Chart

Child 's Name________________ MRN____________ Patient Age_________

Patient Strengths/Interests

Triggers

Reward

Communication

☐ Verbal ☐ Reading ☐ Pictures ☐ Gestures ☐ Other____________________

Special Accommodations

☐ Practice Exam Kit ☐ Squeeze toy ☐ Lead Apron ☐ Bubble Wrap

☐ Pen light ☐ Sunglasses ☐ TV/Tablet ☐ Music

☐ Social Story ☐ Hand Mirror ☐ Other_______________

Visit	1		2		3		4		5	
Date										
	Goal	Performance	Goal	Performance	Goal	Performance	Goal	Performance	Goal	Performance
Other										
Fillings/Crowns										
Radiographs										
Fluoride Varnish										
Rubber Cup Prophy										
Hand Scaling										
Mirror Exam										
Toothbrush Prophy										
Sits in Dental Chair										
Enter Operatory										
Measured By	Dentist	Assistant	Dentist	Assistant	Dentist	Assistant	Dentist	Assistant	Dentist	Assistant

*Behavior 1 =completely unable, 2=able with extreme difficulty, 3=able with moderate difficulty, 4=able with minimal difficulty 5 = able without difficulty

Fig. 6 Sample progress chart

entered the room and discussed the pre-visit questionnaire in detail specifically focusing on communication, triggers, and effective rewards. The family agreed that they would like to have the dentist perform an oral examination that day if possible. The dental team and Jonathan's parents tried to convince him to sit in the dental chair but were unsuccessful. After attempting an exam in the chair, the parents were given a toothbrush to prompt opening. While he was seated in a non-dental chair in the corner of the room, Jonathan opened his mouth and allowed his mother to brush his teeth. After his mother brushed his teeth, he allowed the dentist to brush as well. While brushing the dentist was able to perform a cursory examination of the mouth.

To reinforce positive behaviors, after completing toothbrushing the dentist provided Jonathan with a token to purchase a toy from a vending machine in the lobby.

The dentist then discussed next steps with the parents. They agreed that Jonathan had done very well for a first visit and that it would be worth attempting to teach him to sit in the dental chair for the exam. For the next visit the goal was to have Jonathan sit in the dental chair and open his mouth for a dental mirror. The family was given materials for behavior modeling, including a link to a dental story on the practice website, a photograph of the dental chair that was taken on Jonathan's tablet computer, and a plastic mouth mirror and a disposable mask for home practice. The dentist taught the parents a specific "exam protocol" to perform after brushing each evening. Jonathan was scheduled to return to the clinic in 2 weeks.

In 2 weeks Jonathan returned to the same exam room with the same dentist and assistant. By the time that the dentist entered the room, the patient was already seated in the dental chair. The dentist asked the parent to perform the same hygiene and exam routine they had been practicing at home. Afterward, the dentist repeated the same sequence introducing a dental mirror into the patient's mouth four times for a count of 10 s. The team documented a mixed dentition, generalized crowding, and occlusal attrition with no obvious decay. Immediately after completing the exam, Jonathan was given a token for the toy machine. Jonathan's parents were very happy with how well he did for the dental examination. It was decided that the next visit should be in 1 month and that the goal would be to shape behavior to obtain a panoramic radiograph. Before leaving, Jonathan was shown the panoramic machine, and the family found YouTube videos showing children standing for panoramic radiographs. They planned to watch those at home on the tablet. At the conclusion of the visit, Jonathan was taken for a treat of French fries at a local fast-food restaurant.

Conclusion

- CSHCN are accustomed to receiving educational and behavioral therapies for non-dental reasons.
- The principles of behavior modification include exposure and desensitization. These strategies can be adapted to teach dental skills.
- The dental behavior modification program must be customized for each patient, adapting the dental environment to best suit individual needs.
- Behavior modification requires very little equipment, so it can easily be integrated into practice with minimal setup cost.
- The patient that learns to accept dental care as a child has developed an important life skill. This enables her to receive care over a lifetime and achieve the greatest level of oral health possible.

References

1. Nelson TM, Sheller B, Friedman CS, Bernier R. Educational and therapeutic behavioral approaches to providing dental care for patients with autism spectrum disorder. Spec Care Dentist. 2015;35(3):105–13.
2. Kohlenberg R, Greenberg D, Reymore L, Hass G. Behavior modification and the management of mentally retarded dental patients. ASDC J Dent Child. 1972;39(1):61–7.

3. Orellana LM, Martinez-Sanchis S, Silvestre FJ. Training adults and children with an autism spectrum disorder to be compliant with a clinical dental assessment using a TEACCH-based approach. J Autism Dev Disord. 2014;44(4):776–85.
4. Cuvo A, Godard A, Huckfeldt R, DeMattei R. Training children with autism spectrum disorders to be compliant with an oral assessment. Res Autism Spectr Disord. 2010;4:681–96.
5. Boj JR, Davila JM. A study of behavior modification for developmentally disabled children. ASDC J Dent Child. 1989;56(6):452–7.
6. Entwistle BM, Rudrud EH. Behavioral approaches to toothbrushing programs for handicapped adults. Spec Care Dentist. 1982;2(4):155–60.
7. Gordon D, Terdal L, Sterling E. The use of modeling and desensitization in the treatment of a phobic child patient. ASDC J Dent Child. 1974;41(2):102–5.
8. Maguire KB, Lange B, Sherling M. The use of rehearsal and positive reinforcement in the dental treatment of uncooperative patients with mental retardation. J Dev Phys Disabil. 1996;8(2):167–77.
9. Connick C, Pugliese S, Willette J, Palat M. Desensitization: strengths and limitations of its use in dentistry for the patient with severe and profound mental retardation. ASDC J Dent Child. 2000;67(4):250–5.
10. Lawton L. Providing dental care for special patients: tips for the general dentist. J Am Dent Assoc. 2002;133(12):1666–70.
11. Raposa KA. Behavioral management for patients with intellectual and developmental disorders. Dent Clin N Am. 2009;53(2):359–73, xi.
12. Jaccarino J. Treating the special needs patient with a developmental disability: cerebral palsy, autism and Down syndrome. Dent Assist. 2009;78(6):7–8, 10–1, 34 passim.
13. Greenbaum PE, Melamed BG. Pretreatment modeling. A technique for reducing children's fear in the dental operatory. Dent Clin N Am. 1988;32(4):693–704.
14. Yilmaz S, Ozlu Y, Ekuklu G. The effect of dental training on the reactions of mentally handicapped children's behavior in the dental office. ASDC J Dent Child. 1999;66(3):188–91, 54–5.
15. Fetner M, Cascio CJ, Essick G. Nonverbal patient with autism spectrum disorder and obstructive sleep apnea: use of desensitization to acclimatize to a dental appliance. Pediatr Dent. 2014;36(7):499–501.
16. AlHumaid J, Tesini D, Finkelman M, Loo CY. Effectiveness of the D-TERMINED program of repetitive tasking for children with autism spectrum disorder. J Dent Child (Chic). 2016;83(1):16–21.
17. Klein U, Nowak AJ. Characteristics of patients with autistic disorder (AD) presenting for dental treatment: a survey and chart review. Spec Care Dentist. 1999;19(5):200–7.
18. Lowe O, Lindemann R. Assessment of the autistic patient's dental needs and ability to undergo dental examination. ASDC J Dent Child. 1985;52(1):29–35.
19. DeMattei R, Cuvo A, Maurizio S. Oral assessment of children with an autism spectrum disorder. J Dent Hyg. 2007;81(3):65.
20. Marshall J, Sheller B, Williams BJ, Mancl L, Cowan C. Cooperation predictors for dental patients with autism. Pediatr Dent. 2007;29(5):369–76.
21. Nelson T, Chim A, Sheller BL, McKinney CM, Scott JM. Predicting successful dental examinations for children with autism spectrum disorder in the context of a dental desensitization program. J Am Dent Assoc. 2017;148(7):485–92.
22. Du RY, Yiu CC, Wong VC, McGrath CP. Autism developmental profiles and cooperation with oral health screening. J Autism Dev Disord. 2015;45(9):2758–63.
23. Marshall J, Sheller B, Mancl L, Williams BJ. Parental attitudes regarding behavior guidance of dental patients with autism. Pediatr Dent. 2008;30(5):400–7.
24. Hernandez P, Ikkanda Z. Applied behavior analysis: behavior management of children with autism spectrum disorders in dental environments. J Am Dent Assoc. 2011;142(3):281–7.
25. Greenbaum PE, Turner C, Cook EW 3rd, Melamed BG. Dentists' voice control: effects on children's disruptive and affective behavior. Health Psychol. 1990;9(5):546–58.
26. Backman B, Pilebro C. Visual pedagogy in dentistry for children with autism. ASDC J Dent Child. 1999;66(5):325–31, 294.
27. Association AS-L-H Augmentative and Alternative Communication (AAC). 2017. http://www.asha.org/public/speech/disorders/AAC/. Accessed 5 Sept 2017.

28. Marion IW, Nelson TM, Sheller B, McKinney CM, Scott JM. Dental stories for children with autism. Spec Care Dentist. 2016;36(4):181–6.
29. Fakhruddin KS, El Batawi HY. Effectiveness of audiovisual distraction in behavior modification during dental caries assessment and sealant placement in children with autism spectrum disorder. Dent Res J (Isfahan). 2017;14(3):177–82.
30. Tesini D. The D-termined program of repetitive tasking and familiarization in dentistry. Wellesley, MA: NLM Family Foundation; 2004. https://specializedcare.com/products/d-termined-program-for-patients-with-autism.

Nutritional Considerations for Optimal Oral Health in CSHCN

Elizabeth A. Palmer

Introduction

High-quality nutrition is an important component in the growth and development of a child. Unfortunately, children with special healthcare needs are at increased risk for experiencing nutritional complications that can pose great challenges to maintaining a healthy body and mouth. The sources of the difficulties are numerous—the child's physiological condition itself, the medications and/or diet prescribed to treat the health condition, and the behavioral and psychosocial approaches toward feeding in general. Children with disabilities and chronic conditions may have a decreased ability to consume adequate nutrients (e.g., oral motor dysfunction, cleft lip/palate), an inability to utilize adequate calories (e.g., gastroesophageal reflux), or an increased caloric requirement (e.g., hyperthyroidism). Many CSHCNs take medications in order to manage their medical conditions, which can negatively affect the child's dentition and periodontium. CSHCNs are often on a selective, limited diet either prescribed by the care provider or dictated by the child. There are several diets that limit a child's exposure to specific types of foods in an attempt to manage the symptoms of a disease (e.g., the ketogenic diet for seizure disorder). A self-limited diet may also be dictated by the child's own feeding difficulties (e.g., sensory processing dysfunction). It takes a team approach to address the specific nutritional needs of the child. This may include counseling, therapy (occupational, physical, and/or behavioral), medications, surgery, and alternative feeding approaches. As a dental provider for CSHCN, it is necessary to recognize that the child's diagnosis and associated treatment may bring additional challenges to maintaining oral health. Thus, as key members of the medical team, dental providers are in a prime position to help the child maintain her optimal dentition and periodontium.

E. A. Palmer (✉)
Department of Pediatric Dentistry,
Oregon Health and Science University School of Dentistry, Portland, OR, USA
e-mail: palmerel@ohsu.edu

T. M. Nelson, J. R. Webb (eds.), *Dental Care for Children with Special Needs*,
https://doi.org/10.1007/978-3-030-10483-2_6

Medications and Their Effects on the Dentition

Medications are a very common part of the lives of CSHCN, and while they are necessary, they can pose multiple potential threats to their oral health. It is important to recognize that both the medication itself and the vehicle by which the medicine is delivered may have potential negative side effects.

Many medications used to manage the systemic conditions of CSHCN have clinical implications in the oral cavity. To further complicate the situation, many CSHCNs receive medications for more than one comorbidity, resulting in a complex drug regimen and multiple potential effects. When a CSHCN presents to the dental office, it is important to determine how her medications impact the dentition and periodontium and to work with the family to manage side effects. Strong emphasis should be placed on excellent home oral hygiene practices and diet, as well as frequent dental exams and prophylaxis appointments. The dental provider must also provide relevant educational material to help the patient and her family prepare for the potential short- and long-term side effects of the medications.

CSHCNs with systemic conditions and behavioral diagnoses are typically treated with established classes of medications. Many medications have negative effects on the gingiva, salivary gland function, taste receptors, and oral microbiology. When patients experience such changes in their oral cavity, their nutritional status may be affected. They may avoid certain types of food due to difficulty chewing or swallowing or because the food does not taste good. As the patient's oral healthcare provider, it is paramount to consider these added oral health complications and tailor the patient's care accordingly.

Many medications, such as diuretics (e.g., furosemide) used to treat some cardiac conditions, have the potential for causing xerostomia [1]. It is important to work with the patient in order to best address her possible dry mouth in order to maintain oral health, proper nutritional intake, and a good quality of life. Many other medications alter the patient's ability to taste, so helping her develop and maintain a healthy balanced diet is essential [2]. A few of the most common conditions, the medication classes commonly prescribed to treat them, and their potential oral side effects are summarized in Table 1.

It is also important to consider the long-term effects of medications. Perhaps the best example of the dramatic lifetime effects of medication treatment is that of a patient that has undergone chemotherapy treatment for pediatric cancer. Chemotherapy has several immediate and long-term effects on the oral cavity. While receiving cancer therapy, patients may experience mucositis, xerostomia, stomatitis, bleeding, infection, as well as ulcerative lesions [3]. Depending on the age at which the treatment was initiated, patients treated for pediatric cancer may also suffer long-term dental malformations, including tooth agenesis or malformation, root malformation, malocclusion, and salivary gland malfunction [4]. Children that receive a hematopoietic stem cell transplant are also at risk for the development of oral graft vs. host disease (GVHD) [5]. Oral, esophageal, and stomach chronic GVHD has several clinical manifestations, such as decreased salivary flow, pain,

Table 1 Common diagnoses, medications used to treat them, and potential implications in the oral cavity

Systemic diagnosis	Medication class	Oral cavity implications
Asthma	Inhaled corticosteroids	Stomatitis, candidiasis, xerostomia
	Beta-adrenergic bronchodilators	Xerostomia
Attention deficit hyperactivity disorder	CNS stimulants	Xerostomia, dysgeusia, bruxism, weight gain
	Selective norepinephrine reuptake inhibitors	Xerostomia
	Antihypertensives	Xerostomia, dysphagia, sialadenitis
Autism spectrum disorders	CNS stimulants	Xerostomia, dysgeusia, bruxism
	Selective serotonin reuptake inhibitors	Xerostomia, dysgeusia, bruxism, stomatitis, jaw pain
	Anticonvulsants	Xerostomia, stomatitis
	Antipsychotics	Xerostomia, dysphagia, stomatitis, dysgeusia, tongue/facial edema
	Antihypertensives	Xerostomia, dysphagia, sialadenitis
Cerebral palsy	Antiparkinsonian drugs	Xerostomia
Congenital heart disease	Anticoagulants	Gingival bleeding, petechiae
	Diuretics	Xerostomia
	Beta-blockers	Lichenoid reactions
	ACE inhibitors	Delayed gingival healing
	Calcium channel blockers	Gingival overgrowth
Gastroesophageal reflux disease	Histamine H2-receptor antagonists	Erythema multiforme
	Proton pump inhibitors	Xerostomia, erythema multiforme
Seizure disorders	Anticonvulsants	Gingival bleeding, gingival overgrowth, xerostomia, delayed gingival healing, dysgeusia

atrophy, erythema, lichenoid lesions, mucoceles, ulcerations, pseudomembranes, and/or sensitivity to spicy or acidic foods [6]. For a patient that has been treated with chemotherapeutic medicaments, the long-term effects may last a lifetime. The pediatric dental provider has the ability to address these symptoms and help the patient improve both her nutritional status and quality of life.

Prevention of medication side effects must also include an evaluation of the medicament's delivery system. Due to young age and inability to swallow tablets, oral medications are often delivered to children in a liquid suspension. Oral liquid medicaments are typically sweetened with sucrose in order to decrease the bitter taste of the medication and increase compliance in taking them as directed [7–9]. A recent review of oral liquid medications found that these suspensions contain varying amounts of sucrose, up to 4 g/5 mL [10]. Thus, it is important to explain to the patient and caregiver that exposure to the sugar-sweetened medication, which is often given several times per day, increases the child's risk for the development of dental caries. Children also receive medications via the inhalation delivery route. Medications such as inhaled corticosteroids can cause stomatitis, alteration of the oral flora resulting in candidiasis, and xerostomia.

Limited Diets

A CSHCN is often on a selective, limited diet that makes obtaining proper nutrition difficult. Elimination diets reduce exposure to key food classes in an attempt to manage the symptoms of some systemic diseases (e.g., the ketogenic diet for seizure disorder). These limited diets are either prescribed by the child's care provider or may be implemented by the caregiver without professional recommendation. Four of the most common elimination diets include the ketogenic diet, gluten-free and/or casein-free diet, food additives exclusion diet, and the oligoantigenic diet.

The Ketogenic Diet

The ketogenic diet is a nonpharmacological treatment for seizure disorders that has been prescribed to patients since the 1920s. It is often used either in combination with anticonvulsants or when anticonvulsants are not successful. The ketogenic diet has been demonstrated to be effective in treating several types of seizure disorders including intractable epilepsy, tuberous sclerosis complex, Rett syndrome, Lennox-Gastaut syndrome, lissencephaly, myoclonic-astatic epilepsy, and mitochondrial disorders [11, 12]. More recently, the ketogenic diet has been thought to be a potential treatment option for other neurological disorders such as brain tumors, migraines, and autism spectrum disorder (ASD) [13]. While the ketogenic diet has demonstrated success in a large portion of the patients with seizures, its restrictive nature gives rise to nutritional challenges, as well as difficulty with compliance and long-term maintenance for the patient and her caregivers.

The classical ketogenic diet uses a ratio of 4:1 of total energy from fat to combined protein and carbohydrate. Because the classical ketogenic diet has been thought of as unpalatable, several modified diets including the modified Atkins diet, the medium chain triglyceride diet, and the low glycemic index diet have been demonstrated to also be effective in the treatment of seizures (Table 2). These diets still limit specific types of carbohydrates but have a lower ratio of fat to combined protein and carbohydrate. As a result they are often better tolerated by patients. The mechanism by which these diets work is unknown, but it is theorized that the ketogenic diets generate large quantities of ketone bodies, effectively inducing a metabolic state of ketosis. Ketone bodies interact with multiple molecular targets in the

Table 2 Sample menu for a ketogenic style diet

Breakfast	Ham and cheese omelet Scrambled eggs with mayonnaise
Lunch	Hamburger with red peppers and mushroom Turkey, carrot lettuce wrap
Dinner	Creamy chicken and broccoli Deli meat, cheese, mayonnaise roll-up
Snack	Celery with butter and peanut butter Whole milk string cheese

brain, influencing brain hyperexcitability and hypersynchrony [12, 14]. All ketogenic diets have several possible adverse effects. These include vitamin and mineral deficiency, growth inhibition, gastroesophageal reflux, constipation, kidney stones, and cardiovascular complications. Patients following a ketogenic diet require careful meal planning and vitamin and mineral supplements. For this reason, patients adhering to a strict ketogenic diet are generally monitored very closely by a nutritionist.

A child that is following a ketogenic diet requires individualized dental care. It is important to review the child's diet as well as any supplements she is taking. The child's dentition and gingival health should also be evaluated for signs of vitamin deficiencies such as enamel defects and vitamin D deficiency or bleeding gingiva and vitamin C deficiency [15]. The provider should also evaluate the tooth structure for wear facets characteristic of gastroesophageal reflux. It is critical that dental providers take care not to upset the patient's state of ketosis. For example, a provider should not prescribe liquid suspension pediatric medications that are high in sucrose. In instances where an oral medication is necessitated by the symptoms of the patient, it is essential to consult with the patient's physician or nutritionist that is overseeing the ketogenic regimen. It is also prudent to only recommend those toothpastes and other oral hygiene products that have been approved by the team monitoring the ketogenic diet and avoid use of dental prophylaxis paste and fluoride varnish that may contain sweeteners. The Charlie Foundation for Ketogenic Therapies (https://charliefoundation.org) provides useful information regarding low and no carbohydrate dental products. One advantage of the ketogenic diet is that it is low in carbohydrates and thus not cariogenic in nature. Therefore, the child following it should be at a low caries risk in regard to her food intake.

The Gluten-Free and/or Casein-Free Diet

Food allergies are estimated to be present in 5% of the adult and 8% of the pediatric populations worldwide [16]. Celiac disease is an autoimmune disorder in which gluten, a mixture of proteins isolated from wheat, barley, oats, or rye, causes an immune response in the small intestine. Celiac disease is estimated to be present in about 1% of people worldwide [17]. An allergy to milk proteins is estimated to be present in 1.8% of the United States population [18]. Casein is a protein commonly found in cow's milk and dairy products. Gluten-free and/or casein-free (GFCF) diets are often prescribed to treat people with food sensitivities or allergies to gluten and casein.

GFCF diets are now being studied and employed in an attempt to lessen negative behaviors associated with neurodevelopmental diagnoses, including ASD, attention deficit hyperactivity disorder (ADHD), bipolar disorder, schizophrenia, and psychosis [19, 20]. The link between each diagnosis and the gastrointestinal problems associated with gluten and casein is unknown and is still being evaluated. Current research has only demonstrated weak associations between these diets and improvements in negative behaviors. Thus, while these diets are not strongly endorsed for treatment of negative behaviors, caregivers often implement elimination diets in an attempt to help the child [19].

The provider who has a patient following one or both of these diets should consider frequent nutritional monitoring to ensure the patient is receiving adequate fiber, vitamins, and minerals [21]. Additionally, individuals that have celiac disease and exposure to gluten often present with enamel developmental defects and aphthous ulcers [22].

Other Elimination Diets

There are many other elimination diets, but perhaps two of the most common ones are the food additives exclusion diet and the oligoantigenic diet. The food additives exclusion diet (also known as the Feingold diet) was proposed to eliminate food additives, such as artificial flavors, colors, fragrances, sweeteners, and preservatives as well as naturally occurring salicylates. In the oligoantigenic diet, there is typically an initial elimination phase with the exclusion of most foods except a limited list of hypoallergenic foods. In both diets, if the person has decreased symptoms, then foods may be slowly added back in order to determine which foods are responsible for the adverse physical or behavioral reactions. These diets have been used to improve physical response in people with unknown allergies and to improve behavior in those with neurodevelopmental diagnoses [19].

Dental management of a patient on the food additives exclusion diet or the oligoantigenic diet is similar to the approach taken with someone on the ketogenic diet or the gluten-free and/or casein-free diet. It is important to ensure that the patient is getting adequate nutrition, and consultation with other physicians on the healthcare team may be in order if it appears that supplements may be needed. The oral cavity should be monitored for signs of nutritional deficiency. Prophylaxis paste, fluoride treatment, and home oral hygiene products may all be on the exclusion lists for patients following a strict diet. Therefore, these items should be avoided unless they are cleared by the patient's physician or nutritionist.

In summary, the pediatric dental care provider must be aware of specific requirements related to medically recommended diets, understand that ingredients found in common dental products may affect the diet, and be prepared to consult with the other members of the healthcare team where potential concerns exist.

Feeding Disorders

Feeding is a complex process that requires the successful integration of multiple biologic systems. Because many CSHCNs have medical and developmental conditions that affect these systems, feeding problems that reach clinical significance are common in this population [23]. Feeding difficulties may be associated with medical conditions, oropharyngeal dysfunction, behavioral diagnoses, as well as environmental and caregiver factors.

Feeding difficulties have been reported with an estimated prevalence of 25% in the general pediatric population and in up to 80% of children with developmental disabilities [24, 25]. Physical challenges with feeding such as gastroesophageal reflux and/or oropharyngeal dysphagia are seen in the vast majority of children with moderate-to-severe developmental disability who have feeding difficulties [26]. Within the population of CSHCN, several groups of children are prone to clinically significant feeding challenges:

- Medical conditions such as premature birth
- Craniofacial anomalies (e.g., cleft palate)
- Genetic syndromes (e.g., Russell-Silver syndrome)
- Neurological impairments (e.g., cerebral palsy, sensorineural deafness, severe vision loss) [27, 28]

Feeding difficulties have been reported in up to 89% of children with ASD. This is primarily due to food selectivity that may be related to sensory processing dysfunction, specifically oral sensory sensitivity toward the taste, texture, color, presentation, brand, and/or appearance [29–31].

When a child's feeding difficulty actually hinders her growth and/or emotional development, she may be classified as having a feeding disorder under the DSM-5 (*Diagnostic and Statistical Manual of Mental Disorders*) [32] feeding and eating disorders [33]. The DSM-5 includes three feeding disorder diagnoses: pica, rumination disorder, and avoidant/restrictive food intake disorder.

Types of Feeding Disorder: Pica

Pica is defined as the persistent eating of nonnutritive substances for a period of at least 1 month [32]. The nonfood substances most often described as ingested by children with pica include soil, chalk, plaster, clay, paint, paper, cloth, sand, hair, plastic, coal, insects, wood, pebbles, and animal feces [31]. The eating of nonnutritive substances must be separate from any cultural behavior, for example, there are some African countries in which eating soil is a culturally sanctioned practice. It must also be inappropriate for the developmental level of the child, as it would not include very young children that mouth all sorts of nonfood items. The exact cause of pica is unknown, but in some cases it may present in people experiencing nutritional deficiencies (e.g., iron, zinc, and calcium deficiencies). In such cases, when the deficiency is corrected, the behavior typically resolves. It is also associated with children who have developmental disability and neurodevelopmental diagnoses and thought to be correlated with an inability to use appropriate discriminatory behavior. It has been theorized that such disorders are often an attempt to seek comfort and self-soothe due to emotional deprivation [31].

It is the responsibility of the pediatric dental provider to review each patient's diet and identify potential concerns. Eating nonnutritive substances could be potentially very dangerous (e.g., lead poisoning, parasitic infection, intestinal blockage).

Pica may also have dental consequences. Ingesting fibrous materials may result in fibers becoming trapped in the gingiva and may cause gingivitis or a periodontal abscess. Ingesting hard, abrasive substances may cause excessive dental wear and fracture, as well as potentially causing many other health-related issues. Hence, it is important that the child's feeding disorder is identified quickly so she may be referred for comprehensive assessment and treatment. Additionally, if a patient with a diagnosis of pica is seen in a dental practice, it is best to have minimal loose objects available for her to pick up and ingest (e.g., gauze, cups of prophylaxis paste) and to ensure that someone on the dental team stays with her throughout the appointment to both supervise and engage with the child.

Types of Feeding Disorder: Rumination Disorder

Rumination disorder is a feeding disorder defined as the repeated regurgitation and re-chewing of swallowed or partially digested food [32]. The regurgitation occurs daily and must be differentiated from a child's potential for other gastroesophageal diagnoses (e.g., gastroesophageal reflux) or an eating disorder (e.g., bulimia). Rumination disorder typically develops prior to age one, but it can present initially at any age. It has been proposed that rumination disorder develops as a result of a child's need for stimulation or as the result of stress and anxiety in an attempt to self-soothe. In infants, the behavior tends to resolve spontaneously over time. In older children, particularly those with developmental disability, it may develop into a long-standing habitual behavior as the result of anxiety or other psychiatric symptoms [31]. Infants and children with rumination disorder tend to experience weight loss, malnutrition, infection susceptibility, and even death [34]. Orally, their dentition may present with erosive wear from the frequent stomach acid exposure, and they may have red, inflamed mucosal and gingival tissues.

Types of Feeding Disorder: Avoidant/Restrictive Food Intake Disorder

The diagnosis of avoidant/restrictive food intake disorder (ARFID) describes a feeding disturbance that causes persistent failure to meet appropriate nutritional and/or energy needs. It must be associated with at least one of the following: (1) significant weight loss or limited growth, (2) significant nutritional deficiency, (3) dependence on enteral feeding or oral nutritional supplements, and (4) marked interference with psychosocial functioning [32]. An individual with ARFID may have a disturbance, such as an apparent lack of interest in eating or food, an avoidance based on the sensory characteristics of food, or a fear about the aversive consequences of eating.

Food refusal has a complex etiology. Several studies have demonstrated high rates of comorbid medical diagnoses including gastroesophageal reflux, cardiopulmonary conditions, neurological conditions, food allergies, anatomical anomalies, and delayed gastric emptying [35–37]. The refusal of food is also associated with neurodevelopmental disabilities such as ASD, as well as psychological diagnoses such as anxiety, obsessive-compulsive symptoms, and phobias [38].

Food avoidance based on the sensory characteristics of food is often termed food selectivity. Clinically significant food selectivity is thought to be due to a sensory processing dysfunction in which a child has a limited number and types of foods she will eat. This is based on a sensory sensitivity toward taste, texture, color, presentation, brand, or appearance [29–31]. While this behavior has been described in typically developing children, it occurs at much greater frequency and severity in children with a diagnosis of ASD [39–41]. Additionally, in children with ASD, the more atypical the sensory sensitivity, the more foods are refused [41].

Children that present to the dental office with a known diagnosis of ARFID, sensory processing dysfunction, and/or oral sensory sensitivity will often also refuse dental materials, home oral hygiene products, and even instruments (including the toothbrush) being placed within their mouths. Prior to working with this child, it is important to have a conversation with the child and caregiver about the child's ability to tolerate the stimulation of a toothbrush as well as the various flavors or textures of the prophylaxis paste. If a child is able to use specific toothpaste at home, suggesting that the child bring it to future dental appointments may be helpful in lowering the child's anxiety and improve her ability to tolerate the experience.

Dental Treatment for Children with Feeding Disorders

The dental provider will ideally spend time at each dental visit discussing the child's dietary habits. The child's weight should also be recorded and monitored at each appointment. Because of these conversations and measurements, the pediatric dental provider may be the first clinician to recognize a patient's feeding difficulty. Anomalies in the results of an oral exam such as poor gingival health, severe dental attrition, and wear patterns suggestive of acid erosion should be addressed and followed closely. As feeding difficulties are quite prevalent in CSHCNs, it is important to address feeding habits regularly with each child and her caregiver. When a feeding difficulty or disorder is suspected in a child, it is important to work with the pediatrician to help the child and caregiver obtain resources for assessment and treatment.

Management of Nutritional Challenges

A child's ability to feed is a by-product of her physiologic, motor, and organizational abilities, as well as her environment and caregiver attributes [42]. CSHCNs are at an increased risk for developing disorders in their feeding and experiencing challenges with their growth due to complex medical and/or behavioral comorbidities. Feeding and mealtimes are an important component of physical, mental, emotional, and relational development. Consequently, disruption around feeding can be detrimental to the development of certain children, especially when such disruptions consistently interfere with the nutritional intake. Thus, appropriate diagnosis and treatment is paramount. Evaluation involves nutritional, feeding, behavioral, and medical assessments in order to identify deficiencies in the food ingested by the child, as well as any oral motor dysfunction, behavioral limitations, and medical concerns that could contribute to the nutritional deficiency [43].

Treatment for a child with feeding disorders and resulting undernutrition will likely be multidisciplinary in approach. The care team may include the pediatrician, feeding specialist, occupational therapist, behavioral therapist, gastroenterologist, social worker, speech and language pathologist, developmental pediatrician, and nutritionist. Dietary management of oral motor and behavior feeding disorders may involve frequent feeding with calorie-dense formulas and cereals. The feeding and dietary plan that is prescribed by the child's feeding specialist should be supported by the dental provider regardless of its cariogenic nature, as the highest priority for the child is that she is able to grow and develop appropriately. It is important that the family not receive conflicting information about the child's care from the various health providers. The following examples describe feeding modifications to consider for CSHCN:

- If the child's behavior modification training involves treats, the dental provider should suggest substituting highly cariogenic rewards (e.g., candies) with foods that are less likely to contribute to decay (e.g., sugar-free alternatives). This child will benefit from stressing the importance of a good home oral hygiene program as well as more frequent recall examinations (every 3–4 months).
- A child that is nutritionally deficient may also have frequent feedings with calorie-dense formulas and cereals putting the child at high caries risk. This child may also benefit from stressing the importance of a good home oral hygiene program as well as more frequent recall examinations (every 3–4 months).
- Consider adaptive positioning of the child and utensils while feeding. These same positions may facilitate home hygiene.
- Children that avoid flavors or textures of foods may also be averse to toothpaste. Consider recommending brushing the teeth with just water or, if tolerated, dipping the toothbrush in a fluoride-containing mouthrinse and brushing.
- When children exhibit oral signs of gastroesophageal reflex, the dental provider should discuss the option of prescription medication with the medical team.

Feeding Tubes

When oral feeding is considered unsafe due to oral motor dysfunction or if adequate nutrition cannot be obtained orally, the child may be fed through a feeding tube and/or undergo surgery [43]. Enteral tube feeding can be used as a supplemental or total replacement method for oral eating. There are various types of nonoral feeding methods including nasogastric (NG) tubes, orogastric (OG) tubes, duodenal tubes, gastrostomy (G) tubes, and jejunostomy (J) tubes. NG, OG, and duodenal tubes

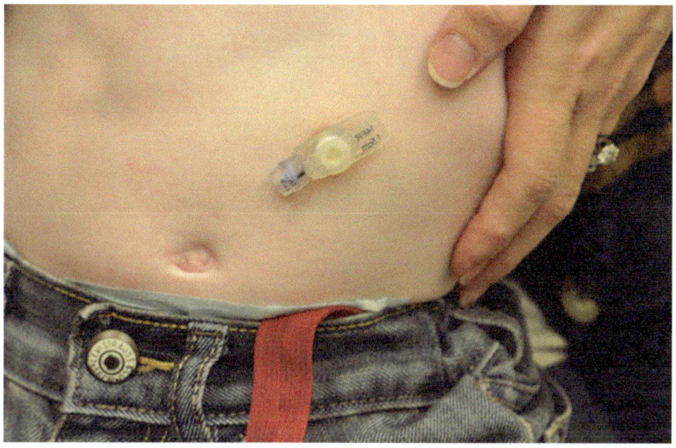

Fig. 1 A gastrostomy tube

have the advantage of nonsurgical placement and are usually prescribed for short-term use. Both G and J tubes require surgical placement, but they also bypass the mouth and nose, so they may result in decreased sensitivity for a child with aversions to contact of her face and head (see Fig. 1). Nutrient-rich formula is provided through the tubes either continuously or in boluses [43].

If the child is able to safely eat orally, an oral feeding plan will be maintained in conjunction with tube feeding. It is important to minimize breaks in oral feeding and stimulation, as this will increase a child's likelihood of an aversive response to oral stimulation. Depending on the reason for the feeding dysfunction, the goal of the child's providers may be to transition to oral eating exclusively, or she may be nutritionally maintained via tube feeding long term. A child that receives the bulk of her nutrition via tube feeding may still have frequent oral "social tastings," during which the child is exposed to foods she finds palatable. These foods may include components of the meals the child's family is eating as well as foods that have minimal nutritional value and are highly cariogenic. For example, ice cream, pudding, crackers, etc. are commonly provided as social tastes to children with feeding tubes. Tasting provides oral stimulation to various food tastes and textures as well as socialization of the child with her family at mealtime. With tasting, the child may or may not swallow the food presented. If the ultimate goal of the treatment is to transition to oral eating, oral exposure to food (e.g., nutrient-dense formula and other foods) will increase over time in volume and frequency. Caries risk may increase depending on the frequency of tastings, and whether or not the child swallows what she eats or holds it in her mouth.

Children with feeding dysfunction due to gastroesophageal reflux for whom medications and feeding modifications have been ineffective may undergo a Nissen fundoplication. A Nissen fundoplication is a surgical procedure in which the gastric fundus is wrapped around the esophagus to tighten the lower esophageal sphincter in order to prevent the reflux of gastric contents (see Fig. 2). The Nissen procedure is often combined with a G-tube placement.

A child being treated for a feeding disorder and undernutrition presents a unique challenge to the dental team. Because it is a medical priority for the patient to gain

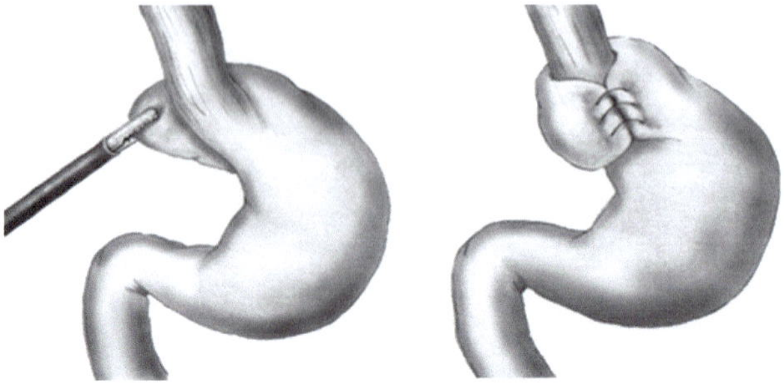

Fig. 2 A Nissen fundoplication. Original Artwork by James P. Gray, M.D. 2007. Released into the public domain by its author, Xopusmagnumx at English Wikipedia, via https://commons.wikimedia.org/wiki/File:Nissen_fundoplication.png. Downloaded 17 Mar 2018

weight, it is important to encourage the family to follow their feeding treatment plan even if it includes frequent oral feedings and/or tastings with cariogenic foods (e.g., the nutritional formula). At the same time, it is essential to educate them about the cariogenic nature of the child's nutritional source. Caregivers should be counseled to brush, rinse, or swab the teeth to keep the child's mouth clean in between food exposures. If a child obtains most/all of her nutrition through a feeding tube, she will be prone to develop gingivitis as well as calculus on all surfaces of the teeth. The clinician may recommend frequent professional dental prophylaxis to limit the amount of calculus that accumulates between appointments.

Before proceeding with any in-office treatment, the patient's ability to safely tolerate dental scaling and prophylaxis should be determined. A medical consult with the child's care providers may be indicated. Caution should be exercised for any child that has been hospitalized for aspiration pneumonia or is unable to cough and clear her airway. During scaling or ultrasonic cleaning, special care should be made to minimize the chance for aspiration. The patient should be positioned in an upright position during the procedure. If the child is receiving protective stabilization (passively or active), it is important to pay attention to the feeding tube's position so as not to disturb or remove it. The dental assistant should isolate all of the loosened calculus and water with the high volume suction in order to prevent any from entering the child's airway. The focus should be on removing the subgingival and supragingival smooth surface calculus. The calculus on the occlusal surfaces of the molars may be reduced, so it does not interfere with occlusion; however, it is thought to act as a natural protective sealant and does not need to be removed [44]. Additionally, a prescription for 0.12% chlorhexidine gluconate (CHX) may be helpful in improving the child's gingival health in between prophylaxis appointments. The CHX may be used in place of toothpaste for children at low risk for dental caries. The caregiver should be instructed to pour a small amount into a cup, to dip the toothbrush in it, and then to apply it to the teeth once daily. A systematic review of chlorhexidine mouthrinse as an adjunctive treatment for gingival health found a large reduction in dental plaque when CHX was used as an adjunct to mechanical oral hygiene procedures for 4–6 weeks and for 6 months. It should be noted that use of CHX for 4 weeks or longer causes extrinsic tooth staining and may contribute to transient taste disturbances [45].

The pediatric dental provider's role in the child's treatment includes the hyper-vigilant monitoring of the oral presentation of the medical conditions and associated treatment, the provision of the appropriate restorative and periodontal treatment in order to maintain the child's oral health, and the proactive promotion of the child's oral and systemic health. The dental provider should pay attention to changes in the child's treatment. For example, a child may have previously been fed primarily via her G-tube with occasional oral tastings and would thus be considered at low risk for dental caries. But at her recent dental visit, it was reported that she has progressed with her feeding therapies and is now eating orally multiple times each day. Her foods are still limited to those that she likes, such as crackers. The long-term plan for her may be to progress to become a primarily orally eater and to either remove the G-tube or to limit its use. The dental provider should support the child's feeding care plan prescribed by her team even though the behaviors and food choices put the child at increased risk for dental decay. It is very important though to discuss with the child and her caregiver the child's increased risk for the development of dental caries and the need for excellent home oral hygiene and possibly more frequent recall exams (e.g., every 3–4 months).

Overweight/Obesity

CSHCN may also have a propensity toward overweight or obesity, defined as abnormal or excessive fat accumulation that presents a risk to health. Currently in the United States, almost one third of the children and adolescents are overweight or obese, and the prevalence has increased in many other developed countries as well. CSHCNs are at a particular risk toward overweight/obesity due to their systemic diagnosis (e.g., Cushing syndrome, Turner syndrome, Prader-Willi syndrome), the restrictive nature of their diet, and/or their limited physical abilities. Additionally, caregivers may be contributing to the weight gain with the use of sweet treats as rewards for desired behaviors.

Overweight and obese children may still be nutritionally deficient due to the limited nutrients contained in their selected foods. It will be important to monitor the oral cavity for poor gingival health and dental caries. Weight and height measurements and BMI should be calculated for all children at their examination appointments. As many of the calorie-dense foods are also often cariogenic, dietary counseling may address both issues. Additionally overweight/obesity adds a significant challenge for sedation. It is prudent to treat a child that is overweight or obese under general anesthesia in a hospital setting instead of employing in-office sedation.

Case-Based Scenario

Lucy, a 6-year-old girl with a known seizure disorder, presented with her mother, Mrs. Jones, to the dental clinic for a new patient evaluation. Lucy appeared healthy and weighed 20 kg. Mrs. Jones reported that Lucy's seizures are managed with daily oral anticonvulsant medication (phenytoin) as well as adherence to a ketogenic diet supplemented with multivitamins. Since starting the diet 1 year ago, Lucy's seizure activity has decreased, and she had not had to use her rescue medication, diazepam. At the time of her dental consultation, Lucy's seizures were primarily absence seizures that still occurred multiple times per week. Lucy was overdue for a regular follow-up appointment with her neurologist, but her mother was not concerned since her overall seizure activity had improved. They have met regularly with Lucy's nutritionist. Lucy's home oral hygiene routine included her mother brushing Lucy's teeth before bed with a pea-sized amount of baking soda and fluoride-containing toothpaste that was approved by her nutritionist. Mrs. Jones noticed that Lucy has swollen gums that bled each time they brushed them. Lucy denied experiencing any pain in her mouth.

Lucy cooperated for a dental exam with a mirror and explorer as well as a radiographic survey. Her extraoral examination revealed that she had competent lip closure, but her lips were dry and cracked. She seemed to have minimal saliva. Intraorally, Lucy had generalized, erythematous, enlarged gingiva that bled easily with gentle manipulation with the explorer. She was in the early mixed dentition with 20 primary teeth and her first permanent molars erupting. The cervical 25% of the clinical crowns of the teeth were covered by gingival tissue. She had minimal plaque and calculus present supragingivally, except a small amount of calculus visible between the mandibular incisors. No dental caries lesions were noted on the visual or radiographic evaluation. Further conversation with Mrs. Jones revealed that Lucy almost always has had dry lips and mouth. Her gingiva has bled for the last few years, and the bleeding seems to be getting worse.

The conversations and examination revealed several key findings and complications to Lucy's oral health:

- Seizures managed with phenytoin, an anticonvulsant that is associated with xerostomia, gingival bleeding, and gingival overgrowth. The patient presented with all three side effects.
- Weight of 20 kg, which was average for her age. She had a healthy appearance; however it was possible that her gingival bleeding may have also been due in part to a vitamin deficiency.
- Overdue for a neurology follow-up appointment.
- Gingivitis, gingival overgrowth, and calculus present.
- Following a ketogenic diet that is low in carbohydrate exposure and thus low caries risk.
- No caries experience.
- Good oral hygiene.

Based on these findings, the following items were discussed with Lucy and her mother:

- The diagnosis of drug-induced gingival overgrowth due to the phenytoin was made. A vitamin deficiency was also discussed as possibly contributing to the bleeding of the gingiva. The medication side effects were discussed with Lucy and her mother including the necessity of excellent oral hygiene in order to minimize the further progression of the symptoms. Lucy was recommended to have an in-office prophylaxis in which the subgingival plaque and calculus are removed with a tentative recall time period of 3 months. It was discussed that the dental team would monitor the gingiva overgrowth at this time with the understanding that a periodontist would be consulted if the symptoms continued to progress.

- To address her xerostomia, it was recommended that Lucy carry a water bottle with her all day so that she is able to wet her mouth as needed. Additionally, Mrs. Jones and Lucy were asked to discuss with their nutritionist possible ketogenic diet-approved saliva substitutes, chewing gums, and mints in order to stimulate saliva production.
- To address her dry lips, it was recommended that Lucy apply a ketogenic diet-approved lip balm.
- To address oral hygiene, it was recommended that Mrs. Jones brush Lucy's teeth twice daily using her approved toothpaste. Given her low caries risk, the dental team opted to refrain from the use of prophylaxis paste or fluoride varnish in office until these products were approved by Lucy's nutritionist.
- Mrs. Jones was asked to bring Lucy's seizure rescue medication to her next appointment.
- The dental provider requested consultation with the neurologist and nutritionist regarding:
  - The examination findings, diagnoses, and recommended treatment plan
  - Verification of anticonvulsant medication type and dosage
  - A nutritional evaluation to rule out a vitamin deficiency
  - The use of 0.12% chlorhexidine gluconate, saliva substitutes, and lip balm while participating in a ketogenic diet
  - A listing of ketogenic diet-approved prophylaxis paste and fluoride varnish for possible future use
  - Lucy's seizure care plan in which the protocol for managing her seizures was described—to be added to her chart and reviewed before each appointment

When Lucy returned to the dental clinic for her prophylaxis appointment, her mother had a conversation with the dental provider. Following the last dental visit, Lucy had visited her neurologist and nutritionist. Both were pleased with her progress. Her daily dietary intake had been monitored for 3 days and was found to be appropriate. Neither provider had any concerns about the prophylaxis appointment, but the nutritionist asked that all 0.12% chlorhexidine gluconate, prophylaxis paste, and fluoride varnish be avoided at this time. The neurologist provided a written seizure care plan for Lucy.

Prior to starting any treatment, the seizure care plan was reviewed with the dental team, Lucy, and her mother. Lucy's mother had her rescue medication ready if needed. Intraoral photographs were taken to document a baseline of the gingival overgrowth. Lucy cooperated well for her dental cleaning. Special attention was made to addressing the subgingival plaque and calculus. She was placed on a 3-month recall plan for prophylaxis.

Conclusions

- CSHCNs are at increased risk for experiencing nutritional challenges due to their complex medical conditions and associated treatments.
- Signs of a child's medical or behavioral conditions and associated treatments are often evident in the dentition and/or periodontium.
- The dental professional is in a key position to recognize that a child is displaying signs for nutritional deficiencies and/or feeding difficulties and should recommend further evaluation when indicated.
- CSHCNs who have nutritional complications due to their medical and/or behavior diagnoses, medication and dietary treatments, and altered feeding experience require careful, individualized treatment plans in order to best meet their specific needs.

References

1. Prasanthi B, Kannan N, Patil R. Effect of diuretics on salivary flow, composition and oral health status: a clinico-biochemical study. Ann Med Health Sci Res. 2014;4(4):549–53.
2. Doty RL, Shah M, Bromley SM. Drug-induced taste disorders. Drug Saf. 2008;31(3):199–215.
3. Scully C, Epstein JB. Oral health care for the cancer patient. Eur J Cancer B Oral Oncol. 1996;32:281–92.
4. American Academy of Pediatrics. Long-term follow-up care for pediatric cancer survivors. Pediatrics. 2009;123:906–15.
5. da Fonseca MA, Hong C. An overview of chronic oral graft-vs-host disease following pediatric hematopoietic stem cell transplantation. Pediatr Dent. 2008;30(2):98–104.
6. Schubert MM, Sullivan KM, Morton TH, Izutsu KT, Peterson DE, Flournoy N, Truelove EL, Sale GE, Buckner CD, Storb R, Thomas D. Oral manifestations of chronic graft-v-host disease. Arch Intern Med. 1984;144(8):1591–5.
7. Kristensen HG. WHO guideline development of paediatric medicines: points to consider in pharmaceutical development. Int J Pharm. 2012;435(2):134–5.
8. Tuleu C. "Formulating better medicines for children"—still paving the road. Int J Pharm. 2012;435(2):99–100.
9. Salunke S, Hempenstall J, Kendall R, Roger B, Mroz C, Nunn T, Tuleu C. European Paediatric Formulation Initiative's (EuPFI) 2nd conference commentary—formulating better medicines for children. Int J Pharm. 2011;419(1–2):235–9.
10. Donaldson M, Goodchild JH, Epstein JB. Sugar content, cariogenicity, and dental concerns with commonly used medications. J Am Dent Assoc. 2015;146(2):129–33.
11. Kossoff EH, Zupec-Kania BA, Amark PE, Ballaban-Gil KR, Christina Bergqvist AG, Blackford R, Buchhalter JR, Caraballo RH, Helen Cross J, Dahlin MG, Donner EJ, Klepper J, Jehle RS, Kim HD, Christiana Liu YM, Nation J, Nordli DR Jr, Pfeifer HH, Rho JM, Stafstrom CE, Thiele EA, Turner Z, Wirrell EC, Wheless JW, Veggiotti P, Vining EP, Charlie Foundation, Practice Committee of the Child Neurology Society, Practice Committee of the Child Neurology Society, International Ketogenic Diet Study Group. Optimal clinical management

of children receiving the ketogenic diet: recommendations of the International Ketogenic Diet Study Group. Epilepsia. 2009;50(2):304–17.
12. Martin K, Jackson CF, Levy RG, Cooper PN. Ketogenic diet and other dietary treatments for epilepsy. Cochrane Database Syst Rev. 2016;(2):CD001903.
13. Verrotti A, Iapadre G, Pisano S, Coppola G. Ketogenic diet and childhood neurological disorders other than epilepsy: an overview. Expert Rev Neurother. 2016;17(5):461–73.
14. Simeone TA, Simeone KA, Stafstrom CE, Rho JM. Do ketone bodies mediate the anti-seizure effects of the ketogenic diet? Neuropharmacology. 2018;133:233–41.
15. Willmott NS, Brayan RA. Case report: scurvy in an epileptic child on a ketogenic diet with oral complications. Eur Arch Paediatr Dent. 2008;9:148–52.
16. Sicherer SH, Sampson HA. Food allergy: epidemiology, pathogenesis, diagnosis, and treatment. J Allergy Clin Immunol. 2014;133:291–307.
17. Rubio-Tapia A, Ludvigsson JF, Brantner TL, Murray JA, Everhart JE. The prevalence of celiac disease in the United States. Am J Gastroenterol. 2012;107(10):1538–44.
18. Liu AH, Jaramillo R, Sicherer SH, Wood RA, Bock SA, Burks AW, Massing M, Cohn RD, Zeldin DC. National prevalence and risk factors for food allergy and relationship to asthma: results from the National Health and Nutrition Examination Survey 2005–2006. J Allergy Clin Immunol. 2010;126:798–806.
19. Ly V, Bottelier M, Hoekstra PJ, Vasquez AA, Buitelaar JK, Rommelse NN. Elimination diets' efficacy and mechanisms in attention deficit hyperactivity disorder and autism spectrum disorder. Eur Child Adolesc Psychiatry. 2017;26:1067–79.
20. Brietzke E, Cerqueira RO, Mansur RB, McIntyre RS. Gluten related illnesses and severe mental disorders: a comprehensive review. Neurosci Biobehav Rev. 2018;84:368–75.
21. Naik RD, Seidner DL, Adams DW. Nutritional consideration in celiac disease and nonceliac gluten sensitivity. Gastroenterol Clin N Am. 2018;47:139–54.
22. Cheng J, Malahias T, Brar P, Minaya MT, Green PH. The association between celiac disease, dental enamel defects, and aphthous ulcers in a United States cohort. J Clin Gastroenterol. 2010;44(3):191–4.
23. Berlin KS, Lobato DJ, Pinkos B, Cerezo CS, LeLeiko NS. Patterns of medical and developmental comorbidities among children presenting with feeding problems: a latent class analysis. J Dev Behav Pediatr. 2011;32(1):41–7.
24. Babbitt RL, Hoch TA, Coe DA, Cataldo MF, Kelly KJ, Stackhouse C, Perman JA. Behavioral assessment and treatment of pediatric feeding disorders. J Dev Behav Pediatr. 1994;15(4):278–91.
25. Manikam R, Perman JA. Pediatric feeding disorders. J Clin Gastroenterol. 2000;30(1):34–46.
26. Schwarz SM, Corredor J, Fisher-Medina J, Cohen J, Rabinowitz S. Diagnosis and treatment of feeding disorders in children with developmental disabilities. Pediatrics. 2001;108(3):671–6.
27. Sullivan PB, Lambert B, Rose M, Ford-Adams M, Johnson A, Griffiths P. Prevalence and severity of feeding and nutritional problems in children with neurological impairment: Oxford Feeding Study. Dev Med Child Neurol. 2000;42(10):674–80.
28. Lifschitz CH. Feeding problems in infants and children. Curr Treat Options Gastroenterol. 2001;4(5):451–7.
29. Ledford JR, Gast DL. Feeding problems in children with autistic spectrum disorders: a review. Focus Autism Other Dev Disabil. 2006;21(3):153–66.
30. Zobel-Lachiusa J, Andrianopoulos MV, Mailloux Z, Cermak SA. Sensory differences and mealtime behavior in children with autism. Am J Occup Ther. 2015;69(5):6905185050.
31. Bryant-Waugh RJ, Piepenstock EHC. Childhood disorders: feeding and related disorders of infancy or early childhood. In: Tasman A, Kay J, Lieberman JA, First MB, Maj M, editors. Psychiatry. 3rd ed. New York: Wiley; 2008. p. 830–46.
32. American Psychiatric Association. Diagnostic and statistical manual of mental disorder. 5th ed. Arlington: American Psychiatric Press; 2013.
33. Eddy KT, Thomas JJ, Hastings E, Edkins K, Lamont E, Nevins CM, Patterson RM, Murray HB, Bryant-Waugh R, Becker AE. Prevalence of DSM-5 avoidant/restrictive food intake disorder in a pediatric gastroenterology healthcare network. Int J Eat Disord. 2015;48(5):464–70.

34. Franco K, Campbell N, Tamburrino M, Evans C. Rumination: the eating disorder of infancy. Child Psychiatry Hum Dev. 1993;24(2):91–7.
35. Field D, Garland M, Williams K. Correlates of specific childhood feeding problems. J Paediatr Child Health. 2003;39(4):299–304.
36. Greer AJ, Gulotta CS, Masler EA, Laud RB. Caregiver stress and outcomes of children with pediatric feeding disorders treated in an intensive interdisciplinary program. J Pediatr Psychol. 2008;33(6):612–20.
37. Williams KE, Field DG, Seiverling L. Food refusal in children: a review of the literature. Res Dev Disabil. 2010;31:625–33.
38. Bryant-Waugh R, Markham L, Kreipe RE, Walsh BT. Feeding and eating disorders in childhood. Int J Eat Disord. 2010;43:98–111.
39. Bandini LG, Anderson SE, Curtin C, Cermak S, Evans EW, Scampini R, Maslin M, Must A. Food selectivity in children with autism spectrum disorders and typically developing children. J Pediatr. 2010;157(2):259–64.
40. Curtin C, Hubbard K, Anderson SE, Mick E, Must A, Bandini LG. Food selectivity, mealtime behavior problems, spousal stress, and family food choices in children with and without autism spectrum disorder. J Autism Dev Disord. 2015;45(10):3308–15.
41. Chistol LT, Bandini LG, Must A, Phillips S, Cermak SA, Curtin C. Sensory sensitivity and food selectivity in children with autism spectrum disorder. J Autism Dev Disord. 2018;48(2):583–91.
42. Wolf LS, Glass RP. Feeding and swallowing disorders in infancy: assessment and management. San Antonio: Therapy Skill Builders; 1992.
43. Jepsen C, Nickel RE. Nutrition and growth. In: Nickel RE, Desch LW, editors. The physician's guide to caring for children with disabilities and chronic conditions. Maryland: Paul H Brooks Publishing Co; 2000. p. 77–98.
44. Owens BM, Sharp KH, Fourmy EE, Phebus JG. Effect of occlusal calculus utilized as a potential "biological sealant" in special needs patients with gastric feeding tubes: a qualitative in vitro contrast to pit and fissure sealant restorations. Gen Dent. 2016;64(4):24–9.
45. James P, Worthington HV, Parnell C, Harding M, Lamont T, Gheung A, Whelton H, Riley P. Chlorhexidine mouthrinse as an adjunctive treatment for gingival health. Cochrane Database Syst Rev. 2017;31:3.

Oral Hygiene and Prevention for CSHCN

Marilynn L. Rothen

Introduction

Children with special healthcare needs (CSHCN) are at higher risk for oral diseases than their typically developing peers [1]. This is particularly true for dental caries. Multiple caries risk assessment tools, including caries management by risk assessment (CAMBRA) and those developed by the American Academy of Pediatric Dentistry (AAPD), the American Dental Association (ADA), and the American Academy of Pediatrics (AAP), consider special healthcare needs in children less than 6 years of age a risk factor for developing caries. These children are at higher risk than typically developing peers, and they often present greater clinical challenges. Therefore, it is especially important to start prevention early in life. When providing care to CSHCN, clinicians must take into consideration the type and degree of disability and the age of the child. As with typically developing children, the caregiver plays a very important role in prevention and oral hygiene. This chapter will address techniques clinicians can use when working with CSHCN and their caregivers. These include developing the clinician/caregiver relationship, home and professional fluoride application, dietary modification, hygiene devices, and strategies for home care.

M. L. Rothen (✉)
Department of Oral Health Sciences, University of Washington School of Dentistry, Seattle, WA, USA
e-mail: rothen@uw.edu

T. M. Nelson, J. R. Webb (eds.), *Dental Care for Children with Special Needs*, https://doi.org/10.1007/978-3-030-10483-2_7

Fostering the Therapeutic Relationship

The clinician and caregiver are partners in a therapeutic relationship that is focused on the health of the CSHCN. This requires the clinician to personalize the information and guidance delivered to each individual patient and caregiver. Treating CSHCN is an interprofessional activity. The clinician must first become familiar with the child's medical condition, social history, network of other providers, and educational or training programs that affect the child's care. Much of this information can be gathered in pre-visit questionnaires and augmented through in-person interviews. Once the clinician has learned key information about the child, he can turn to ascertaining what the caregiver and CSHCN presently know and do in the area of oral hygiene. This is an opportunity to seek input from caregivers who are the experts on their child.

It may be that the caregiver has limited understanding of the significance of daily oral hygiene to the prevention of dental diseases. The caregiver may not be effective at his own oral self-care, so helping him to understand the objectives of daily oral hygiene may be an important first step to initiating effective oral care for the patient. However, many caregivers are aware of the importance of oral hygiene, and instead they primarily need assistance developing skills to address the physical, cognitive, and behavioral challenges presented by CSHCN. This will better enable them to incorporate oral care into a complex daily routine [2].

Regardless of each patient's individual circumstances, there are three key prevention concepts we seek to maximize:

1. Regular fluoride use
2. Reducing the cariogenic potential of the patient's diet
3. Daily removal of plaque biofilm

Fluoride: Prevention and Treatment of Dental Caries

Dental Caries

Dental caries is on the rise in children 2–5 years old. The process starts with the eruption of the first tooth around the age of 6 months [1, 3]. It is for this reason that the AAPD recommends that all children establish a dental home by age 1. Caries requires the presence of teeth for bacterial adherence and a diet high in carbohydrates, which allows cariogenic bacteria to predominate in the biofilm on the teeth. It is helpful for caregivers to understand that dental caries is a preventable condition and to have a basic understanding of this infectious disease process. Many may not be aware that the bacteria that cause caries are transmitted to the child by the primary caregiver(s) through the sharing of saliva from kissing, food tasting, and sharing of utensils, etc. Caregivers may also not fully understand the role of carbohydrates, frequency of consumption, and acid-producing bacteria in the disease process—or how aggressive caries can be in primary teeth that have thinner enamel than their permanent counterparts.

Lift the Lip

Dental caries in primary teeth frequently appears first near the gingival margin of maxillary incisors. Therefore, caregivers should be shown how to examine the teeth for signs of caries by lifting the upper lip. They can play an important role in monitoring the child's oral health by regularly performing the "lift the lip" activity. Chairside tools with photos that demonstrate the stages of caries, beginning with white spot lesions at the gingival margin, can assist providers in teaching caregivers about early signs of caries (Fig. 1).

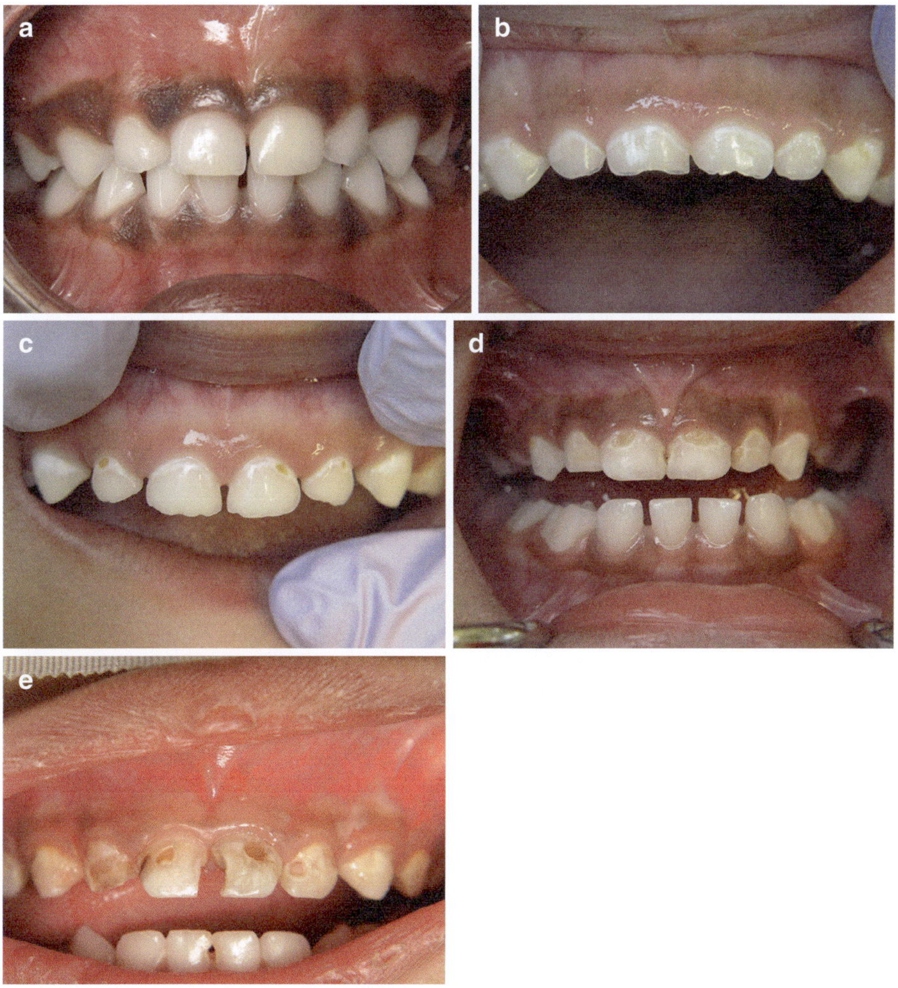

Fig. 1 Progression of dental caries in primary teeth. (**a**) Healthy teeth, (**b**) white spot lesions, (**c**) early caries, (**d**) moderate caries, (**e**) severe caries. Note abscess above tooth #F

Water Fluoridation

A clinician caring for a CSHCN needs to ascertain whether the child is benefiting from community water fluoridation. In areas with optimal community water fluoridation (CWF) of 0.7 mg/L, population studies show that the availability of fluoride from this source provides up to a 25% reduction in dental caries [4]. Children benefit from this source of fluoride when it is used for drinking, preparing food, and used in infant formula. Ask if the child drinks water regularly, and determine the source of the water. For most bottled water, the fluoride content is well below the recommended level of 0.7 mg/L, and fluoride content is not required to be printed on packaging unless it has been added. Commonly used home carbon water filters do not remove fluoride. However, the use of osmotic filters and distillation will remove fluoride. If the child drinks tap water, it is important to determine if the water is fluoridated optimally. The local water department can be contacted for this information, and well water can be tested by the health department. The Centers for Disease Control and Prevention (CDC) maintains a website, My Water's Fluoride, where one can determine fluoride levels by county for participating states (https://nccd.cdc.gov/DOH_MWF/default/default.aspx).

Fluoride Supplementation

If an assessment of the drinking water available to a CSHCN reveals that he is not receiving water with an optimal level of fluoride, other means of fluoride supplementation should be considered. According to CDC guidelines, fluoride supplements should only be prescribed to children without access to fluoridated water, and the American Dental Association (ADA) indicates that fluoride supplements should only be prescribed to children at high risk of dental caries [5, 6]. Having special needs is a risk factor for dental caries, so fluoride supplementation may be appropriate for CSHCN without access to fluoridated drinking water.

Fluoride supplements may be prescribed in the form of drops or tablets, depending on the physical and developmental age of the child. These are administered by the caregiver, requiring minimal cooperation from the child. However, unlike CWF, fluoride supplementation requires compliance on the part of a busy caregiver. The prescription must be filled on a regular basis, and the fluoride supplement must be administered daily. Table 1 indicates the ADA recommended daily dose of fluoride supplementation based on the age of the child and the fluoride concentration in drinking water [6].

Table 1 Dietary fluoride supplementation schedule

Age	Fluoride concentration in drinking water		
	<0.3 ppm F[a]	0.3–0.6 ppm F	>0.6 ppm F
Birth to 6 months	0	0	0
6 months to 3 years	0.25 mg/day	0	0
3 to 6 years	0.50 mg/day	0.25 mg/day	0
6 to 16 years	1.00 mg/day	0.50 mg/day	0

[a]ppm F: parts per million fluoride (1.0 ppm = 1 mg/L)
Reprinted with permission from Elsevier

Fluoride Toothpaste: Over-the-Counter (OTC)

The only ingredient in toothpaste that has been proven to prevent dental caries is fluoride [7, 8]. Fluoride toothpaste for caries prevention in primary teeth is supported by a Cochrane review of literature in 2010 and two more recent reviews [7, 9, 10]. Fluoride is present in more than 90% of over-the-counter (OTC) toothpaste in the United States [11, 12]. OTC toothpastes have a concentration of 1000–1100 parts per million (ppm) fluoride, in the form of sodium fluoride, stannous fluoride, or sodium monofluorophosphate. All have demonstrated equivalent caries prevention [9].

Some OTC toothpastes are marketed as fluoride-free for children age 2 years and younger. This may lead some parents or caregivers to believe that children under age 2 should not use fluoride toothpaste. However, all children can benefit from the use of the proper amount of fluoride toothpaste from the time the first tooth erupts. This is especially true for CSHCN who frequently have an elevated risk for dental caries.

When teeth first begin to erupt, they should be brushed daily with the proper amount of fluoride toothpaste. Children under age 3 should have a smear of toothpaste, not more than the size of a grain of rice, applied to their toothbrush. If a child is 3–6 years of age, the amount of toothpaste on the brush should be the size of a pea (Fig. 2). Fluoride toothpaste is more effective at caries prevention when applied twice daily than when used only once per day [13–15]. Therefore, it is prudent to develop the habit of brushing after breakfast and before bed. It is commonly recommended that typically developing children should be supervised through age 6 when using fluoride toothpaste. For CSHCN, the need for oral hygiene supervision and/or assistance should be considered according to the child's developmental age. All children should be encouraged to spit out the excess and not rinse after brushing. This allows a small amount of fluoride to be retained in the mouth during sleep when salivation decreases and when medication use may increase dry mouth [16].

Parents concerned about the risk of fluorosis may be informed that the risk has been shown to be low when the proper amount of fluoride toothpaste is used under supervision. This is true for areas with CWF where the child drinks tap water [17].

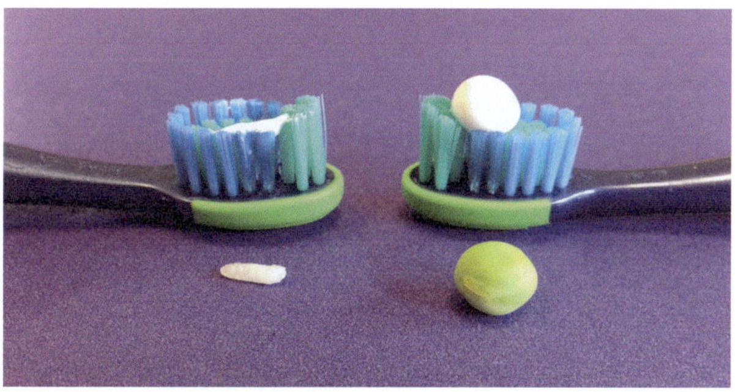

Fig. 2 Smear/grain of rice versus pea-sized amount of toothpaste

5000 PPM Fluoride Toothpaste
Disp: One tube
Sig: Place a pea-sized amount of toothpaste onto toothbrush. Brush onto all tooth surfaces in the morning and at night. Spit, do not rinse.

Fig. 3 Sample 5000 PPM toothpaste prescription

Parents and caregivers of CSHCN should understand that the risk of the dental caries, a potentially disfiguring disease, is greater than the risk of fluorosis.

Some CSHCN may accumulate calculus rapidly, particularly those who rely on gastrostomy tube feedings. These children may benefit from the use of a tartar control fluoride toothpaste. The anti-calculus agents in these toothpastes vary widely and include triclosan with or without polyvinyl methyl ether (PVM)/maleic acid (MA) copolymer and crystal growth inhibitors such as pyrophosphate with or without PVM/MA copolymer, sodium hexametaphosphate, polyaspartate, zinc citrate, and zinc chloride [18].

Fluoride Toothpaste: Prescription Strength

For children age 6 and older with an elevated risk of dental caries, a prescription fluoride toothpaste or gel with 5000 ppm sodium fluoride content may be recommended (Fig. 3). This is only appropriate for children who are capable of spitting out the excess. Avoid giving the child water to rinse after brushing as this will decrease the benefit of the intervention and increase the likelihood of swallowing the toothpaste. Inform caregivers about the importance of supervision when using a prescription fluoride toothpaste. A pea-size is the proper amount for either the gel or toothpaste formulation.

Fluoride Rinses: Over-the-Counter and Prescription

Fluoride is available as a rinse in either an OTC strength of 0.05% or a prescription strength of 0.2% fluoride. Fluoride rinsing is not recommended for children under age 6 due to their inability to adequately spit after swishing. While this remains true for CSHCN, for those that do not tolerate the use of toothpaste or gel due to gagging, foaming, or taste sensitivities, daily fluoride application may be achieved by dipping a toothbrush in a fluoride rinse and brushing the child's teeth. Recommendation of either an OTC or a prescription strength fluoride rinse should be determined by the child's developmental and chronological age and level of risk for dental caries.

Fluoride Trays

The application of prescription strength fluoride gel daily in custom trays is used by high-risk patients, particularly those with inadequate salivary flow due to head and neck radiation therapy. Trays may be similarly considered for children age 6 or older if the child is able to tolerate holding trays in the mouth for 5 min and able to spit out the excess fluoride on removal. It is preferable not to rinse afterwards and to use the fluoride trays just prior to sleep. Demonstrate the use of a cotton swab to spread a drop (less than a pea) of fluoride gel in each tray. The use of fluoride trays in children requires supervision and may not be practical for children with behavioral issues.

Fluoride Treatment: In-Office

Fluoride Varnish

Topical fluoride varnish application has become a staple of in-office prevention routines. The majority of varnishes available in the United States are a 5% sodium fluoride formulation, equivalent to 22,600 ppm of fluoride ion in a colophony/resin base. It is available in multi-use tubes or in unit doses of 0.25 mL for patients in the primary dentition and 0.4 mL for the mixed or adult dentition. The original formulation, still found in multi-use tubes, is amber colored, while most unit doses are now white/tooth colored and come in a variety of flavors. A 2.5% sodium fluoride varnish is recently available in 12 mL bottles or 0.3 mL unit doses and is a shellac-based, white liquid formulation. While resin-based varnishes work best when applied to dry teeth, with the shellac-based product, it is not critical to fully dry the teeth.

Fluoride varnish is cleared for the treatment of dentin hypersensitivity by the Food and Drug Administration (FDA). It is used "off-label" to prevent or treat dental caries. It is safe for use with children 0–6 years of age, and recommendations for professionally applied topical fluoride are based on the risk level of the child [19]. CSHCN at moderate risk for dental caries should have fluoride varnish application at regular 6-month intervals, and those at high risk will benefit from application every 3 months.

The application process is simple and well tolerated even by young children. Prophylaxis prior to treatment is not necessary. Both varnish formulations will set on contact with moisture, adhering to the tooth surfaces and releasing fluoride over the next several hours. Therefore, clinicians generally instruct patients not to brush the teeth until the following day.

Povidone-Iodine Treatment Prior to Fluoride Varnish Application

In high-risk populations, the application of the antiseptic 10% povidone-iodine (PVP-I) has been shown to reduce *Streptococcus mutans* and reduce the incidence of dental caries in primary and permanent teeth [20–22]. After ascertaining that the child does not have an allergy to iodine, the teeth are dried, and a cotton-tipped applicator is used to swab 1–2 mL PVP-I on the teeth. The excess is wiped away with gauze, followed directly by fluoride varnish application to the dry teeth.

Silver Diamine Fluoride

Silver diamine fluoride (SDF) was cleared for treatment of dentin hypersensitivity by the FDA in 2014 and like fluoride varnish is used off-label to treat or prevent dental caries. SDF became available in the United States in 2015 in a 38% liquid formulation containing 25% silver, 5% fluoride, and 8% ammonia in water. In 2018, a 38% SDF kit that includes potassium iodide received approval for marketing in the United States. The two-step procedure, application of SDF followed immediately by application of potassium iodide, is designed to reduce the staining associated with SDF. Because CSHCN frequently present with behavioral and medical management challenges, it may be possible to apply SDF to slow or arrest dental caries and delay or avoid restorative treatment requiring sedation or treatment in a hospital setting.

While SDF is generally thought of as a treatment for dental caries, it has been shown to prevent the development of caries lesions in non-affected teeth when applied only to existing lesions [23]. It can also be used to prevent the development of caries lesions in the pits and fissures of posterior teeth [24]. For that reason, it is recommended as a preventive agent for children at high risk for dental caries [25]. CSHCN can benefit from application of SDF to the occlusal surfaces of both primary and permanent molars as they begin to erupt as a primary preventive measure. Dental sealants have been shown to be somewhat more effective than SDF for prevention of dental caries in molar pits and fissures. However, their use may be limited in CSHCN because the effectiveness of traditional sealants is technique sensitive requiring good moisture control, which is usually accomplished with a cooperative patient, a dental assistant, and a fully erupted tooth. Additionally, sealant application is substantially more costly than SDF application. Application of SDF to the pits and fissures of erupting posterior teeth will not limit application of glass ionomer sealants (used when cooperation and isolation do not allow for traditional sealant placement) or later application of traditional sealants when eruption of the tooth permits adequate moisture control and the child has learned to cooperate. Protocols for application of SDF are discussed in Chap. 9, "Alternative Caries Management Strategies."

Diet: Important Considerations for Reducing Cariogenic Bacteria

Caregivers are likely aware that too much sugar can contribute to dental caries. However, they may not be aware that carbohydrates in foods such as crackers, pasta, fruit juices, or dried fruit contain sugar and starches that can contribute to caries, especially if daily plaque removal is challenging and suboptimal. Creating an awareness of the types of foods and drinks that are most likely to contribute to dental caries is the first step in working with families on establishing a diet conducive to good oral health. Additionally, it is important for parents and caregivers to be aware of how the frequency and timing of food and drink consumption contributes to the caries process.

It may be new information for caregivers that many processed foods, even foods that do not taste sweet, contain sugar or starch and can promote caries. Once caregivers can identify cariogenic foods and beverages, it is important for them to understand that if these are consumed with meals, the potential for them to cause dental caries is greatly diminished. It is equally important for oral healthcare providers to know that many CSHCN have conditions that require a diet of high-carbohydrate foods as an important source of nutrition for the child to thrive (e.g., use of nutrition drinks/protein shakes to maintain weight). Medical providers may not have a good understanding of the dental caries process and the relationship of food choices to dental health. Consultations with other care providers may be necessary to help develop dietary regimens that meet nutritional needs for these children and minimize the contribution of diet to dental caries. As oral health impacts systemic health, dietary habits that lead to increased oral disease may adversely affect the chronic condition and the health of the CSHCN. This illustrates the importance of working with caregivers to better understand all aspects of the child's healthcare needs and to help the caregiver balance nutritional and oral health needs.

Depending on individual patient requirements, providers may offer dietary advice such as:

- Whenever possible, consume foods containing sugar or starch with meals.
- Avoid using sweet treats as rewards or for positive reinforcement.
- Continuous snacking is unhealthy for the teeth; therefore snacking should be limited to discrete times (ideally <3 times/day).
- When possible, choose nutritious snacks such as nuts, fresh fruits and vegetables, or string cheese.
- Sugar-sweetened beverages are harmful to teeth, and even 100% fruit juice should be limited to no juice before age 1, 4 ounces per day for children aged 1–3 years, 4–6 ounces per day for children aged 4–6 years, and not more than 8 ounces per day for children older than 7 years.
- For children who are regularly nursing or drinking from a bottle, progressively diluting cariogenic liquid with water until finally the child is receiving only water in the bottle may be helpful.
- Transitioning from the bottle or breast-feeding to the use of an uncovered cup at meals or with snacks may be a solution to the at-will consumption of cariogenic liquids permitted by bottles and sippy cups.
- Brush after meals and snacks when possible; if not practical rinse with water.

CSHCN are frequently subject to dietary modification because of chronic health conditions and that may make the above recommendations problematic. Clinicians need to familiarize themselves with the nutritional requirements of the child's condition, for example:

- Congenital heart disease, cystic fibrosis, and the secondary infections seen in AIDS/HIV and cancer lead to a hypermetabolic state that requires dietary modification to meet the energy and protein requirements for growth [26]. Children with these chronic conditions will need more frequent meals and snacks with energy-dense foods to meet their nutritional requirements.
- Food selectivity or conditions associated with decreased appetite further challenge the caregiver to provide adequate nutrition. The incentive to select foods

that the child is willing to eat may override optimal choices for nutrition and good oral health.
- Children with regular nausea and vomiting (e.g., chemotherapy treatment) should avoid beverages that cause additional erosion.
- A soft food diet may be required in some instances. Children with cystic fibrosis and cancer may find chewing tiring [26]. Cancer treatment may induce mucositis, and AIDS/HIV may result in candida infections, oral ulcers, and inflammation.

Many medications for children have a high sugar content. This may not be a concern for an acute illness when taken for a short duration, but for children with chronic conditions, a daily regimen of sugar-sweetened medications may contribute to caries risk. Clinicians should advise caregivers to avoid administering medication before bed if possible and instead recommend that medications be taken with meals unless the directions specify otherwise. Children should rinse with water after taking sugar-sweetened medications.

Additionally, these medications may cause xerostomia, the sensation of dry mouth. Compensation for dry mouth may increase the consumption of sweetened beverages, while at the same time, oral health suffers from the loss of the protective functions of saliva and its ability to clear foods from the mouth, neutralize acids, and remineralize teeth, due to inadequate saliva flow. Clinicians can assist with the management of xerostomia for CSHCN in much the same way that they assist other patients. Alternative medications can be discussed with the patient's physician. Saliva stimulants may be recommended such as sipping sugar-free liquids and sucking ice chips or sugarless lozenges or gum if age appropriate. Swabbing or rinsing several times a day with a solution of half a teaspoon each of salt and baking soda to a cup of warm water may help return the oral environment to a neutral pH. There are over-the-counter saliva substitutes to moisten the oral tissues that can be swabbed on prior to eating or bed. Daily mechanical plaque removal with a fluoride toothpaste reduces the increased risk of dental caries from the combined effect of sugar-sweetened medications and xerostomia and may help reduce gingival enlargement caused by some medications prescribed for CSHCN.

Xylitol is a naturally occurring sugar substitute that is safe for use by children with diabetes. It is not metabolized by cariogenic bacteria; therefore products sweetened with xylitol are approved to be labeled sugar-free by the FDA. Recommending xylitol gum and lozenges, if age and condition appropriate, can assist with saliva stimulation for those experiencing xerostomia and may provide some protection against the development of dental caries when a minimum of 6 grams is consumed per day, divided over at least three administrations [27]. When making their recommendations, clinicians should be aware that the cost of xylitol products is often higher than other sugar-free or sugar-sweetened choices.

Early dental visits are opportunities to provide anticipatory guidance to caregivers that will help foster dietary habits conducive to good oral health, such as advising nighttime bottles be filled only with water and not cariogenic liquids. Clinicians also need to be prepared to assist caregivers with practical strategies for making behavior and dietary changes when necessary. Acknowledging that there may be lapses in the effort to make even modest changes can help caregivers to identify barriers to reaching their goal.

Oral Hygiene Devices

Toothbrushes

The toothbrush is perhaps the simplest and most important oral hygiene device. Both manual and electric toothbrushes can be good options for CSHCN, though the vibration of the electric toothbrush may not be tolerated by some children. On the other hand, CSHCN who are sensory seeking may enjoy a powered brush. Caregivers should select a soft-bristled brush with a head size small enough to access tight spaces in the back of the mouth. A systematic brushing technique that cleans all tooth surfaces should be demonstrated to caregivers, with emphasis on cleaning the gingival margin where plaque formation begins on smooth tooth surfaces. The demonstration should be followed by the caregiver brushing the teeth of the child, if possible. Having the caregiver demonstrate his understanding of the technique will allow the clinician to assist with important adaptations to assure that all tooth surfaces are cleaned. Additionally, the demonstration may reveal challenges the clinician can address that would otherwise have gone unnoticed.

For example, even the ergonomic handles of today's toothbrushes may not be easy for a CSHCN to grasp. Toothbrush handles can be enlarged by securing a sponge or foam around the handle with rubber bands. A bicycle handle or tennis ball can serve the same purpose. In some cases, the same Velcro devise that straps to a child's hand to assist in holding a utensil for eating may be used to hold a toothbrush or a simple rubber band may also do the job. Figure 4 illustrates these adaptations.

Both patients and caregivers may find that an electric toothbrush simplifies the brushing technique by automatically performing the brushing motion along the gingival margin. However, the caregiver needs to understand how the technique differs with the electric brush for it to be effective. If an electric toothbrush is used, encourage the caregiver to bring the brush to the appointment. This enables the clinician to offer the child something he is familiar with and allows for technique coaching during the dental visit.

If angulation is a problem, especially when the child has limited opening, the neck of some manual toothbrushes can be bent to the proper angle by running them under hot water. If the child has difficulty holding the mouth open for tooth brushing, several tongue blades wrapped together and turned on edge can serve as a mouth prop for the child to rest the teeth on while brushing. There are foam mouth props for this purpose available online and three-sided toothbrushes in child and regular size. The "Surround" toothbrush is helpful when the opening is limited as it cleans the lingual, buccal, and occlusal surfaces simultaneously (Fig. 5). Advise caregivers that toothbrushes should not be shared and a new manual toothbrush should be used every 3 months or following a contagious illness.

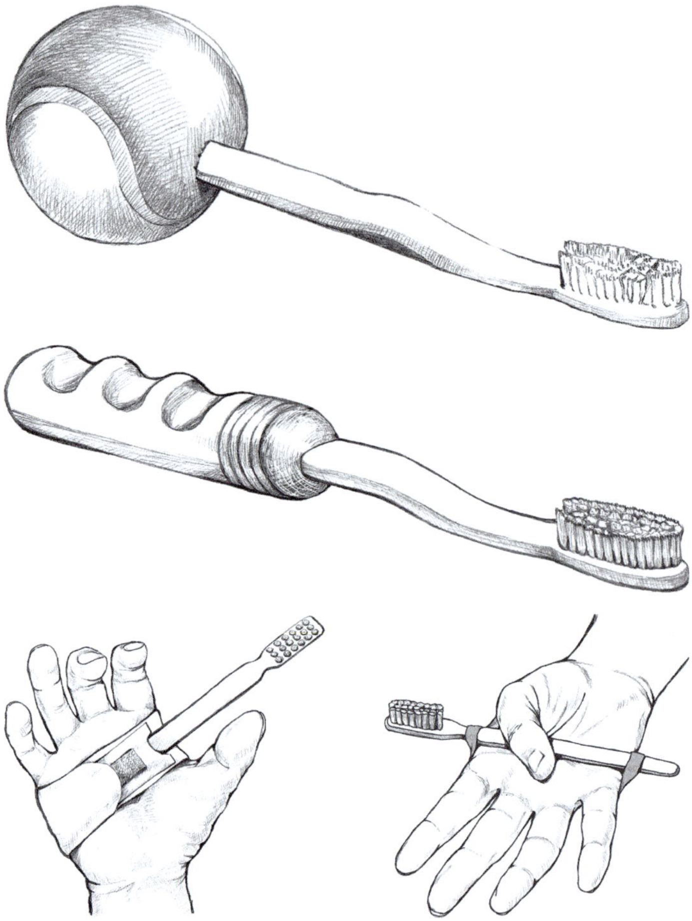

Fig. 4 Toothbrushes adapted for CSHCN

Interproximal Cleaning

While a thorough toothbrushing that delivers fluoride daily is the most essential aspect of oral hygiene, cleaning between the teeth is highly desirable and can be accomplished by a variety of devices. Flossing the child's teeth is the most common method. The caregiver may use a length of floss wrapped around his fingers to remove the plaque between any teeth with contacts. This method of flossing takes considerable skill, and clinicians should observe the caregiver's technique to make certain that the gingiva is not injured inadvertently and that the technique is effective at food and plaque removal. Flossing aids such as floss handles or floss picks, especially those designed for children, can facilitate this process (Fig. 6). Caregivers may need to experiment to find the right device to access all teeth. It may help the caregiver to learn to use these devices in his mouth in order to appreciate how to

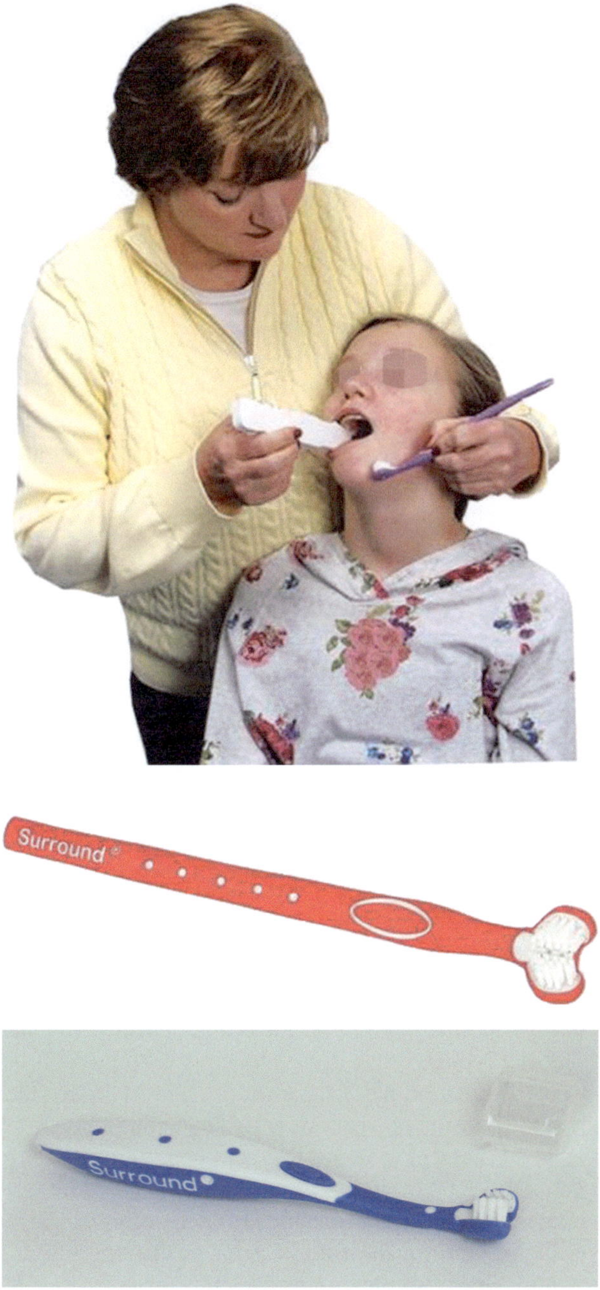

Fig. 5 Caregiver using foam Open Wide® Mouth Rest; Surround® three-sided adult and toddler toothbrushes

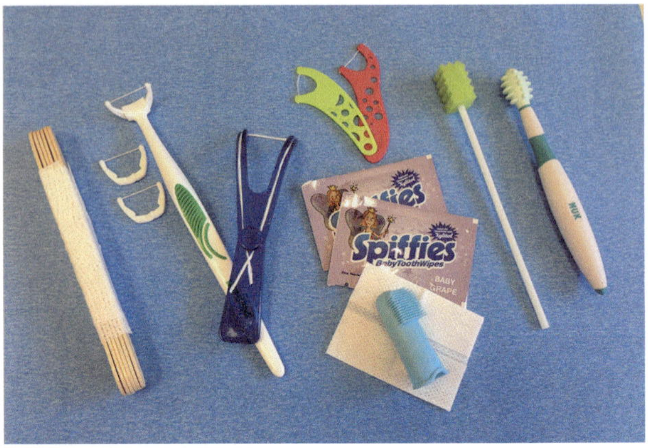

Fig. 6 Oral hygiene aids: wrapped tongue blades for mouth prop, floss handles, kids' flossers, finger brush on tooth wipe, sponge/foam brush, and NUK massage brush

apply the technique to the child. Flossing aids may also be useful when it is not safe for the caregiver to place his fingers in the child's mouth, and the device should be unlikely to break if the child bites down.

Tooth Wipes and Finger Brushes

Infants may initially be introduced to daily mouth cleaning with a wet washcloth or gauze. Xylitol tooth wipes or finger brushes that slip over the end of a finger may also be used (Fig. 6). Tooth wipes are designed as a one-time use, disposable device. The child should be introduced to daily toothbrushing with fluoride toothpaste when the first teeth erupt, but these aids may be convenient for cleaning the teeth at other times such as after between-meal snacks especially following consumption of energy-dense foods or when away from home.

Sponge/Foam Brushes

Sponge brushes are available plain, with flavoring, dentifrice, glycerin, or sodium bicarbonate added. If a sponge brush is used to apply toothpaste, it is recommended that the caregiver apply the toothpaste separately to be certain that the child receives a fluoridated toothpaste in the correct amount. The sponge brushes available with sodium bicarbonate are helpful to neutralize acid conditions in the mouth for children with acid reflux (GERD) or problems with nausea and vomiting. Foam brushes with glycerin come with lemon flavoring and are used as moisturizers for dry mouth conditions. By placing them in the freezer prior to use, the child may find them pleasant in the same manner as sucking on ice chips or popsicles. Sponge brushes are useful as applicators for these various agents and for palliative care, but do not replace toothbrushing for plaque removal (Fig. 6).

Chlorhexidine Gluconate (CHX) Rinse

Chlorhexidine gluconate (CHX) is an antimicrobial rinse that may be prescribed when bacterial plaque control is not optimal. It has been shown to reduce dental plaque and gingivitis [28, 29]. Among CSHCN, those with diabetes and trisomy 21 are prone to developing gingivitis and periodontal disease due to a compromised immune system [30]. CHX is available in an alcohol-based or water-based formula. The water-based formula is recommended for children. Additionally, alcohol has a drying effect on the oral tissues. The product instructions are to rinse for 30 s with 15 mL (half a capful) of CHX twice daily. The substantivity of CHX, that is, its ability to bind to the oral tissues for slow release, is approximately 12 h. Because of these binding properties, caregivers and patients using CHX need to be instructed to establish a routine that avoids rinsing with CHX within 1 h of toothpaste use, as the positive cations of CHX bind the negative fluoride ions. The regimen recommended when addressing chronic conditions such as gingivitis or periodontal disease is daily rinsing for 1 week each month with professional evaluation after 6 months of use. If children have swallowing difficulties or are unable to spit, CHX can be swabbed on the teeth either with a sponge/foam brush, a toothbrush, or by cotton swab. Caregivers may apply it by spraying each side of the mouth.

Oral Hygiene Strategies

The clinician's role goes beyond educating the caregiver about prevention of oral diseases and instruction in oral hygiene techniques. He will want to work closely with caregivers for their input in developing an individualized home oral hygiene plan. This will include strategies to accomplish desired goals with input from the caregiver. Caregivers need support and encouragement to increase their confidence as they develop and implement oral hygiene routines for CSHCN. The clinician will be called on to assist in problem-solving unique circumstances, overcoming barriers that interfere with goals, and encouraging continued performance in spite of challenges.

Research indicates that caregivers of CSHCN desire simple oral hygiene goals and a primary challenge they face is incorporating oral hygiene into the child's daily routine [2]. Providers should praise caregivers for bringing the child in for professional services and inform them that you are pleased to be able to work with them to provide care and develop the most workable plan for performing daily oral hygiene. Seek input from caregivers regarding goals that they believe can be accomplished, and work with caregivers to identify barriers to those goals and strategies that facilitate achieving them. Interestingly, the same research shows that caregivers indicate having oral hygiene supplies handy is important, but they did not emphasize the need for special supplies that are adapted to meet functional limitations of CSHCN. Understanding the importance of oral health is also not a common motivator for caregivers of CSHCN [2]. Lack of knowledge may not be the problem; it may be that other barriers get in the way of achieving good oral health for the child in their care. Therefore, it appears that the clinician's ability to assist caregivers in developing simple, practical strategies is of primary importance. This requires knowledge about the CSHCN and compassion for the challenges faced by the child and caregiver. See Table 2 for age-specific oral hygiene strategies.

Table 2 Age-specific oral hygiene strategies

Age	Strategies
Infants and toddlers: 0 up to 3 years	Pre-eruption: wipe the mouth gently with a damp washcloth or gauze or commercially available wipes with xylitol to introduce the child to the cleaning procedure
	As soon as the first tooth erupts, brush the teeth daily with an infant-size toothbrush to clean all surfaces of teeth
	Use a "smear" or "grain of rice" amount of fluoride toothpaste, twice daily
	"Lift the lip" to facilitate brushing and check for early signs of caries
	Focus on brushing the gingival margin
	Use the knee-to-knee position for home hygiene
	Up to the age of 6, implement a routine that incorporates caregiver brushing after the child has done it himself
Young children: 3 up to 6 years	The goal is twice-daily delivery of fluoride toothpaste to the oral cavity
	The amount of fluoride toothpaste is now pea-size
	Encourage the child to spit out excess toothpaste, but not to rinse, so a small amount of fluoride remains in the oral cavity
	Under age 6, children should avoid mouthwashes as they are not capable of adequately spitting out after swishing
	For CSHCN who do not tolerate toothpaste because of foaming, gagging, or taste sensitivity, dip the toothbrush in OTC or prescription fluoride rinse, and then brush the teeth
	For children who don't tolerate foaming toothpaste, choose products that do not contain sodium laurel sulfate (e.g., Biotene, OraNurse Unflavored Toothpaste, ClōSYS, Sensodyne PRONAMEL)
	Establish routines that are practical for the child and family
Children: 6 up to 12 years	Children in this age group have a mixed dentition, with the challenge of cleaning an increasing number of teeth whose positions change as they erupt
	Brush teeth twice daily with a pea-sized amount of fluoride toothpaste
	The child should spit out excess toothpaste, but not rinse
	Adult caregivers should assist with and supervise brushing
	A good gauge as to whether a child in this age range is ready for independent toothbrushing is whether the child has the fine motor skills to tie shoelaces. If not, the caregiver should continue to brush the child's teeth after the child has had his turn
	With the eruption of permanent teeth, the caregiver should be shown how to floss the child's teeth if that is not already being done. The closed contacts between permanent teeth make it important to remove interproximal plaque and reduce the risk for dental caries and gingivitis

Table 2 (continued)

Age	Strategies
Adolescents: 12–18 years	Adolescence is marked by increasing independence and broader socialization. It may begin as early as 10 years of age in the general population and be delayed past age 12 in CSHCN
	Many CSHCN will face the usual adolescent risks to oral health including traumatic injuries, tobacco, alcohol, and/or drug use and poor nutritional choices
	Poor oral hygiene and hormonal changes put adolescents at increased risk for periodontal disease compared to younger age children
	Consider more frequent periodontal recall for CSHCN with conditions such as diabetes or trisomy 21 that put them at higher risk for periodontal disease
	Consider CHX use twice daily for 1 week each month if gingival conditions are poor
	Consider fluoride supplements up to 16 years of age if the adolescent is not benefiting from community water fluoridation and is at high risk for dental caries [31]
	A prescription for 5000 PPM toothpaste may benefit high caries-risk adolescents
	OTC or prescription fluoride mouth rinse may be an alternative to prescription toothpaste
	Work with the caregiver and adolescent to make modest changes such as eliminating one sugar-sweetened beverage a day/week and establishing a small reward system for meeting that goal

Positions to Enhance Home Oral Hygiene

As with typically developing children in the pre-cooperative stage, positioning the CSHCN is critical for effective toothbrushing and interproximal cleaning. The clinician will want to demonstrate options for the caregiver based on the age and condition of the child. Have the caregiver support the head and body in various positions, and work with the caregiver and child to determine what will be most practical for them.

Infants and very young children can be held in the lap or in the knee-to-knee position. The knee-to-knee position requires the assistance of another person who holds the child as if hugging the child with the child's legs wrapped around the waist. The assistant's knees form a table with the caregiver who will brush the teeth. The assistant lays the child back into the caregiver's lap and holds the child's hands, while the caregiver brushes the teeth (Fig. 7).

As children grow older, other positions may be helpful to facilitate cooperation and provide the caregiver with a good view of the oral cavity.

- The caregiver sits on the bed or a couch, and the child lays with his head on the caregiver's lap.
- The child lays on the floor, using pillows as needed for comfort of the child and caregiver.
- The caregiver kneels on the floor behind the child and places the child's head on his lap, while the child stretches out on the floor.

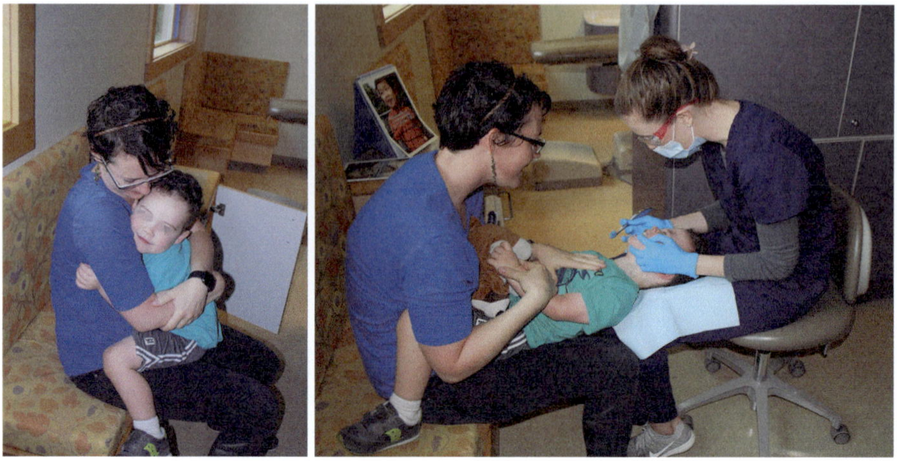

Fig. 7 The knee-to-knee position for toothbrushing and examination

- A beanbag chair may be molded to allow a child to be supported in a comfortable reclined position.
- The child sits in a chair, the head tilted back, while the caregiver stands behind and supports the child's head against his body with one arm.
- Alternatively, the caregiver can sit in a chair, and the child sits on the floor with the head tilted back between the caregiver's knees. In this position, the caregiver can gently secure the child's head with the knees and the child's arms behind the caregiver's legs to keep the child still and the hands from interfering with toothbrushing.
- Children in wheelchairs may have their teeth brushed while remaining in the wheelchair. The child tilts the head back, while the caregiver stands or sits behind the child and supports the child's head against their body with one arm to brush the child's teeth. It may be that the wheelchair has support for the child's head and can be tipped back for a good view of the tooth surfaces to be brushed. Be sure to lock the wheels of the wheelchair (Fig. 8).

Cooperation Strategies

Caregivers trying to establish a new habit or routine for a CSHCN may encounter resistance. Behavior challenges may be due to child anxiety caused by the new activity. To improve cooperation, suggest that the caregiver use the "tell-show-do" approach and slowly introduce oral hygiene aids and activities. The caregiver should "tell" the child what they are going to do and describe how it will feel in positive terms before doing it. They can "show" the child each step before performing it in the child's mouth or even demonstrate it in their own. For example, the child can feel and hold the toothbrush prior to brushing. When they "do" toothbrushing, it

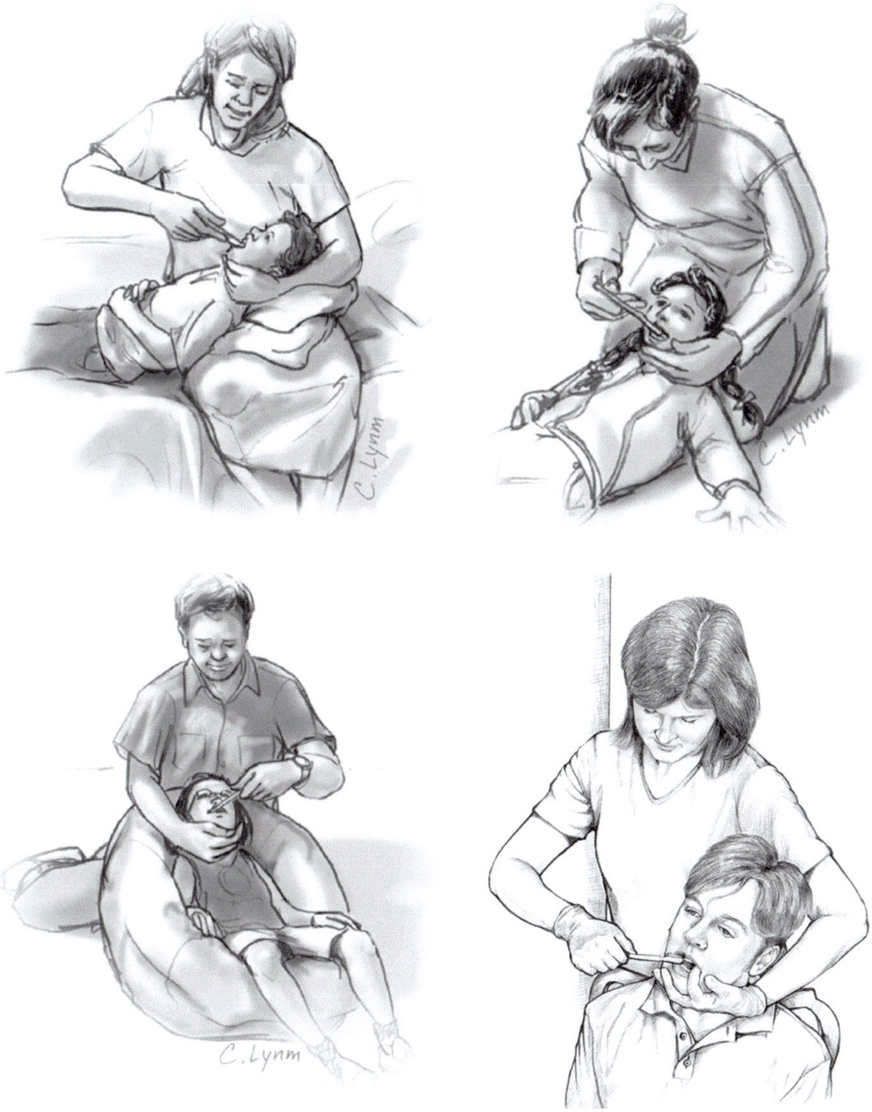

Fig. 8 Positions for oral hygiene. Illustrations courtesy of C. Lynm, adapted and used with permission from Perlman SP, Friedman C, Kaufhold GH. 1996. Special Smiles: A Guide to Good Oral Health for Persons with Special Needs. Washington, DC: Special Olympics, Healthy Athletes, Special Smiles; Boston University

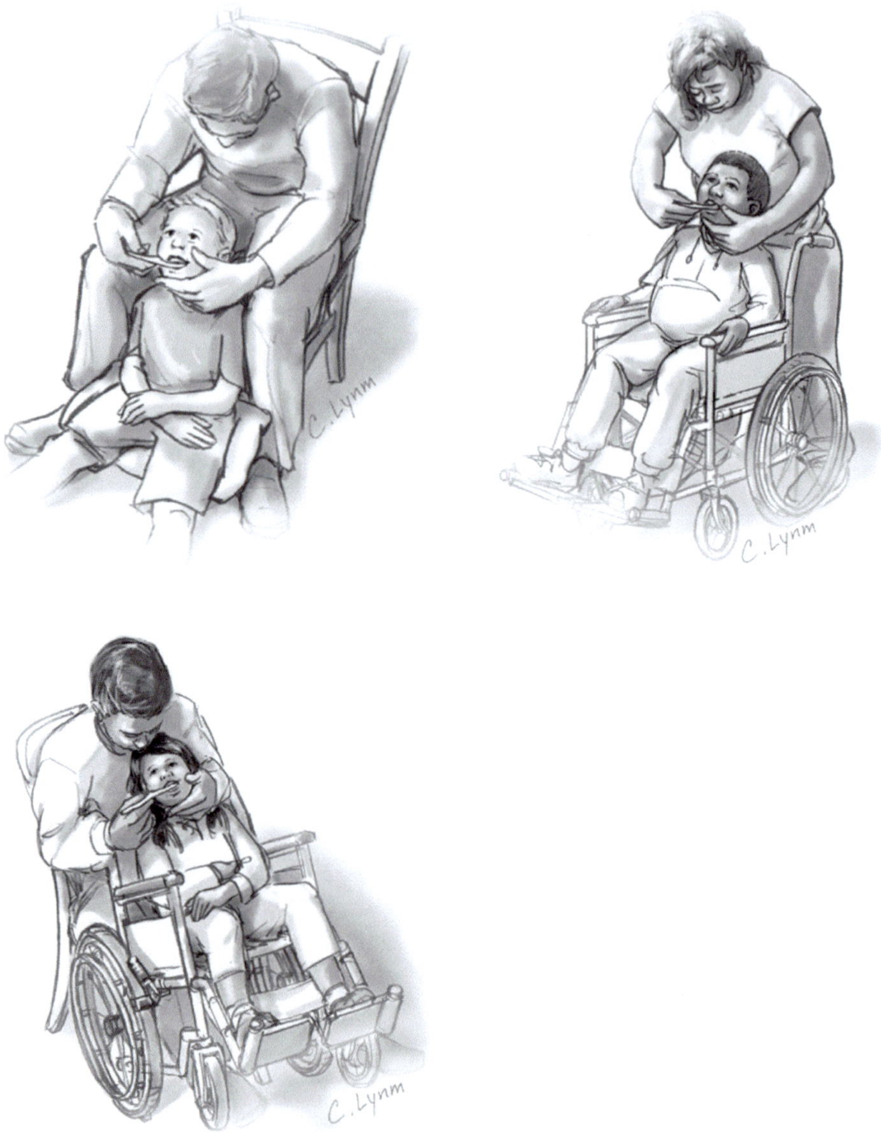

Fig. 8 (continued)

should be performed following the same steps used in "tell" and "show" for consistency. The caregiver will want to reinforce positive behaviors, initially praising the child for even minimal cooperation. The caregiver knows best how much patience is required when teaching a new skill or activity to a CSHCN but will appreciate the clinician's support and empathy.

Routine is frequently important for CSHCN, so home oral hygiene should be performed at the same time, in the same place, and following the same routine every day. The location for toothbrushing will be based on comfort and convenience for the child and caregiver. Holding a "preferred item," such as a favorite stuffed animal as part of the routine, may provide comfort to the child. Social stories, visual sequencing cards, timers, and toothbrushing tablet apps can also be useful (see Chapter "Desensitization and Therapeutic Behavioral Approaches to Dental Care"). After breakfast and before bed are optimal times for home hygiene, but timing is less important than finding a time that is practical for the family. Work with the caregiver to determine a protected time where the best-laid plans are not likely to go sideways. For example, oral hygiene can be performed at the kitchen table following a meal substituting a bowl for the bathroom sink. Ask the caregiver what might interfere with the time they propose.

Will the child be too tired?
Will other children need the caregiver's attention?
Is there someone else available to assist?
Is another time more likely to work?

For CSHCN with a hyperactive bite and gag reflex, introducing oral hygiene aids slowly may be helpful. A mouth prop may help the child by allowing him to relax his teeth on the prop. In the case of a strong gag reflex, the child may be more comfortable having the teeth brushed before breakfast when the stomach is empty. It may also help to avoid use of a foaming toothpaste. Suggest either a non-foaming fluoride toothpaste such as Biotene, OraNurse Unflavored Toothpaste, ClōSYS, or Sensodyne PRONAMEL, or dip the toothbrush in a fluoride rinse to brush the teeth.

Food pouching is common for some CSHCN (Fig. 9). After meals and medications, caregivers should be advised to check the mouth for retained food or medication particles. If pouching occurs regularly, it will increase the risk for caries. Have the child rinse with water following the meal if he is capable of doing so. A finger sweep, sponge/foam brush, cotton swab, or the NUK massage brush can be used to remove the retained food or medication from the vestibule if the child is not able to rinse (Fig. 6).

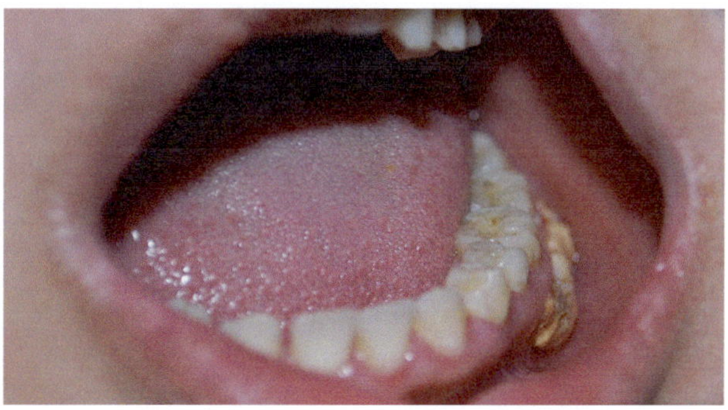

Fig. 9 Food pouching

Case-Based Scenario

Jonathan, the 8-year-old boy with trisomy 21 introduced in chapter "Desensitization and Therapeutic Behavioral Approaches to Dental Care," and his parents have established a relationship with the dental providers. Following an introductory visit where Jonathan allowed his mother and then the dentist to brush his teeth sitting in a chair in the corner of a quiet room, the family used behavior modeling at home for 2 weeks to prepare Jonathan for a mirror-only dental examination. At that second visit, the examination revealed a classic mixed dentition, generalized crowding, and occlusal attrition with no obvious carious lesions. The dental provider praised the parents for the work they had done to prepare Jonathan for the examination visit and for the care they were providing him at home.

On Jonathan's third visit, following a successful panoramic radiograph, the dental provider began discussion with the parents about the three main areas of prevention to be incorporated into Jonathan's home oral care plan: exposure to fluoride, minimizing the cariogenic potential of Jonathan's diet, and adequate plaque removal. Prior to this discussion, the dental provider reviewed the pre-appointment questionnaire the parents had completed and confirmed that Jonathan's family lives in an area with community water fluoridation and that he had also begun to participate in an Individualized Education Program (IEP) at the school he attends for children with intellectual disabilities.

The discussion with the parents began by asking what they are currently doing to care for Jonathan's teeth with the preamble that they have been very successful to date as he is caries-free. The parents shared that they brush his teeth at least once per day with a fluoride toothpaste, usually after breakfast, as cooperation before bed when he is tired is poor. They use only a small amount of a non-foaming fluoride toothpaste because Jonathan has difficulty spitting and rinsing. After experimenting with numerous toothpastes to find one that Jonathan would tolerate, they settled on the non-foaming (sodium laurel sulfate-free) toothpaste, as it seemed to relieve his burning tongue sensation. The parents were informed that using a pea-sized amount of toothpaste is the correct amount for Jonathan's age and that having a small amount of the fluoride toothpaste remain in the mouth provides protection from dental caries. They were encouraged to continue having him spit out the excess, but not to rinse.

For the next dental visit in 1 month, Jonathan's parents prepared him for a fluoride varnish application using the behavior modeling technique they had used to prepare him for an examination. At the appointment, prior to fluoride application, Jonathan's mother brushed his teeth at the sink simulating the way his teeth are brushed at home. This allowed observation of the technique and positioning used. It was noted that his mother was challenged to reach the lingual surfaces due to macroglossia and hypertonic muscle movement around the oral cavity that is typical for patients with trisomy 21.

Following application of fluoride varnish, the dental provider learned about Jonathan's diet and beverage consumption from his parents. At age 8 they were still able to control most of Jonathan's eating habits, so snacks were limited, and they avoided sweets and sugar-sweetened beverages (SSB), drinking milk with meals and water at other times. However, they were not aware that crackers and pretzels had cariogenic potential and were advised to have him drink water after those snacks or to substitute healthy snacks such as nuts, fresh fruits and vegetables, or cheese when possible. Use of tap water was reinforced, but concern was expressed about Jonathan choosing SSB as his independence increased. His parents were advised to monitor these potential changes to his diet as alterations to the home oral care plan might be needed, including a prescription strength fluoride toothpaste.

While keeping the parents' goals in mind and strategies simple, the dental provider noted that the plan for future visits would include working with the parents to incorporate the following in order of priority: a second toothbrushing during the day, adapting the toothbrush and/or brushing technique to reach the gingival margin of the lingual surfaces, and interdental cleaning. Additionally, Jonathan's growing independence meant that he was learning to brush his own teeth. In the future, discussion about including oral self-care skills in IEP would be important to assist Jonathan in developing and practicing oral self-care routines. The dental provider also considered enlisting the help of his occupational therapist to suggest tools or technique modifications to assist him in performing oral hygiene activities. Noting that the risk for periodontal disease is increased in patients with trisomy 21 due to alterations in the immune system, Jonathan's ability to accomplish adequate plaque removal on his own as he becomes a more independent adolescent would become increasingly important.

Conclusion

Clinicians work closely with caregivers to prevent oral diseases in CSHCN by developing an individualized home oral hygiene plan tailored to the child's condition and developmental age. There are three main areas of prevention to be incorporated into the plan, each with assessments and options for the clinician to consider:

- *Regular exposure to fluoride including at home and in office*: Consider fluoride in drinking water, OTC toothpaste, prescription toothpaste, fluoride varnish, and silver diamine fluoride.
- *Minimize the cariogenic potential of the CSHCN's diet when possible in balance with the child's unique nutritional needs*: Advise consuming sugar and starch with meals, choosing nutritious snacks, reducing sugar-sweetened beverages, avoiding bottles that contain anything other than water, and taking sweetened medications with meals, and consider xylitol, saliva substitutes, and sodium bicarbonate to assist with xerostomia.
- *Adequate plaque removal with devices and strategies that work for the CSHCN and the caregiver*: Focus on practical oral hygiene goals that can be incorporated into the child's daily routine, select proper size toothbrushes, teach proper

brushing technique, employ flossing and brushing aids to facilitate hygiene measures, emphasize a regular oral hygiene routine, and teach the caregiver how to assist and supervise home care efforts.

Clinicians have the opportunity to play a significant role in assisting the caregiver and CSHCN with the development of oral hygiene habits that can prevent disease and improve the quality of life for CSHCN.

Useful Resources and Web Links

The National Institute of Dental and Craniofacial Research (NIDCR) of the National Institutes of Health (NIH) has a useful publication series for clinicians and caregivers, titled *Practical Oral Care for People with Developmental Disabilities* available at the following website: https://catalog.nidcr.nih.gov/OrderPublications/

National Institute of Dental and Craniofacial Research. Developmental Disabilities. https://www.nidcr.nih.gov/health-info/developmental-disabilities/more-info

National Maternal and Child Oral Health Resource Center, Georgetown University. Special Care: An Oral Health Professionals Guide to Serving Children with Special Health Care Needs. https://www.mchoralhealth.org/SpecialCare/

Association of State and Territorial Dental Directors (ASTDD). Maternal and Child Oral Health. https://www.astdd.org/maternal-and-child-health/

References

1. U.S. Department of Health and Human Services. Oral health in America: a report of the surgeon general. Rockville, MD: U.S. Department of Health and Human Services, National Institute of Dental and Craniofacial Research, National Institutes of Health; 2000.
2. Campanaro M, Huebner CE, Davis BE. Facilitators and barriers to twice daily tooth brushing among children with special health care needs. Spec Care Dentist. 2014;34:185–92.
3. Dye BA, Tan S, Smith V, Lewis BG, Barker LK, Thornton-Evans G, et al. Trends in oral health status: United States, 1988–1994 and 1999–2004. Vital Health Stat 11. 2007;(248):1–92.
4. Center for Disease Control and Prevention (CDC). Community Water Fluoridation. Available at: https://www.cdc.gov/fluoridation/index.html. Page last updated: 21 Feb 2018. Page accessed: 17 Jun 2018.
5. Center for Disease Control and Prevention (CDC). Recommendations for using fluoride to prevent and control dental caries in the United States. MMWR Morb Mortal Wkly Rep. 2001;50(RR14):1–42.
6. Rozier RG, Adair S, Graham F, et al. Evidence-based clinical recommendations on the prescription of dietary fluoride supplements for caries prevention: a report of the American Dental Association Council on Scientific Affairs. J Am Dent Assoc. 2010;141:1480–9.
7. Wright JT, Hanson N, Ristic H, Whall CW, Estrich CG, Zentz RR. Fluoride toothpaste efficacy and safety in children younger than 6 years: a systematic review. J Am Dent Assoc. 2014;145:182–9. https://doi.org/10.14219/jada.2013.37.
8. Chi DL, Tut O, Milgrom P. Cluster-randomized xylitol toothpaste trial for early childhood caries prevention. J Dent Child. 2014;81:27–32.

9. Walsh T, Worthington HV, Glenny AM, Appelbe P, Marinho VC, Shi X. Fluoride toothpastes of different concentrations for preventing dental caries in children and adolescents. Cochrane Database Syst Rev. 2010;20:CD007868.
10. Dos Santos AP, Nadanovsky P, de Oliveira BH. A systematic review and meta-analysis of the effects of fluoride toothpastes on the prevention of dental caries in the primary dentition of preschool children. Community Dent Oral Epidemiol. 2013;41:1–12.
11. Marinho VC, Higgins JP, Sheiham A, Logan S. Fluoride toothpastes for preventing dental caries in children and adolescents. Cochrane Database Syst Rev. 2003;1:CD002278.
12. Beltrán-Aguilar ED, Barker LK, Canto MT, Dye BA, Gooch BF, Griffin SO, et al. Surveillance for dental caries, dental sealants, tooth retention, edentulism, and enamel fluorosis—United States, 1988–1994 and 1999–2002. MMWR Surveill Summ. 2005;54(3):1–43.
13. Pitts N, Duckworth R, Marsh MP, Mutti B, Parnell C, Zero D. Post-brushing rinsing for the control of dental caries: exploration of the available evidence to establish what advice we should give our patients. Br Dent J. 2012;212:315–20.
14. Twetman S. Caries prevention with fluoride toothpaste in children: an update. Eur Arch Paediatr Dent. 2009;10:162–7.
15. Rothen M, Cunha-Cruz J, Zhou L, Mancl L, Jones JS, Berg J, on behalf of the Northwest PRECEDENT network. Oral hygiene behaviors and caries experience in Northwest PRECEDENT patients. Community Dent Oral Epidemiol. 2014;42:526–35.
16. Chestnutt IG, Schafer F, Jacobson APM, Stephen KW. The influence of toothbrushing frequency and postbrushing rinsing on caries experience in a caries clinical trial. Community Dent Oral Epidemiol. 1998;26:406–11.
17. US Department of Health and Human Services. Public Health Service recommendation for fluoride concentration in drinking water for prevention of dental caries. Federal Register 80 FR 24936. 2015 May 1. https://federalregister.gov/a/2015-10201. Accessed 24 Feb 2018.
18. van Loveren C, Duckworth RM. Anti-calculus and whitening toothpastes. In: van Loveren C, editor. Toothpastes. Basel: Karger; 2013. p. 61–74.
19. Weyant RJ, Tracy SL, Anselmo TT, Beltran-Aquilar ED, Donly KJ, Frese WA, et al. Topical fluoride for cares prevention: executive summary of the updated clinical recommendations and supporting systematic review. J Am Dent Assoc. 2013;14:1279–91.
20. Berkowitz RJ, Koo H, McDermott MP, Whelehan MT, Ragusa P, Kopycka-Kedzierawski DT, et al. Adjunctive chemotherapeutic suppression of mutans streptococci in the setting of severe early childhood caries: an exploratory study. J Public Health Dent. 2009;69:163–7. https://doi.org/10.1111/j.1752-7325.2009.00118.x.
21. Lopez L, Berkowitz R, Spiekerman C, Weinstein P. Topical antimicrobial therapy in the prevention of early childhood caries: a follow-up report. Pediatr Dent. 2002;24:204–6.
22. Tut OK, Milgrom P. Topical iodine and fluoride varnish combined is more effective than fluoride varnish alone for protecting erupting first permanent molars: a retrospective cohort study. J Public Health Dent. 2010;70:249–52. https://doi.org/10.1111/j.1752-7325.2010.00163.x.
23. Chu CH, Lo ECM, Lin HC. Effectiveness of silver diamine fluoride varnish in arresting dentin caries in Chinese pre-school children. J Dent Res. 2002;81:767–70.
24. Llodra JC, Rodriguez A, Ferrer B, Menardia V, Ramos T, Morato M. Efficacy of silver diamine fluoride for caries reduction in primary teeth and first permanent molars of schoolchildren: 36-month clinical trial. J Dent Res. 2005;84:721–4.
25. Horst JA, Ellenikiotis H, Milgrom PL. UCSF Protocol for caries arrest using silver diamine fluoride: rationale, indications and consent. J Calif Dent Assoc. 2016;44:16–28.
26. Moursi AM, Fernandez JB, Daronch M, Zee L, Jones CL. Nutrition and oral health consideration in children with special health care needs: implications for oral health care providers. Pediatr Dent. 2010;32:333–42.
27. Mäkinen KK. Sugar alcohol sweeteners as alternatives to sugar with special consideration of xylitol. Med Princ Pract. 2011;20:303–20.
28. Gunsolley JC. A meta-analysis of six-month studies of antiplaque and antigingivitis agents. J Am Dent Assoc. 2006;137:1649–57.

29. Chibinski AC, Pochapski MT, Farago PV, Santos FA, Czlusniak GD. Clinical evaluation of chlorhexidine for the control of dental biofilm in children with special needs. Community Dent Health. 2011;28:222–6.
30. Abanto J, Ciamponi AL, Francischini E, Murakami C, de Rezende NP, Gallottini M. Medical problems and oral care of patients with Down syndrome: a literature review. Spec Care Dentist. 2011;31:197–203.
31. American Academy of Pediatric Dentistry Clinical Affairs Committee. Guideline on adolescent oral health care. Pediatr Dent. 2015;37:49–56.

Common Oral Conditions in Children with Special Needs

Evelina Kratunova and Marcio A. da Fonseca

Introduction

Children with special healthcare needs (CSHCN) are surviving longer due to medical, pharmaceutical, and technological advances made in the last few decades. Many diseases that once were fatal have become chronic, manageable conditions. Unfortunately, many of the therapeutic modalities used in the management of those conditions may lead to significant oral conditions that can impact a patient's quality of life. Given the varied etiologies of health conditions, the differing abilities of patients to cooperate, and the side effects and potential interactions of drugs, the dental professional is usually faced with a challenge—in order to treat an oral health condition, one needs to consider how the patient's overall care is affected by delivery of dental care. Therefore, a care plan has to be very specific to each situation encountered. This chapter will review the most common oral conditions seen in patients with special needs and discuss general recommendations for care.

Self-Injurious Behavior

Self-injurious behavior (SIB) is a behavioral disturbance with intentional harm to one's own body without suicidal intent [1]. It includes self-biting, scratching, pulling, cutting, rubbing, hitting, inserting objects in the body, eye poking, head banging, skin picking, tooth self-extraction, self-mutilation/amputation, and interference with wound healing [1, 2].

SIB is more commonly seen in children with autism spectrum disorder (ASD), visual impairment, overactive/impulsive behavior, sensory processing difficulties,

E. Kratunova, MDSc, DChDent (✉) · M. A. da Fonseca, DDS, MS
Department of Pediatric Dentistry, College of Dentistry, University of Illinois at Chicago, Chicago, IL, USA
e-mail: evekrat@uic.edu; marcio@uic.edu

T. M. Nelson, J. R. Webb (eds.), *Dental Care for Children with Special Needs*,
https://doi.org/10.1007/978-3-030-10483-2_8

sleep disorder, and anxiety [2–4]. It is also observed in children with certain medical conditions and genetic syndromes, such as familial dysautonomia, congenital insensitivity to pain, and Lesch–Nyhan, fragile X, Down, Prader–Willi, Smith–Magenis, cri-du-chat, Cornelia de Lange, and Lowe syndromes [2–4]. Pain and discomfort may directly cause self-injury, i.e., children with chronic pain self-injure near the site of pain in an attempt to remove the painful experience [3, 4]. SIB can also be learned through social reinforcement. This indicates that the patient's home and school environments have significant influence on behavior [2]. Patients in a comatose state and those with neurological injuries may present neuropathological chewing, an uncoordinated activity of masticatory muscles, leading to clenching spams, biting, gnawing, and bruxing. The overall prevalence of SIB is difficult to determine; however, it has been noted to be 27.7% in ASD [5] and approximately 5% in children with severe intellectual disability [4]. It generally increases with age and the degree of intellectual impairment [3].

SIB does not resolve without intervention, and management of oral self-injury is a challenge for the dental practitioner. Management depends on (1) the etiology of SIB, (2) the patient's medical history, and (3) the severity, frequency, and method of inflicting injury [1]. Therefore, there is no standard technique to treat oral self-injury; treatment is tailored to each patient's presentation. Therapeutic options include behavioral modification, medications, use of intraoral appliances, and surgery [1]. Management of oral SIB with appliances is dependent on the patient's and the caretakers' ability and/or willingness to contribute to the treatment and the patient's health status. The appliance must [6]:

1. Reflect soft tissues away from the occlusal table.
2. Not cause additional injury to the patient.
3. Allow full range of mandibular movement.
4. Allow good oral hygiene.
5. Withstand breakage and displacement forces over an indefinite period of time.
6. Allow healing of traumatized tissues.
7. Have a good retention.
8. Be easily fabricated, inserted, and removed by the dental provider and caretaker.

Many different appliances have been described with varying degrees of success, the most common being a soft mouthguard. It may be possible to remove the appliance once the habit has stopped, but, in many cases, it may have to be placed for extended periods of time.

Bruxism

Bruxism is defined as a repetitive jaw muscle activity characterized by clenching or grinding of the teeth and/or by bracing or thrusting of the mandible, occurring either during sleep ("sleep bruxism") or during waking hours ("awake bruxism") [7]. The pathophysiology is unknown; the most accepted theory describes it as a neuromotor dysregulation disorder [8]. The condition can lead to deleterious health effects, such as orofacial pain, masseter hypertrophy, tooth wear, tooth fracture, restoration and implant failure, and tooth loss [7, 9, 10]. A diagnostic grading system for bruxism has been proposed as:

Possible (based on self-report, report of a caretaker/partner, and/or the anamnestic part of a clinical exam)
Probable (self-report and clinical inspection)
Definite (self-report, clinical examination, and a polysomnographic recording) [7]

The gold standard for diagnosis of sleep bruxism is a polysomnographic study with video and audio recordings because it evaluates muscle activity that characterizes bruxism, "rhythmic masticatory muscle activity" [9]. The dentist can also prescribe easy-to-use electromyographic devices for use during sleep to evaluate muscle activity [10].

Bruxism is a common occurrence in children, but most outgrow the condition. Its prevalence is difficult to determine and tends to decrease with age, and it is reported to range from 6 to 50% in patients younger than 12 years old [11, 12]. Bruxism can be subdivided in primary idiopathic and secondary iatrogenic (as a manifestation of neurological disorders, psychiatric sleep disorders, developmental disabilities, and dystonias) [8–10]. Sleep disturbances, functional and parafunctional habits, psychosocial factors, and secondhand smoking are considered risk factors for sleep bruxism in children [13].

There is no definitive treatment or cure for bruxism, and it is important to recognize the reasons behind each patient's habit in order to choose an effective treatment modality [9, 10]. Grinding and equilibration of teeth and occlusal rehabilitation do not eliminate bruxism [9, 10]. Mouthguards can be used to protect the teeth but they will not stop or cure the condition [8, 9]. When considering intraoral appliances for children with bruxism, particularly those with complex health issues, the dentist must exercise caution as described in the management of oral SIB. Currently, there is no pharmacological protocol for treatment or management of bruxism [9]. Several drugs, such as buspirone, clonazepam, clonidine, and hydroxyzine, have been tried, but there is insufficient evidence of their effectiveness [8, 9, 12]. Botulinum toxin has been used with some success in children and adults, but the exact dose, duration, and frequency of use have yet to be determined [10, 14]. Cognitive and behavioral approaches (stress reduction, counseling, lifestyle changes, etc.) show promise, but at this point, there are many limitations to their application [9, 10].

Gingival Overgrowth

Gingival overgrowth (GO) is a generalized or localized enlargement of the gingival tissues that affects both sexes equally [15, 16]. It develops slowly within the marginal and attached gingiva and/or the interdental papilla but does not spread beyond the mucogingival junction [15, 16]. GO is caused by excessive accumulation of extracellular matrix proteins, type I collagen being the most common. The term GO has replaced "gingival hyperplasia," which represents an increase in cell number, and "gingival hypertrophy," an increase in the size of the cells [15, 16]. Both are histological diagnoses that do not adequately describe the different pathological processes within the periodontal tissues [15]. In severe cases, the condition can result in soft tissue covering the crowns of the teeth. This leads to problems in function (mastication, speech), esthetics (diastemas, tooth displacement, retention of primary teeth), and periodontal health. It can lead to significant decrease in patient quality of life [16].

Local and systemic factors can contribute to the disease process [15].

Local factors that can lead to GO are dental plaque, trauma, odontogenic and/or periodontal abscesses, mouth breathing, incompetent lips, prostheses, orthodontic appliances, implants, poorly contoured restorations, pathologies (fibrous epulis, pyogenic granulomas, peripheral giant cell granuloma), or a combination of these factors [15].

Systemic factors that cause GO include immunological and hormonal responses to pregnancy and puberty (due to an increase in circulating progesterone and estrogen), drugs, systemic diseases, vitamin C deficiency (scurvy), non-syndromic genetic factors (hereditary gingival fibromatosis), and rare genetic diseases and syndromes [15, 16]. It can also be idiopathic [16].

Immunosuppressant drugs (cyclosporine), calcium channel blockers (nifedipine, diltiazem, verapamil), and antiepileptic medications (phenytoin) can induce GO [15, 16]. Overgrowth caused by these medications is clinically similar (a granular or pebbly surface, coalescing to form lobules), typically appears in the anterior segments 3 months after the start of therapy, and does not lead to tooth mobility and attachment loss [15]. A synergistic effect is seen when the drugs are used in combination, and lack of optimal oral hygiene can exacerbate the process. Some systemic diseases and conditions that may present GO include leukemias (particularly acute myeloid leukemia), granulomatous diseases (Crohn's disease, sarcoidosis), malignant neoplasms (melanoma, non-Hodgkin's lymphoma, sarcomas, metastatic tumors), and neurofibromatosis [15].

The diagnosis of GO is based on the patient's history and clinical presentation [1, 2]. Histopathological evaluation of the affected tissue is considered if resolution of the overgrowth is not achieved after initial therapy [15]. Treatment varies depending on the etiology of the GO and extent of disease progression. Discontinuation or lowering of the dose of the causative drug can result in improvement or even resolution of the condition [15]. Scaling and good oral hygiene may reduce or resolve the overgrowth, but surgical intervention, with a scalpel, laser, or electrocautery, may be warranted in severe cases [15]. Rinses with 0.12% chlorhexidine twice a day for 2 weeks can be used as an adjunct measure [15]. Recurrence is common (Fig. 1).

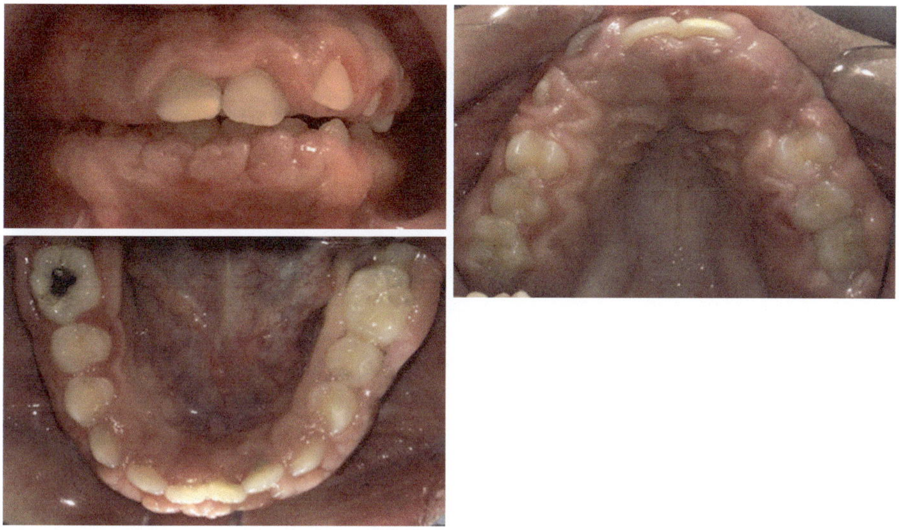

Fig. 1 Intraoral photographs (anterior view, maxillary arch, and mandibular arch), showing GO in a 13-year-old female with developmental delay and epilepsy, who is taking long-term seizure medication divalproex (compound of sodium valproate and valproic acid)

Oral Candidiasis

Candida is a fungus found in the gastrointestinal tract, vaginal tract, skin, and mucous membranes [17, 18]. Infections by *Candida* may occur in neonates, infants, in immunocompromised individuals, in cases of breakdown of skin or mucosal barriers, in patients with xerostomia, in malnutrition (particularly vitamin B12 or folate deficiencies), during changes in the normal flora caused by medical treatment (e.g., chronic use of antibiotics, corticosteroids, chemotherapy), and in patients wearing dental prostheses or appliances [17–19]. Poor oral hygiene and dental caries are also associated with an increased presence of *C. albicans*, which is the most common species [17, 19]. Most yeasts in the mouth are found in the tongue, palate, and buccal mucosa [19].

The growth of *Candida* can lead to different types of candidiasis, which is the most frequent fungal oral infection in humans [19]. The diagnosis of superficial candidiasis is usually based on its typical clinical appearance, but objective assays, such as biopsy, exfoliative cytology, and cultures, can be done [19].

Pseudomembranous candidiasis (thrush) is frequently seen in children [18]. It presents as superficial white/yellow plaques on the labial and buccal mucosa, hard and soft palate, tongue, and oropharynx and can be easily wiped off, leaving a raw underlying surface [18, 19].

Nystatin ointment 100,000 U/g
Disp: 15 – 30 g tube
Sig: apply to affected areas after meals and before bedtime for 14 days

Ketoconazole (Nizoral) cream 2%
Disp: 15 g tube
Sig: apply to affected areas daily at bedtime

Fig. 2 A sample prescription for treatment of angular cheilitis

Erythematous or atrophic candidiasis presents as bright red macular lesions that can occasionally cause a burning sensation in the tongue [18]. Both types of candidiasis can be treated with topical therapies, such as gentian violet or topical nystatin in infants, and nystatin or clotrimazole for older children [18].

Angular cheilitis is a mixed bacterial–fungal infection of the corners of the mouth, leading to painful cracking, fissuring, erythema, and bleeding [17, 19]. It can be treated with an antifungal cream or ointment three times a day (Fig. 2).

Both nystatin and clotrimazole can contain a lot of sucrose, which may contribute to the development of dental caries, especially in patients with xerostomia.

Occasionally the practitioner will encounter a more resistant form of the infection (hyperplastic candidiasis) or one that does not respond to therapy. In these cases, systemic therapy should be initiated, and a tissue biopsy can be considered due to potential for malignant transformation [19]. Deep fungal infections, such as invasive aspergillosis, histoplasmosis, and mucormycosis, usually affect immunosuppressed patients and can be life-threatening. They must be managed aggressively with tissue debridement and systemic antifungal medications.

Disinfection of dental appliances or prostheses, as well as toothbrushes and denture brushes, is important to prevent candidiasis. The acrylic porosity allows for fungal contamination, and the microclimate underneath the appliance provides an ideal environment for yeast growth [19]. A sodium hypochlorite solution (one part household bleach in ten parts of water) can be used to disinfect dental aids, prostheses, and appliances that do not have metal parts [19].

Dental Erosion

Dental erosion (DE) is defined as an irreversible loss of tooth structure associated with chemical dissolution of hydroxyapatite crystals, caused by extrinsic or intrinsic acids, without involvement of cariogenic microorganisms or acid produced by plaque bacteria [20]. DE often coexists with or can be aggravated by *attrition* (tooth-to-tooth grinding) and *abrasion* (tooth to other surfaces abnormal mechanical contact) [20]. The effects of DE can range from tooth sensitivity and reduced esthetics to occlusal discrepancies, pulp exposure, and associated periapical pathology [20, 21]. Its prevalence has not been established, but it is known to increase with age [22]. DE is more common in primary teeth due to their thinner and less mineralized hard structures [23] and in certain groups of CSHCN (e.g., cerebral palsy, trisomy 21, and GERD (gastroesophageal reflux disease)) [24, 25].

The interaction of chemical (acidic substances), behavioral, and biologic factors with tooth surfaces over time determines development and severity of DE [26]. *Intrinsic sources* of acid include GERD, frequent vomiting, eating disorders, chronic regurgitation, and rumination [21, 27, 28]. *Extrinsic sources* include medicaments (e.g., effervescent or chewable tablets) and dietary products (fruit juice, carbonated and sports drinks, acidic foods), which are now recognized as the leading cause of erosive lesions in children and adolescents [21, 29–31]. Carbonated drinks typically contain citric acid, phosphoric acid, and sodium citrate, which all have high erosive potential [30].

Behavioral factors include eating, drinking, or swallowing practices that increase the frequency or prolong the contact of dietary products in the mouth [20, 21, 28]. CSHCN who require frequent intake of high-calorie products and rehydrating drinks due to nutritional needs may hold or pouch foods in the mouth for a long period of time. This may lead to DE and dental caries. The timing of exposure also has influence on the erosive effect. Drinks used in a bottle during sleep times have a high tendency to cause DE because low salivary flow decreases protection against erosion. Similarly, at times of dehydration (e.g., during sports practice), the dry oral tissues are more vulnerable to the destructive activity of acidic beverages [29].

Biological factors, such as saliva, can also change the individual's risk for DE. Saliva has important protective functions including formation of dental pellicle, buffering capacity, clearance, and remineralization activity. Therefore, reduction of the salivary flow rate is directly associated with decrease in bicarbonate levels that can lead to lower buffering capacity and pH [20, 21, 26]. Certain medications (e.g., antiemetics, antihistamines, tranquilizers, and antiparkinsonian drugs) can also decrease the salivary flow. A direct correlation between drugs used to treat asthma and DE has not been consistently confirmed [21, 32, 33].

Erosive lesions produced by gastric acid characteristically start on the palatal surfaces of maxillary incisors and later affect maxillary premolars and molars. In advanced stages, DE can involve occlusal surfaces and mandibular teeth [21, 28]. As a result of the erosive process, the enamel becomes thinner, silky, glazed, and with less pronounced tooth surface anatomy [21, 26]. A characteristic cupping of cusp tips and incisal edges occurs as DE progresses, and over time chipping of the thinned enamel can occur. At later stages, dentin exposure and loss of occlusal morphology may appear. Erosive lesions are usually wide and shallow, with hard, smooth surfaces and rounded boundaries [21, 27].

The diagnosis of DE is based on a thorough evaluation of the patient's medical and dental history as well as on clinical examination of the lesion appearance and pattern of tooth surface loss. A comprehensive dietary analysis may be required to establish extrinsic acid sources. If an intrinsic source or xerostomia is suspected, a prompt referral to the patient's physician is necessary because an effective medical therapy can limit the associated risk factors and complement dental management.

Prevention efforts can be customized to each patient and should be directed at control and limitation of the known DE etiology [20, 21]. Medical referral can help with management of GERD, modification of dietary choices, and reduction of harmful habits and behaviors. Dental management involves enhancement of protective factors and improvement of salivary mechanisms. Topical application of fluoride agents and remineralizing products [e.g., casein phosphopeptide–amorphous calcium phosphate (CPP–ACP)] [22] can improve the resistance of the tooth structures to acidic challenges. Regular patient recall for professional fluoride therapy and prescription of high-concentration (5000 ppm) fluoride toothpaste can also help prevent DE [21, 27, 28].

Oral rehabilitation is indicated for restoration of dental defects, alleviation of tooth sensitivity, pulpal symptomatology, and restoration of occlusion and vertical dimension. In both primary and permanent dentitions, small lesions can be managed with composite resin restorations, while larger defects in posterior teeth may require preformed metal crowns. Resin-modified glass ionomer cements also present a restorative choice in CSHCN due to the ease of placement and continuous fluoride release. Another advantage is that tooth preparation can be minimal. Deciduous incisors can be treated with strip crowns or prefabricated esthetic crowns (zirconia or pre-veneered stainless-steel crowns). Anterior permanent teeth with advanced DE can be managed with direct composite veneers or adult strip crowns. In the permanent dentition, restorative interventions should only be initiated after adequate assessment of occlusal clearance in intercuspal position [28]. In cases of advanced DE with insufficient clearance, rehabilitation of the occlusal vertical dimension can be required. After reaching skeletal maturity, permanent restorative solutions, such as porcelain crowns and veneers, become available. An interdisciplinary approach with involvement of a restorative specialist and orthodontist may also be necessary in severe cases of DE.

Xerostomia

Normal salivary function is essential for good oral health. Saliva is a vital component in protection against oral infection, tooth remineralization, and digestion; it also supports chewing, swallowing, and speech [34]. It has been estimated that healthy children have stimulated salivary flow rate of at least 1 ml/min, a value that is greater than the adult norm (0.7 ml/min) [35]. Xerostomia, or dry mouth, refers to the subjective perception of reduced moisture in oral cavity. Potential causes of xerostomia include mouth breathing, dehydration, medications, salivary gland disorders, or medical conditions affecting salivation [36]. These risk factors are more common in pediatric patients with special needs, for whom xerostomia can be a frequent oral health concern.

Dry mouth can be a transient or persistent sign of dehydration, which may occur in diarrhea (due to food intolerance, Crohn's disease, bacterial or viral infection) or vomiting (due to psychogenic or eating disorders) [36]. Children with diabetes mellitus can present with complaints of xerostomia because of polyuria, especially if glycemic control is poor [37]. Patients who are mouth breathers usually present dry mucosa in the hard palate and the anterior maxilla [36]. Xerostomia is also a known side effect of certain medications, such as anticholinergics, antidepressants, antipsychotic agents, diuretics, antihypertensive drugs, sedatives, anxiolytics, muscle relaxants, analgesics (opioids and nonsteroidal anti-inflammatories), bronchodilators, and antihistamines [38]. Furthermore, cytotoxic chemotherapeutic drugs used in children with malignancies damage the acinar salivary gland cells and directly decrease the salivary output. Similarly, radiotherapy with local field or total body irradiation can cause xerostomia that may last long after cancer treatment [36, 39]. Disorders that directly affect the salivary glands and lead to impaired function include Sjogren's syndrome, ectodermal dysplasia, partial or total salivary gland agenesis, and HIV infection. The parotid gland is most frequently affected in children [36, 38].

The diagnosis of xerostomia can be established after a thorough medical history evaluation and clinical examination. Attention should be given to associated symptoms and reported medications. Usual patient complaints include dry mouth, altered taste, and difficulty with swallowing and speaking. In epidemiological studies, various standardized questionnaires have been proposed to aid clinical diagnosis [40]. Objective chairside methods include measuring stimulated and unstimulated salivary flow by spitting or suctioning methods and absorbent tips [36]. Samples for biologic, microbiological, immunologic, and chemical analyses may be required as well as the use of imaging modalities (radiography, sialography, computed tomography, magnetic resonance, or radionuclide imaging) [36, 40]. In CSHCN with behavioral challenges, performing clinical testing may be difficult. Pathognomonic signs can be helpful in making a diagnosis of hyposalivation. These may include frothy or sticky saliva, lack of pooling in floor of mouth, depapillation of the dorsum of the tongue, glassy oral mucosa and palate, smooth gingival architecture, and fissured tongue (Fig. 3) [41]. Patients with xerostomia are at increased risk of rampant caries and dental erosion.

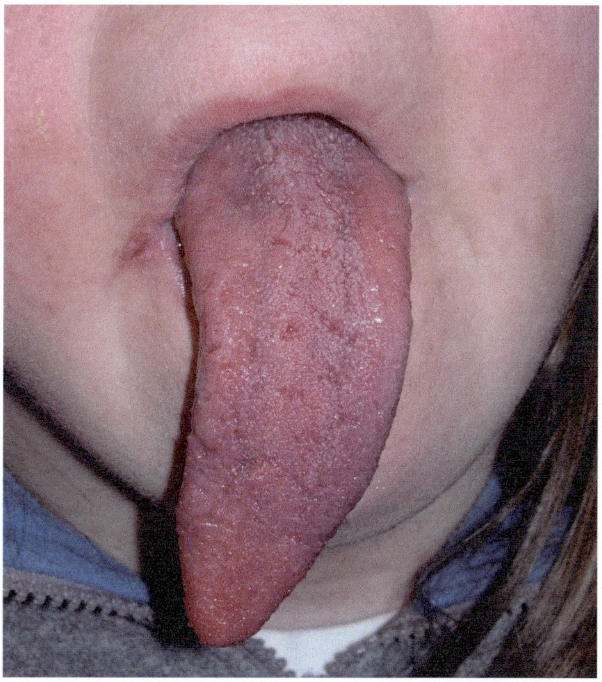

Fig. 3 Macroglossia, angular cheilitis, and fissured tongue in a patient with Trisomy 21

Management strategies for xerostomia aim to reduce symptoms and increase salivary flow rate. These measures should be customized according to the specific etiology and individual risk factors. Assuring appropriate hydration levels through frequent intake of fluids and increase in humidity levels during sleep is important. Patients should also avoid irritating oral hygiene products and foods with a hard consistency or strong flavors. Sugar-free chewing gum and xylitol candy are useful to stimulate salivation [40, 42]. Lemon drops should be used judiciously because of the potential to develop dental caries. Management of mouth breathing (e.g., orthodontic therapy for malocclusions, tonsillectomy and adenoidectomy, exercise and physiotherapy for facial muscle hypotonia) should be done in applicable cases. Pharmacological management includes prescription of mucosal lubricants, saliva substitutes, and saliva stimulants (systemic and oral sialagogues) [40, 42]. Saliva substitutes contain minerals (fluoride, calcium, and phosphate) and carboxymethylcellulose or hydroxyethylcellulose, which increase viscosity and imitate natural saliva without altering the existing flow [40]. In cases where the patient's regular medications are causing hyposalivation, the dental professional should consult with the patient's physician. The physician may be able to provide a replacement medication with a less xerogenic potential or consider a dose reduction to levels that do not cause dry mouth [36, 40].

Sialorrhea

Sialorrhea (drooling or ptyalism) refers to unintentional saliva leakage outside of the mouth [43]. It is a debilitating and challenging symptom in CSHCN. Drooling is considered normal physiological phenomenon in healthy infants. It typically diminishes by 1.5–3 years of age, at the time of maturation of orofacial motor functions [43]. Persisting beyond age of 4 years, the salivary incontinence is deemed pathological [44].

Sialorrhea can be either a sign of overproduction of saliva (hypersalivation) or caused by dysfunctions in the orofacial neuromuscular systems responsible for normal swallowing [45].

Healthy swallowing reflex is essential for the continuous saliva clearance from the oral cavity. The mechanism of swallowing results from a series of coordinated movements of orofacial structures, including skeletal muscles (tongue, masticatory, and palatal complex), smooth muscles (pharynx, esophagus), and bones (mandible, hyoid) [46]. It consists of oral, pharyngeal, and esophageal phase, each with different neurological regulation [43]. The medial temporal lobes and limbic system of the cerebral cortex are responsible for the voluntary control of the oral phase. The swallowing center in medulla oblongata and pons is active during the pharyngeal swallow. Cranial nerves V, VII, IX, and X play a part by carrying impulses to salivary nuclei [43]. The autonomic nervous system also coordinates both the pharyngeal and esophageal phases [46]. Medical conditions leading to impairment of any orofacial structure or neurological regulator can cause sialorrhea. Drooling can be an isolated entity or present in concurrence with other disorders. Common etiology associated with drooling is summarized in Table 1 [43, 47].

Table 1 Etiology associated with sialorrhea

Neurological conditions	Syndromes	Orofacial deficits	Other
• Cerebral palsy • Amyotrophic lateral sclerosis • Cerebrovascular trauma/accident • Stroke • Parkinson's disease • Congenital suprabulbar paralysis • Encephalitis • Hypoxic encephalopathy • Severe mental retardation • Hydrocephalus	• Down syndrome • Worster–Drought syndrome • Landau–Kleffner syndrome • Angelman's syndrome • Freeman–Sheldon syndrome • Moebius syndrome	• Severe malocclusion (anterior open bite, increased overjet) • Tongue thrust • Lip incompetency (poor muscle control) • Congenital or acquired tongue deformities • Advanced dental ridge resorption	• Idiopathic • Side effect of therapeutic medication—clozapine • Painful swallowing caused by infectious diseases (herpes virus, coxsackie virus, etc.) • Unfavorable head posture • Nasal obstruction

Sialorrhea is a relatively common clinical complaint in CSHCN [47]. About 28% of children with neurological conditions permanently suffer from drooling [48]. Neurologic diseases cause sialorrhea by the mechanism of impaired swallowing. Examples are cerebral palsy, amyotrophic lateral sclerosis, cerebrovascular trauma, stroke, Parkinson's disease, congenital suprabulbar paralysis, some forms of encephalitis, hypoxic encephalopathy, severe mental retardation, and hydrocephalus [49]. In children, drooling is most typical for cerebral palsy with reported 58% of the patients affected [50]. In adults, saliva incontinence is observed in Parkinson's disease at a rate of about 47% [51].

Hypersalivation can be idiopathic or caused by side effects of therapeutic medication. The antipsychotic drug clozapine is known to cause saliva overproduction in 30–80% of the patents [52]. Cases of drooling associated with difficulties in swallowing can be observed even in patients with reduced saliva output [49]. Sialorrhea can occur in some rare syndromes including Moebius syndrome, Angelman syndrome, Freeman–Sheldon syndrome, or Landau–Kleffner syndrome [43, 47].

Regardless of its etiology, drooling is problematic and distressful for patients and caregivers. It can lead to clinical, functional, and social impairment. The constant wetting of the skin and clothing is associated with physical discomfort, requirement for continuous care, and social stigma. Drooling can cause perioral skin irritation and infection (*Candida albicans*). It interferes with speech and mastication and leads to loss of fluid and electrolytes. Patients who drool due to dysphagia are also at increased risk of aspiration and aspiration pneumonia [43, 47].

It is recognized that management of sialorrhea is challenging and typically requires interdisciplinary approach. Appropriate treatment modalities include conservative and invasive methods, which should be chosen carefully with consideration to the specific etiology of the problem. The available management options are summarized in Table 2 [47, 53].

Table 2 Common treatment modalities for drooling

Conservative methods
• *Oral motor therapy*—aims at developing and/or improving oral motor skills (lip continence, sucking, tongue and jaw movements). It can be done in conjunction with appropriate speech therapy and physiotherapy. "Chin cup" appliance, placing pressure on the chin to achieve anterior oral seal, has been described useful in specific cases
• *Behavioral modification via biofeedback*—aims at training patients to swallow when prompt by an auditory signal. Utilizes a series of exercises combined with auditory electromyography feedback with electrodes placed on the orbicularis oris muscle. It is recommended for older children (8 years of age and older) with good intellectual function, well-motivated, and with moderate drooling problems
• *Orofacial regulation therapy*—involves the use of various custom-made or prefabricated functional appliances with vestibular and/or lingual stimulators ("buttons" and "beads" added to standard acrylic base plates), acting as active components that induce movements of the oral musculature. For example, a lingual button that stimulates sucking strengthens hypotonic perioral musculature and helps to achieve tongue retrusion
Therapeutic medication and minimally invasive methods
• *Anticholinergic medicaments* (cholinergic muscarinic receptor antagonists), such as atropine, scopolamine/hyoscine, and glycopyrronium bromide can be prescribed to reduce the saliva production
Oral or topical (dermal patch) application can be considered
Contraindicated in patients with cardiac disease, pyloric obstruction, glaucoma, paralytic ileus, and prostate hypertrophy
The dose should be considered carefully as these drugs can lead to dry mouth, constipation, blurred vision, urinary retention, irritability, and confusion
Systemic side effects and potential drug-to-drug interactions should be evaluated before use
• *Botulinum toxin injections*
The botulinum toxin is a potent neurotoxin that blocks the release of acetylcholine
Three types A and one type B botulinum toxin (onabotulinumtoxinA, abobotulinumtoxinA, incobotulinumtoxinA, and rimabotulinumtoxinB) are used therapeutically
The injections are given percutaneously in the parotid and submandibular glands
Ultrasound guidance can improve the efficacy and safety of the application. Sedation or general anesthesia may be required for managing behavior in young children
The result typically lasts between 6 weeks and 6 months
Side effects include facial and muscle weakness (due to diffusion of the botulinum toxin in into masseter or pharyngeal muscles) with associated difficulty of chewing, swallowing, and risk of aspiration, risk of local infection or hematoma at the side of injection, salivary duct calculi, and facial nerve injury
Surgical management
• Surgery is irreversible and should be undertaken only in severe cases where other alternatives have been proved unsuccessful
• Various surgical procedures have been proposed, utilizing three main approaches
Interventions leading to reduction of saliva production: transtympanic neurectomy, salivary gland excision, and blocking the flow of saliva into the mouth (duct ligation)
Procedures rerouting the site of saliva ejection in the oral cavity: bilateral submandibular gland relocation, duct ligation, combination of submandibular gland duct relocation, and sublingual gland excision
Combinations of the above-described methods

Addressing situational factors, such as unfavorable head position, airway issues, and/or orthodontic anomalies, is first line of management [47]. A medical consultation for possible correction of the cause or altering prescribed medication should also be considered in applicable cases. The management modalities for drooling are introduced gradually from conservative and minimally invasive to more aggressive options, depending on patient response and severity of the issue. Physiological modalities, such as oral motor therapy, behavior modification, or orofacial regulation therapy, may prove sufficient in alleviating sialorrhea in certain cases [47]. If these approaches fail, anticholinergic medication or injections with botulinum toxin can be explored. Surgical interventions are irreversible and should be undertaken only in severe cases where other alternatives have been proven unsuccessful. Radiotherapy to salivary glands to reduce saliva production is not recommended in children due to increased risk of malignancies. Regular dental recall is paramount in all cases and particularly where the management of drooling involves significant reduction in salivary output.

Temporomandibular Disorders

Temporomandibular disorder (TMD) is a group of conditions affecting the temporomandibular joint (TMJ), the muscles of mastication, and the associated anatomical structures [54]. The umbrella term encompasses various masticatory system dysfunctions including muscle disorders, inflammatory and degenerative TMJ problems, and disk displacements (Table 3). Typical symptoms portray pain in the affected anatomical structures, headaches, joint sounds, deviations, and restrictions of the TMJ movements [55, 56].

TMDs are more common in adults, and the prevalence is known to increase with age. Signs and symptoms are reported with various frequencies in children, with an estimated overall prevalence range of 16–68% [56–58]. There is a lack of data in special needs populations; however, they frequently present with conditions associated with the TMD etiology (Table 4) and may be more at risk for the disorder. For

Table 3 Masticatory system dysfunctions

Temporomandibular joint disorders	Masticatory muscle disorders
• Arthralgia—synovitis, capsulitis, retrodiscitis • Disk displacement—with or without reduction • Joint hypermobility—subluxation, luxation • Joint hypomobility—fibrous changes, ankylosis • Osteoarthritis • Systemic arthritis • Neoplasms • Fractures	• Orofacial muscle pain—myalgia, tendonitis, myositis, spasm • Central disorders—centrally mediated myalgia, fibromyalgia • Dyskinesia, dystonia • Contracture • Hypertrophy • Neoplasm

Table 4 Common etiologies of temporomandibular disorders

Traumatic injuries to the lower jaw • Force impact to the chin Fractures of the mandible—particularly unilateral and bilateral intracapsular or subcondylar fractures • Inadequate management resulting in ankylosis (prolonged immobilization) or facial asymmetry
Microtrauma from parafunctional habits: • Bruxism • Clenching • Hyperextension • Repetitive habitual behaviors associated with overloading of the TMJ
Anatomical specifics: • Craniofacial anomalies • Congenital deformities and developmental abnormalities (aplasia or hypoplasia of the mandibular condyle) • Anatomical malformations/abnormalities of the mandibular fossa, condyle, ramus, and disk • Steep articular eminence of the temporal bone • Malocclusions Skeletal anterior open bite Posterior crossbite Class III malocclusion Overjet greater than 6 mm
Systemic causes • Connective tissue diseases: Rheumatoid arthritis Systemic lupus erythematosus Juvenile idiopathic arthritis Psoriatic arthritis • Joint hypermobility (e.g. Ehler–Danlos syndrome) • Genetic susceptibility
Psychosocial factors—may cause parafunctional habits • Emotional stress • Depression, anxiety • Sleep dysfunction

example, signs and symptoms related to TMJ issues were found to be significantly more common in a group of adolescents with intellectual disability than in matched healthy controls [59].

The etiology of TMD is complex with implicated functional, structural, and psychological causes. The multifactorial nature of TMD makes direct correlation between symptoms and diagnosis difficult. Changes affecting single or multiple teeth, occlusal relationships, periodontal ligament, TMJ, or masticatory muscles along with systemic and psychosocial problems can reduce the temporomandibular apparatus adaptive ability and lead to TMD [60, 61].

Diagnosis is established upon taking a thorough patient history, clinical assessment, and imaging tests (panoramic and lateral cephalometric radiographs, computed TMJ tomography, cone beam computed tomography, and magnetic resonance imaging). Standardized questionnaires for TMD screening have been proposed for detailing of symptom information [56, 60]. Physical evaluation consists of palpation of the masticatory and cervical muscles for areas of tenderness, palpation of the TMJ lateral capsule for condyle positioning, auscultation of joint sounds, and assessment of the mandibular range of movements (in maximum opening, lateral, and protrusive excursion). Achieving an accurate diagnosis is essential for successful management [60, 61].

TMD management strategies are focused on reduction/elimination of pain, improvement of function, and ultimately of the patient's quality of life [62, 63]. These include reversible (conservative) and irreversible methods of care. The treatment can be further categorized into active, requiring patient participation, and passive, which is independent of compliance. Often, due to the multifactorial etiology of TMD, complex management is required rather than a single therapeutic modality. Conservative approaches include:

- Patient education and behavioral management—such as modifying habits, training in relaxation, conscious avoidance of excessive jaw movements, and strategies to improve sleep
- Physical therapy—such as muscle exercise regimens, application of transcutaneous electrical nerve stimulation, massage, thermo-/coolant therapy, iontophoresis, and ultrasound
- Therapeutic medication—nonsteroidal anti-inflammatories, muscle relaxants, and anxiolytics
- Occlusal splints, which reduce parafunctional habits due to occlusion alteration, providing orthopedic stability of the TMJ [62, 63]

Pharmacological therapy should be discussed in advance with the patient's healthcare provider. Comorbidities and potential drug interactions should be taken into consideration. Occlusal adjustments and orthodontic/orthognathic management are irreversible treatment modalities. Occlusal discrepancies of single teeth or tooth groups can be adjusted with selective hard surface grinding or dental restorations (intracoronal or full coverage solutions).

Orthodontic therapy can eliminate malocclusions that may compound TMD [62, 63]. In cases of craniofacial deformities, complex orthognathic and plastic surgery may be required for successful management. In selected cases with muscular etiology, botulinum toxin A injections can be considered for muscle relaxation [64].

Some TMD disorders can be progressive, so early diagnosis and management of the TMD is important in CSHCN who are still growing. Early intervention may help limit irreversible changes, abnormal craniofacial growth, or mandibular dysfunction into adult life [63].

Hypodontia and Hyperdontia

Hypodontia and hyperdontia are developmental dental anomalies that affect the normal number in a dentition. These defects are consequence of the action of various etiological factors (genetic and environmental) during the initiation and proliferation stage of tooth development [65].

Hyperdontia defines a dentition with teeth in excess of the normal number, also known as supernumerary teeth (SN) [66]. It is hypothesized that localized areas of increased dental lamina activity may cause either its lingual extension to develop an accessory tooth bud (supplemental SN) or its epithelial remnants to proliferate (rudimentary SN) [66, 67]. SN appear more often in family members, indicating genetic predisposition. Incidence in primary dentition is estimated to be 0.3–0.8% (with no gender predilection), and in the permanent dentition, it is 0.1–3.8%, where males are twice as likely to be affected as females [68]. It has been reported that SN commonly occur along with other developmental tooth anomalies, *dens in dente* and *macrodontia* in particular [66, 68]. Increased prevalence of SN is seen in patients with cleidocranial dysplasia, Gardner's syndrome, and cleft lip and palate. Other syndromes with high SN association are Goldenhar, Hallermann–Streiff, incontinentia pigmenti, oro-facial-digital syndrome type I, Ellis–Van Creveld, Ehlers–Danlos type III, Marfan, Nance–Horan, and trichorhinophalangeal syndrome 1 [66].

SN may appear in singles or multiples, with unilateral or bilateral presentation. Hyperdontia can develop in any part of the jaws, more frequently in the anterior maxilla, followed by the mandibular premolar areas. SN are classified by location and morphology (Table 5) [65–68]. The eruption path (normal, altered, or impacted) depends on tooth orientation and morphology [69]. Up to 34% of permanent SN will erupt, compared with 73% of primary SN [67].

Diagnosis is based on patient history, clinical examination, and imaging. Asymptomatic SN may be an incidental radiographic finding. Common clinical situations that may prompt SN investigation are unilateral persistence of deciduous teeth, failure of eruption of successor, wide diastema, or malposition of maxillary incisors [68]. Three-dimensional localization of SN can be established with standard radiographs using the vertical and/or horizontal parallax technique or from cone beam computed tomography. SN may negatively affect

Table 5 Classification of supernumerary teeth

Morphology	Location
Conical • Triangular or conical (peg) shape • Located between upper central incisors *Tuberculate* • Barrel-shaped appearance • Located palatal to maxillary incisors *Supplemental* • Shape and size of a normal tooth • Located at end of tooth series *Odontome/Odontoma* (hamartoma) • Compound: composed of tooth-like structures • Complex: mass of disordered mature dental tissues	*Mesiodens* • Palatal to maxillary incisors • Rarely in buccal or horizontal position *Paramolar* • Rudimentary SN molar • Buccal or palatal to last molar in arch *Distomolar* • Rudimentary SN molar • Located distal to last molar in arch *Parapremolar* • Similar shape and size to a premolar • Located in premolar region

adjacent teeth and structures and can also develop their own clinical complications (Table 6) [66, 68–70].

Indications and timing for treatment are based on SN orientation and position, patient age, and associated complications. Conservative management, including monitoring and periodic radiographic assessment, is considered in asymptomatic cases with SN and unaffected adjacent structures. Management decisions regarding erupted SN are based on their morphology, alignment, and arch space requirements [65, 67]. Routine extraction is typically undertaken; however, supplemental erupted SN of proper shape and size may be kept if associated with a healthy and functional dentition. Patients with impacted and/or multiple SN are managed using an interdisciplinary approach. This may involve input from pediatric dentists, orthodontists, and oral surgeons. Surgical extraction is recommended for unerupted SN causing complications. Evidence demonstrates that 91% of teeth with impeded eruption due to SN will erupt spontaneously within 18 months of SN removal [71]. Otherwise, such teeth may require bonded gold chain and orthodontic traction. There is controversy about the ideal time for removal of impacted SN. Some authors advocate early intervention to prevent risk of complications, while others are concerned with potential surgical damage to adjacent immature teeth. Recent literature supports removal of anterior region SN at 6–7 years of age [72]. In patients with cleft palate, SN in the cleft area are extracted at the time of bone graft surgery for cleft closure. Once diagnosed cases should be observed for additional late forming SN [65, 68].

Congenitally missing teeth (CMT) result from developmental dental agenesis.

- *Hypodontia* is the presence of five or fewer teeth.
- *Oligodontia* is defined as six or more missing teeth (excluding wisdom teeth).
- *Anodontia* indicates complete absence of teeth [73].

Tooth agenesis can be caused by physical obstruction of the dental lamina, lack of sufficient space for tooth development, or failure in initiation of the underlying

Table 6 Clinical complications of supernumerary teeth

Problems with adjacent teeth/ structures	Problems with supernumerary teeth
Adjacent permanent teeth • Delayed or impeded eruption • Malposition, displacement • Dilacerations/ root development problems • Root resorption Space related issues • Overcrowding, space opening (wide diastema) • Obstacle for sufficient space closure during orthodontic treatment	• Cyst formation (4–9% of impacted SN) • Migration into the nasal cavity, maxillary sinus, or hard palate (rare) • Late-forming SN: patients with early history of anterior SN may have additional late developing SN particularly in premolar region (incidence of 24%)

mesenchyme. Genetic and local factors are implicated in the trigger, but the exact etiology remains unclear [74]. Examples of local factors include radiation and chemotherapy at early age, hormonal and metabolic local disturbances, osteomyelitis, trauma, and accidental removal of successors. CMT may occur as part of a genetic syndrome or as non-syndromic isolated trait [75]. Hypodontia is relatively common, whereas non-syndromic oligo-/anodontia are rare. The prevalence of hypodontia is 0.1–2.4% in the primary and 0.15–16.2% in permanent dentitions [75]. Maxillary and mandibular lateral incisors are the most frequently missing deciduous teeth. Mandibular second premolars, maxillary lateral incisors, maxillary second premolars, and mandibular incisors are commonly affected permanent teeth [73]. Deciduous hypodontia usually is associated with hypodontia in the secondary dentition and may also affect other tooth groups [74, 76]. Hypodontia often presents together with microdontia. Missing maxillary lateral incisors are linked to ectopic maxillary canines, both with similar genetic pattern [76]. Hypodontia is also associated with other dental anomalies including delayed formation and eruption of teeth, short roots, infraocclusion of primary molars, ectopic eruption of teeth, taurodontism, rotation of incisors and premolars, and developmental enamel defects [73, 75]. Over 80 different syndromes/conditions have CMT, such as ectodermal dysplasias (the most common reason for syndromic oligodontias), Van der Woude syndrome, oro-facial-digital syndrome type I, Rieger syndrome, incontinentia pigmenti, Down syndrome, and cleft lip and palate [73, 75].

Diagnosis of CMT is based on patient and family history combined with clinical and radiographic examination to confirm tooth absence beyond the time of expected developmental age range. Cases with multiple CMT should be further investigated for potential syndromic etiology (if previously undiagnosed) with an appropriate referral to medical and genetic services. Alveolar processes in the areas of CMT may be underdeveloped, narrow, with reduced vertical height, and lower face height. Microdontia associated with hypodontia has poorer abutment potential for restorations. Retained primary teeth without successors may develop attrition and/or become submerged, allowing for tipping of the adjacent teeth or over-eruption of the opposing teeth [73, 77].

Depending on the severity, CMT can present a treatment challenge and require a well-coordinated interdisciplinary team approach. Hypo-/oligodontia can also negatively affect the patient's oral health-related quality of life [73]. Specialist expertise from pediatric dentistry, orthodontics, prosthodontics, oral surgery, and psychology may be required in complex cases. Management strategies include maintenance of the existing dentition, facilitation of oral functions (mastication, speech), and improvement of dental esthetics. Restorative options depend on the patient's age, severity of the condition, required timing of interventions, orthodontic management, and financial factors. Fixed and long-term restorations are considered upon completion of patient's growth. Removable partial dentures, composite veneers, and resin-bonded bridges are available interim options. Space management in hypodontia is essential [74, 77]. Treatment of jaw relationship problems, overcrowding and space distribution should be completed before considering final restorations and implant placements. Some early interceptive measures may alleviate potential problems. Once growth is complete, implants and implant-supported prostheses can be planned [73, 77].

Developmental Defects of Enamel

Developmental defects of enamel (DDE) refer to a group of qualitative and quantitative enamel abnormalities caused by aberrations in amelogenesis. These conditions represent irreversible changes, as once mineralized the enamel structure cannot remodel [78]. Enamel phenotypes depend on severity, onset, and duration of the disturbance and are often associated with multiple causes [79].

Various genetic, epigenetic, and environmental (local and systemic) factors can disturb normal developmental enamel pathways [79]. DDE can be caused by sporadic mutations of *genes* coding for matrix proteins, or it can be part of inherited systemic conditions—where multiple structures of common origin are affected [80]. Furthermore, DDE can be related to congenital disorders that have a similar genetic pathway to amelogenesis (e.g., parathyroid gland abnormalities) [78]. Genetic factors produce generalized defects that are unrelated to particular periods of tooth formation. *Epigenetics* refers to external influences that can regulate gene expression. Acquired DDE are the result of local and systemic *environmental insults*, such as infection, medicaments, exposure to chemicals, trauma, metabolic disturbances, and radiation (Table 7) [78, 79]. Local environmental factors are

Table 7 Acquired (environmental) risk factors for dental developmental defects

	Systemic		
Local	Prenatal	Perinatal	Postnatal
• Local trauma (intrusion/avulsion of predecessor) • Tooth in line of jaw fracture • Instrumental pressure trauma during laryngoscopy • Electric burns • Ankylosis of predecessor • Long-lasting periradicular infection of predecessor • Congenital epulis • Teeth in area of clefts • Therapeutic irradiation	• Anemia, Pregnancy toxemia • Pregnancy toxemia • Cardiac disease • Congenital syphilis • *Cytomegalovirus* infections • Rubella infections • Maternal diabetes • Fluoride (excess) • Thalidomide • Hypoxia • Malnutrition, vitamin A and D deficiency • Vitamin A and D deficiency • Renal disease • Urinary tract infections	• Low birth weight • Prematurity • Neonatal asphyxia • Hypocalcemia • Respiratory distress syndrome • Tetanus • Traumatic birth injuries • Bile duct defects • Breech presentation • Erythroblastosis fetalis • Hemolytic disorder • Hepatitis	• Adrenal, thyroid, hypothyroid hyper-/hypofunction • Cytotoxic medications • Fluoride (excess) • Poliomyelitis • Encephalitis • Pneumonia • Otitis media • Endocrinopathies, neurological disorders • Neurological disorders • Congenital cardiac disease • Gastrointestinal disturbances • Intestinal lymphangiectasis • Measles • Mumps • Diphtheria • Chickenpox • Nephrotic syndrome • Renal dysfunction • Sickle cell anemia • Vitamin A, C, and D deficiency • Vitamin D intoxication

associated with DDE of a single tooth or groups of adjacent teeth and tend to have asymmetrical distribution in the dentition. Systemic factors (prenatal, perinatal, and postnatal) produce chronological defects, which depend on the timing of the insult. Affected teeth develop concurrently, thus showing a symmetric distribution. With long-standing systemic causes, the resultant enamel defect will be generalized [79]. CSHCN have increased risk of the DDE due to many potential risk factors.

Despite the array of potential causes, DDE have limited phenotype expressions [78].

Enamel hypoplasia is DDE with reduced enamel quantity. It presents as pits, grooves, or wider areas of thin or missing enamel and is caused by disturbance of the stage of matrix formation and secretion [78].

Enamel hypomineralization is a qualitative defect with deficiency in mineral content evident as diffuse or demarcated opacities (altered enamel translucency) with white, yellow, or brown discoloration, affecting various tooth surface areas [78].

Hypomineralization results from abnormal processes of mineralization and maturation (inadequate removal of matrix proteins) [78]. Due to a structural weakness, teeth with enamel hypomineralization are vulnerable to posteruptive enamel breakdown (PEB) that leads to further loss of enamel and can clinically resemble a hypoplastic defect. Distinction between the two types of DDE is based on assessment of areas with lack of enamel. In PEB, the remaining structure is softer with sharp borders of the defect, while hypoplastic enamel tends to appear of harder consistency and smoother margins.

Amelogenesis imperfecta (AI) is a group of inherited heterogeneous conditions affecting the structure and appearance of the dental enamel in a uniform manner of all teeth in both dentitions. AI can be expressed as hypoplasia, hypomineralization, or a combination of the two. Some AI variants are less clinically evident in the primary dentition [81]. Conditions associated with AI include tricho-dento-osseous syndrome, cone-rod dystrophy, Kohlschutter syndrome, McGibbon syndrome, vitamin D-resistant rickets, and autoimmune polyendocrinopathy [81].

Examples of acquired DDE with systemic origin include fluorosis, molar incisor hypomineralization (MIH), and chronological hypoplasia. Fluorosis is a qualitative DDE, resulting from an increase in fluoride concentration within the microenvironment of the ameloblasts during enamel formation. MIH is a hypomineralization defect that affects (1) permanent first molars and incisors and (2) primary second molars and canines.

The clinical diagnosis of DDE includes taking a careful family and patient history, medical background (identification of potential systemic disturbances), pedigree plotting (suspected genetic factors), intraoral examination of hard tissues, and identification of possible DDE phenotypes. Radiographic assessment can provide evidence by comparing the radiopacity of affected enamel in comparison with adjacent hard structures. Hypomineralized DDE tend to have radiolucency closer to that of dentine or bone, whereas hypoplastic enamel has a more radiopaque appearance—similar to normal tooth structure.

Patient complaints of DDE include reduced esthetics, sensitive teeth, and loss of tooth structure due to wear or PEB. The severe generalized DDE types may also have significant psychosocial impact on a patient's well-being. Early diagnosis and a clear care plan are important for an optimal outcome. Cases of AI or other generalized DDE may require interdisciplinary management involving a pediatric dentist, orthodontist, and restorative specialist. Early preventative regimens should be established, as the defective and rough enamel structure inherently presents with increased risk for plaque accumulation, caries development, and compromised gingival health [78]. Professional application of topical fluorides, use of toothpaste with optimum levels fluoride, CPP–ACP products, and dietary modification must be implemented early. Rigorous hygiene instruction with professional maintenance is important for the success of future orthodontic and restorative treatment.

The main aims of oral rehabilitation are improving esthetics, reducing sensitivity, correcting or maintaining vertical dimension, and restoring masticatory function. Localized DDE may require fewer interventions with restoration limited to affected surfaces with basic dental materials. Generalized DDE may involve more planning. Typically, preformed metal crowns offer a durable restorative option that can be placed for severely affected posterior teeth in a single visit. For anterior teeth, direct composite veneers, composite strip crowns, or prefabricated esthetic crowns offer durable and effective solutions. Bonding with adhesive restorations may present as a challenge in some qualitative DDE. Pre-treating of qualitative DDE with 5% sodium hypochlorite may produce better results due to removal of acid-insoluble proteins surrounding the crystals in the defective enamel [82]. Minimal interventions, such as microabrasion or bleaching, can be sufficient for esthetic improvement in mild cases.

Case-Based Scenario

A 16-year-old Caucasian male presented for dental assessment at a hospital-based specialist dental clinic [83]. The patient was referred by his neurologist for management of a cheek-biting habit with a history of a 10-month duration and previous unsuccessful treatment attempts. The chief complaint was pain and persistent ulceration of the lining of the patient's left cheek caused by self-injury.

The medical background included bilateral thalamic venous angiomas, hydrocephalus with ventriculoperitoneal shunt, significant developmental delay, increased body mass index (overweight), and spasticity. He also had a history of brain hemorrhage and utilized a wheelchair. The list of regular medications was comprised of baclofen, olanzapine, fluvoxamine, and bupropion hydrochloride. No known drug allergies were reported.

The extraoral examination revealed dystonic posturing of the neck with an associated reduced ability of the oral musculature to perform voluntary movements. Intraorally, the patient presented with poor oral hygiene, generalized plaque-induced gingivitis, and permanent dentition with multiple carious lesions. He showed Class I malocclusion with moderate overcrowding in both arches, normal overjet, and no overbite.

The examination of the left buccal mucosa revealed an open ulceration consistent with soft tissue trauma caused by persistent, uncontrolled biting (Fig. 4). This self-injurious behavior (SIB) resulted in pain and functional disturbances of normal eating and swallowing. Previous attempts to limit the biting habit included an acrylic occlusal splint and composite resin buildups of occlusal surfaces of the maxillary premolars and molars. However, the patient's strong biting force had led to breakage of both the acrylic splint and the buildups.

After clinical examination, thorough professional oral hygiene, and instructions for appropriate home care, a treatment plan was customized to achieve a complete oral rehabilitation. To address the biting habit, a modified Hawley appliance with lateral shields to protect the buccal mucosa was custom designed (Figs. 5 and 6).

Alginate impressions were obtained at the initial visit, and the appliance was delivered at the subsequent appointment. The primary retention of the modified Hawley retainer was achieved via a labial bow and ball clasps. The shields and the bow were reinforced with extra solder and acrylic placed on the internal surface of the shields. The patient showed adequate dental cooperation and was able to wear the appliance as instructed (at all times, including eating with removal only for cleaning). Healing of the ulceration was noted at the 1-week follow-up and the lesion fully resolved after a month (Fig. 7). The patient continued to return to the clinic for restorative and preventive dental care, including reassessment of retainer use and SIB. At his last visit, the parent reported that the patient had discontinued the wear of the appliance for over a week and the SIB had not returned.

The customized Hawley retainer proved to work well in this case and resulted in limiting the patient's uncontrolled biting habit. The use of such an appliance may be reduced after resolution of the self-injurious behavior, with reimplementation at any sign of SIB relapse [83].

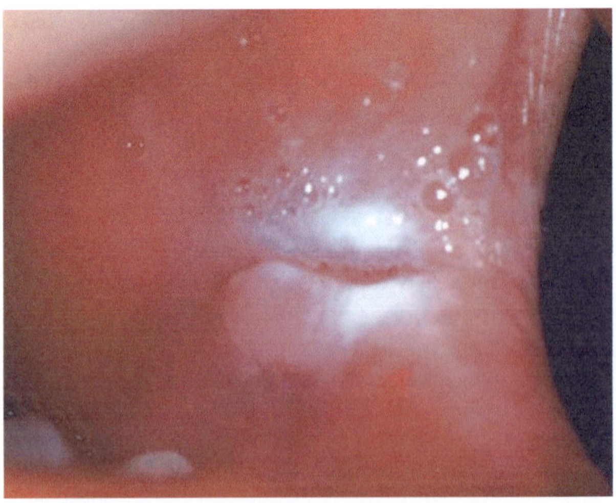

Fig. 4 Intraoral view of the traumatic ulceration of the left buccal mucosa caused by the patient's SIB

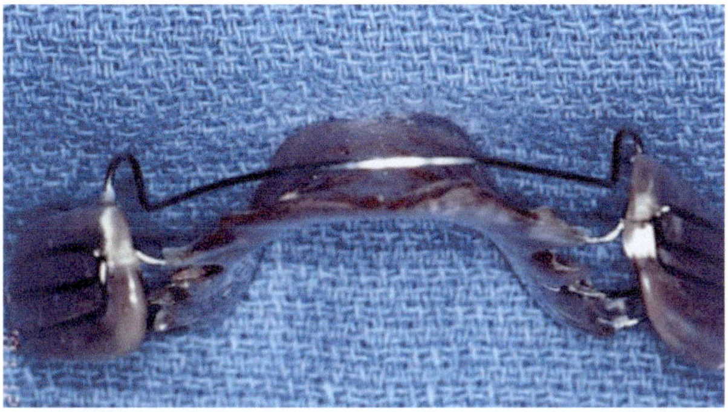

Fig. 5 Modified Hawley retainer with custom design to limit the patient's SIB

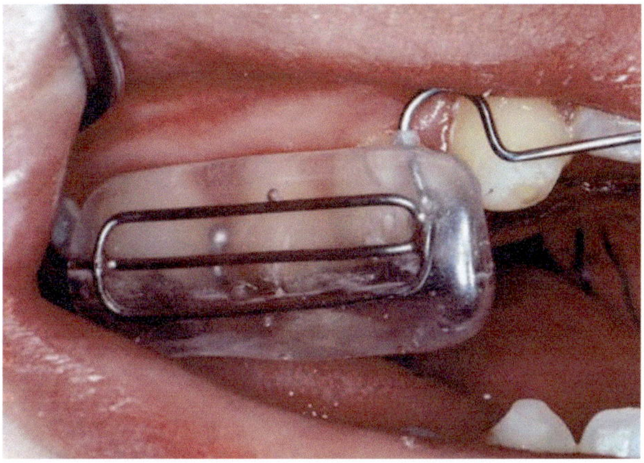

Fig. 6 Intraoral view of the appliance in use

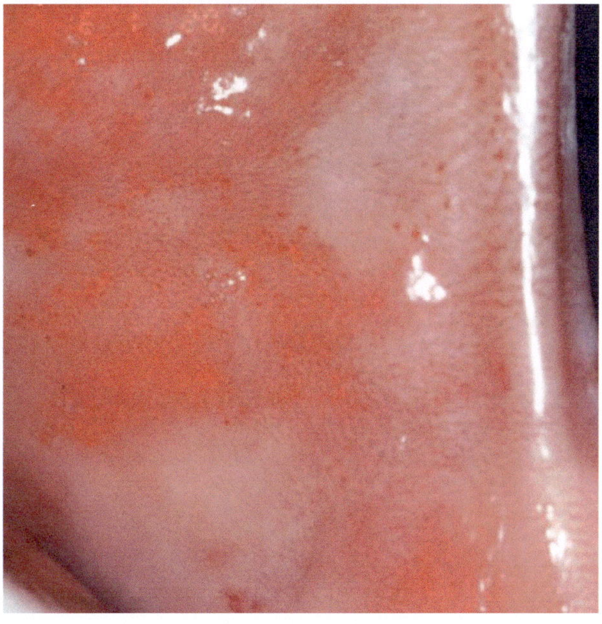

Fig. 7 Healed buccal mucosa after 28 days of appliance use

Conclusion

- Due to complexity of their medical background or side effects of clinical therapy, CSHCN experience more frequently than non-disabled counterparts, oral conditions characterized with persistent and challenging issues.
- The management of these oral conditions commonly requires consideration of specific etiology, appropriate multilevel planning, and interdisciplinary approach to therapy.
- Collaboration with the patient's physician is essential in preventing complications of oral care.
- Dental professionals are key members of the team of healthcare providers for CSHCN and play a paramount role in enhancing the patient's quality of life through management of the oral conditions and providing oral health education.

References

1. Cannavale R, Itro A, Campisi G, Compilato D, Colella G. Oral self-injuries: clinical findings in a series of 19 patients. Med Oral Patol Oral Cir Bucal. 2015;20:e123–9.
2. Arron K, Oliver C, Moss J, Berg K, Burbidge C. The prevalence and phenomenology of self-injurious behavior and aggressive behavior in genetic syndromes. J Intellect Disabil Res. 2011;55(Part 2):109–20.
3. Oliver C, Richards C. Practitioner Review: self-injurious behavior in children with developmental delay. J Child Psychol Psychiatry. 2015;56:1042–54.
4. Oliver C, Licence L, Richards C. Self-injurious behavior in people with intellectual disability and autism spectrum disorder. Curr Opin Psychiatry. 2017;30:97–101.
5. Soke GN, Rosenberg SA, Hamman RF, et al. Brief Report: prevalence of self-injurious behaviors among children with autism spectrum disorder—a population-based study. J Autism Dev Disord. 2016;46:3607–14.
6. Hanson GE, Ogle RG, Giron L. A tongue stent for prevention of oral trauma in the comatose patient. Crit Care Med. 1975;3:200–3.
7. Lobbezoo F, Ahlberg J, Glaros AG, et al. Bruxism defined and graded: an international consensus. J Oral Rehabil. 2013;40:2–4.
8. Clark GT, Ram S. Orofacial movement disorders. Oral Maxillofac Surg Clin North Am. 2016;28:397–407.
9. Castrillon EE, Ou K-L, Wang K, Zhang J, Zhou X, Svensson P. Sleep bruxism: an updated review of an old problem. Acta Odontol Scand. 2016;74:328–34.
10. Goldstein RE, Clark WA. The clinical management of bruxism. J Am Dent Assoc. 2017;148:387–91.
11. Machado E, Dal-Fabbro C, Cunali PA, Kaizer OB. Prevalence of sleep bruxism in children: a systematic review. Dental Press J Orthod. 2014;19(6):54–61. https://doi.org/10.1590/2176-9451.19.6.054-061.oar.
12. Castroflorio T, Bargellini A, Rossini G, Cugliari G, Rainoldi A, Deregibus A. Risk factors related to bruxism in children: a systematic literature review. Arch Oral Biol. 2015;60:1618–24.
13. Macedo CR, Macedo EC, Torloni MR, Silva AB, Prado GF. Pharmacotherapy for sleep bruxism. Cochrane Database Syst Rev. 2014;23:CD005578. https://doi.org/10.1002/14651858.CD005578.pub2.
14. Monroy PG, da Fonseca MA. The use of botulinum toxin-A in the treatment of severe bruxism in a patient with autism: a case report. Spec Care Dentist. 2006;26:37–9.

15. Beaumont J, Chesterman J, Kellet M, Durey K. Gingival overgrowth: part 1: aetiology and clinical diagnosis. Br Dent J. 2017;222:85–91.
16. Gawron K, Lazarz-Bartyzel K, Potempa J, Chomyszyn-Gajewska M. Gingival fibromatosis: clinical, molecular and therapeutic issues. Orphanet J Rare Dis. 2016;11:9.
17. Telles DR, Karki N, Marshall MW. Oral fungal infections—diagnosis and management. Dent Clin N Am. 2017;61:319–49.
18. Pinto A, Haberland CM, Baker S. Pediatric soft tissue oral lesions. Dent Clin N Am. 2014;58:437–53.
19. Muzyka BC, Epifanio RN. Update on oral fungal infections. Dent Clin N Am. 2013;57:561–81.
20. Lussi A, Carvalho TS. Erosive tooth wear: a multifactorial condition of growing concern and increasing knowledge. Monogr Oral Sci. 2014;25:1–15.
21. Taji S, Seow WK. A literature review of dental erosion in children. Aust Dent J. 2010;55:358–67.
22. Zawaideh FI, Owais AI, Mushtaha S. Effect of CPP-ACP or a potassium nitrate sodium fluoride dentifrice on enamel erosion prevention. J Clin Pediatr Dent. 2017;41(2):135–40. https://doi.org/10.17796/1053-4628-41.2.135.
23. Jaeggi T, Lussi A. Prevalence, incidence and distribution of erosion. Monogr Oral Sci. 2014;25:55–73.
24. Carvalho TS, Lussi A, Jaeggi T, Gambon DL. Erosive tooth wear in children. Monogr Oral Sci. 2014;25:262–78.
25. Shaw L, Weatherill S, Smith A. Tooth wear in children: an investigation of etiological factors in children with cerebral palsy and gastroesophageal reflux. J Dent Child. 1998;65:484–6.
26. Bell EJ, Kaidonis J, Townsend GC. Tooth wear in children with Down syndrome. Aust Dent J. 2002;47:30–5.
27. Lussi A, Jaeggi T. Erosion—diagnosis and risk factors. Clin Oral Investig. 2008;12(Suppl 1):S5–S13.
28. O'Sullivan E, Milosevic A. UK national clinical guidelines in paediatric dentistry: diagnosis, prevention and management of dental erosion. Int J Paediatr Dent. 2008;18(Suppl 1):29–38.
29. Bartlett D. Intrinsic causes of erosion. Monogr Oral Sci. 2006;20:119–39.
30. Lussi A, Jaeggi T, Zero D. The role of diet in the aetiology of dental erosion. Caries Res. 2004;38(Suppl 1):34–44.
31. Seow WK, Thong KM. Erosive effects of common beverages on extracted premolar teeth. Aust Dent J. 2005;50:173–8.
32. Hunter L, Patel S, Rees J. The in vitro erosive potential of a range of baby drinks. Int J Paediatr Dent. 2009;19:325–9.
33. Dugmore CR, Rock WP. Asthma and tooth erosion: is there an association? Int J Paediatr Dent. 2003;13:417–24.
34. Carpenter GH. The secretion, components, and properties of saliva. Annu Rev Food Sci Technol. 2013;4:267–76.
35. Dawes C. How much saliva is enough for avoidance of xerostomia? Caries Res. 2004;38:236–40.
36. Walsh LJ. Dry mouth: a clinical problem for children and young adults. Int Dent SA. 2007;9:48–58.
37. Murrah VA. Diabetes mellitus and associated oral manifestations: a review. J Oral Pathol. 1985;14:271–81.
38. Guggenheimer J, Moore PA. Xerostomia: etiology, recognition and treatment. J Am Dent Assoc. 2003;134:61–9.
39. Majorana A, Schubert MM, Porta F, Ugazio AG, Sapelli PL. Oral complications of pediatric hematopoietic cell transplantation: diagnosis and management. Support Care Cancer. 2000;8:353–65.
40. Villa A, Connell CL, Abati S. Diagnosis and management of xerostomia and hyposalivation. Ther Clin Risk Manag. 2014;11:45–51.
41. Osailan S, Pramanik R, Shirodaria S, Challacombe SJ, Proctor GB. Investigating the relationship between hyposalivation and mucosal wetness. Oral Dis. 2011;17:109–14.
42. Visvanathan V, Nix P. Managing the patient presenting with xerostomia: a review. Int J Clin Pract. 2010;64:404–7.

43. Lakraj AA, Moghimi N, Jabbari B. Sialorrhea: anatomy, pathophysiology and treatment with emphasis on the role of botulinum toxins. Toxins (Basel). 2013;5(5):1010–31.
44. Hamdy S, Aziz Q, Rothwell JC, Hobson A, Barlow J, Thompson DG. Cranial nerve modulation of human cortical swallowing motor pathways. Am J Phys. 1997;272(4):G802–8.
45. Silvestre-Rangil J, Silvestre FJ, Puente-Sandoval A, Requeni-Bernal J, Simó-Ruiz JM. Clinical-therapeutic management of drooling: review and update. Med Oral Patol Oral Cir Bucal. 2011;16(6):e763–6.
46. Jestrović I, Coyle JL, Sejdić E. Decoding human swallowing via electroencephalography: a state-of-the-art review. J Neural Eng. 2015;12(5):051001. https://doi.org/10.1088/1741-2560/12/5/051001.
47. Meningaud JP, Pitak-Arnnop P, Chikhani L, Bertrand JC. Drooling of saliva: a review of the etiology and management options. Oral Surg Oral Med Oral Pathol Oral Radiol Endod. 2006;101:48–57.
48. Sullivan PB, Lambert B, Rose M, Ford-Adams M, Johnson A, Griffiths P. Prevalence and severity of feeding and nutritional problems in children with neurological impairment: Oxford Feeding Study. Dev Med Child Neurol. 2000;42:674–80.
49. Tahmassebi JF, Curzon ME. The cause of drooling in children with cerebral palsy—hypersalivation or swallowing defect? Int J Paediatr Dent. 2003;13:106–11.
50. Tahmassebi JF, Curzon ME. Prevalence of drooling in children with cerebral palsy attending special schools. Dev Med Child Neurol. 2003;45:613–7.
51. Hyson HC, Johnson A, Jog MS. Survey of sialorrhea in parkinsonian patients in southwestern Ontario. Can J Neurol Sci. 2001;28:S46–7.
52. Hung CC, Fu PK, Wang HY, Chan CH, Lan TH. Treatment effects of traditional Chinese medicines suoquan pill and wuling powder on clozapine-induced hypersalivation in patients with schizophrenia: study protocol of a randomized, placebo-controlled trial. J Chin Integr Med. 2011;9:495–502.
53. Nunn JH. Drooling: review of the literature and proposals for management. J Oral Rehabil. 2000;27(9):735–43.
54. Poveda Roda R, Bagan JV, Díaz Fernández JM, Hernández Bazán S, Jiménez Soriano Y. Review of temporomandibular joint pathology part I: classification, epidemiology and risk factors. Med Oral Patol Oral Cir Bucal. 2007;12:E292–8.
55. Laskin DM. Temporomandibular disorders: a term past its time? J Am Dent Assoc. 2008;139:124–8.
56. da Sena MF, Mesquita KS, Santos FR, Silva FW, Serrano KV. Prevalence of temporomandibular dysfunction in children and adolescents. Rev Paul Pediatr. 2013;31:538–45.
57. Godoy F, Rosenblatt A, Godoy-Bezerra J. Temporomandibular disorders and associated factors in Brazilian teenagers: a cross-sectional study. Int J Prosthodont. 2007;20:599–604.
58. Sönmez H, Sari S, Oksak Oray G, Camdeviren H. Prevalence of temporomandibular dysfunction in Turkish children with mixed and permanent dentition. J Oral Rehabil. 2001;28:280–5.
59. Tanboga I, Durhan MA, Durmus B, Marks LA. Temporomandibular disorders in young people with an intellectual disability: prevalence of signs and symptoms. Eur J Paediatr Dent. 2014;15:349–54.
60. American Academy of Pediatric Dentistry. Guideline on acquired temporomandibular disorders in infants, children, and adolescents. Pediatr Dent. 2016;38:308–14.
61. Thilander B, Rubio G, Pena L, De Mayorga C. Prevalence of temporomandibular dysfunction and its association with malocclusion in children and adolescents: an epidemiologic study related to specified stages of dental development. Angle Orthod. 2002;72:146–54.
62. American Academy of Orofacial Pain. Orofacial Pain. In: deLeeuw R, Klasser GD, editors. Guidelines for assessment, diagnosis, and management. Chicago: Quintessence Publishing; 2013. p. 5.
63. Howard JA. Temporomandibular joint disorders in children. Dent Clin N Am. 2013;57:99–127.
64. Dym H, Israel H. Diagnosis and treatment of temporomandibular disorders. Dent Clin N Am. 2012;56:149–61.

65. Klein OD, Oberoi S, Huysseune A, Hovorakova M, Peterka M, Peterkova R. Developmental disorders of the dentition: an update. Am J Med Genet C Semin Med Genet. 2013;163C:318–32.
66. Fleming PS, Xavier GM, DiBiase AT, Cobourne MT. Revisiting the supernumerary: the epidemiological and molecular basis of extra teeth. Br Dent J. 2010;208:25–30.
67. Rajab LD, Hamdan MAM. Supernumerary teeth: review of the literature and a survey of 152 cases. Int J Paediatr Dent. 2002;12:244–54.
68. Shah A, Gill DS, Tredwin C, Naini FB. Diagnosis and management of supernumerary teeth. Dent Update. 2008;35:510–2, 514–6, 519–20.
69. Hall A, Onn A. The development of supernumerary teeth in the mandible in cases with a history of supernumeraries in the pre-maxillary region. J Orthod. 2006;33:250–5.
70. Brook AH, Elcock C, al-Sharood MH, McKeown HF, Khalaf K, Smith RN. Further studies of a model for the etiology of anomalies of tooth number and size in humans. Connect Tissue Res. 2002;43:289–95.
71. Leyland L, Batra P, Wong F, Llewelyn R. A retrospective evaluation of the eruption of impacted permanent incisors after extraction of supernumerary teeth. J Clin Pediatr Dent. 2006;30:225–31.
72. Omer RS, Anthonappa RP, King NM. Determination of the optimum time for surgical removal of unerupted anterior supernumerary teeth. Pediatr Dent. 2010;32:14–20.
73. Rakhshan V. Congenitally missing teeth (hypodontia): a review of the literature concerning the etiology, prevalence, risk factors, patterns and treatment. Dent Res J (Isfahan). 2015;12(1):13.
74. Larmour CJ, Mossey PA, Thind BS, Forgie AH, Stirrups DR. Hypodontia—a retrospective review of prevalence and etiology. Part I. Quintessence Int. 2005;36:263–70.
75. AlShahrani I, Togoo RA, AlQarni MA. A review of hypodontia: classification, prevalence, etiology, associated anomalies, clinical implications and treatment options. World J Dent. 2013;4:117–25.
76. Pirinen S, Arte S, Apajalahti S. Palatal displacement of canine is genetic and related to congenital absence of teeth. J Dent Res. 1996;75:1742–6.
77. Nunn JH, Carter NE, Gillgrass TJ, Hobson RS, Jepson NJ, Meechan JG, Nohl FS. The interdisciplinary management of hypodontia: background and role of paediatric dentistry. Br Dent J. 2003;194:245–51.
78. Seow WK. Developmental defects of enamel and dentine: challenges for basic science research and clinical management. Aust Dent J. 2014;59(Suppl 1):143–54.
79. Brook AH. Multilevel complex interactions between genetic, epigenetic and environmental factors in the aetiology of anomalies of dental development. Arch Oral Biol. 2009;54S:S3–S17.
80. Freiman A, Borsuk D, Barankin B, Sperber GH, Krafchik B. Dental manifestations of dermatologic conditions. J Am Acad Dermatol. 2009;60:289–98.
81. Crawford PJ, Aldred M, Bloch-Zupan A. Amelogenesis imperfecta. Orphanet J Rare Dis. 2007;2:17.
82. Saroglu I, Aras S, Oztas D. Effect of deproteinization on composite bond strength in hypocalcified amelogenesis imperfecta. Oral Dis. 2006;12:305–8.
83. Silva DR, da Fonseca MA. Self-injurious behavior as a challenge for the dental practice: a case report. Pediatr Dent. 2003;25(1):62–6.

Medical Management of Dental Caries

Elise W. Sarvas

Introduction

Modern dentistry is undergoing a paradigm shift from surgical management of caries to medical management. This new approach is of particular interest to clinicians working with medically complex populations, as it more closely mirrors the medical care their patients are already receiving and allows for dental care to be minimally invasive.

Primary, Secondary, and Tertiary Care

In medicine, care is conceptualized into three broad levels: primary, secondary, and tertiary. For example, primary care of non-insulin-dependent diabetes mellitus includes preventive measures such as eating a healthy diet, maintaining an appropriate body weight, and regular exercise. Secondary care for this disease includes intervention with medications such as metformin or sulfonylureas. If the disease continues to progress, tertiary care in the form of surgery (e.g., bariatric procedure to maintain body weight or limb amputation) may be necessary. From the dental profession's barber-surgeon origins until the late twentieth century, dentistry has been concerned primarily with tertiary treatment of oral disease sequelae. As more of the infectious process was understood, the profession embraced a medical model to manage the disease (Fig. 1). A key component of the medical management of caries movement is assessing the patient's caries risk and prescribing primary, secondary, and tertiary dental care options as appropriate within the context of the individual's health-care needs.

E. W. Sarvas (✉)
Division of Pediatric Dentistry, Department of Developmental and Surgical Sciences, University of Minnesota, Minneapolis, MN, USA

T. M. Nelson, J. R. Webb (eds.), *Dental Care for Children with Special Needs*,
https://doi.org/10.1007/978-3-030-10483-2_9

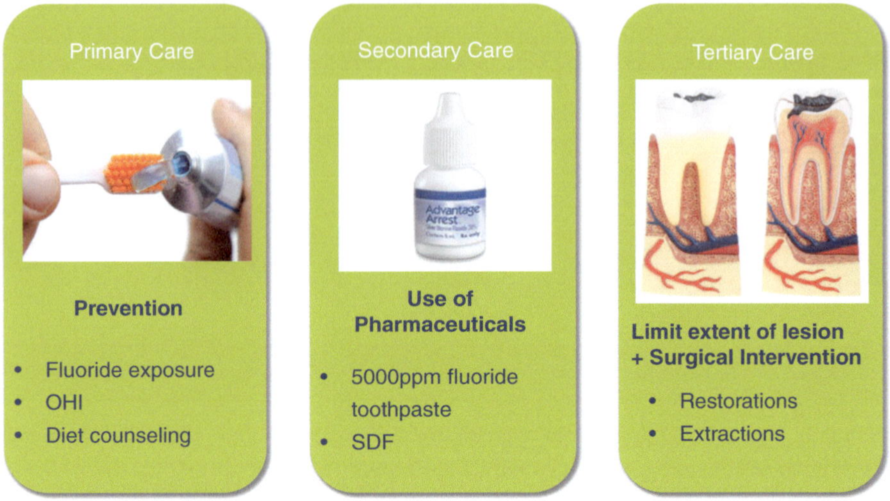

Fig. 1 Medical management of dental disease

Primary Dental Care

A thorough caries risk assessment of an individual is the first step in primary dental care. Multiple risk assessment tools are available for dental practitioners, and all automatically place children with special health-care needs (CSHCNs) into moderate- or high-risk categories [1–3]. Not all CSHCNs are at high risk of developing dental caries, and prevention programs should be tailored to their individual risk factors. Identifying individual risk factors such as the need for a cariogenic diet, use of medications that may be dosed in sugary suspensions or cause xerostomia, inability to maintain optimal oral hygiene, decreased salivary buffering capacity, and other condition-specific caries risk factors can help oral health-care providers identify successful prevention strategies.

Secondary Dental Care

Secondary care in the form of minimally invasive medicaments is an emerging field in dentistry. These pharmaceuticals aim to keep existing lesions from progressing. Fluoride varnish application for white spot lesions is one of the most common chemotherapeutics used for this purpose. Other medicaments include chlorhexidine rinses, which are bactericidal and bacteriostatic and reduce pellicle formation. Recently a "new old medicine," silver diamine fluoride (SDF), has regained favor for its antimicrobial and caries-arresting properties. SDF differs from other chemotherapeutics because it successfully stops a cavitated lesion from progressing, while the other available medicaments work best before a lesion is fully cavitated. Future research will hopefully continue to add secondary care adjuncts to the dental arsenal.

Secondary care can allow a clinician to delay dental treatment in the context of an individual's overall health care. Emergency dental care is fortuitously a rare event. Certain conditions such as an avulsed permanent tooth or facial cellulitis that compromise the airway need immediate attention. For all other issues, the clinician may have the ability to delay treatment until an individual's other medical complexities are stable [4]. Individuals with special health-care needs face a lifetime of adjunctive therapies. These can range from routine care such as occupational and speech therapy or frequent infusions of antibiotics to more acute care needs such as radiation or chemotherapy. These health-care needs may, in the short term, supersede the need for routine dental care, and the clinician should be prepared to watchfully delay routine dental treatment needs. Techniques may include using secondary chemotherapeutics to delay or arrest disease in addition to minimally invasive treatments to avoid more invasive dental procedures under sedation or general anesthesia.

Tertiary Dental Care

While it is desirable to treat dental disease using primary and secondary prevention, this is not always possible to avoid or delay restorative dental care. Dental needs that require acute surgical attention include odontogenic abscesses, caries, or trauma that severely compromise oral form and function and other systemic conditions that necessitate immediate resolution of oral disease (e.g., pending heart transplant, initiation of oncology treatment). Additionally, social considerations such as distance a family travels to the clinic, limited parent availability for dental appointments, and other family logistics may make multiple prevention or minimally invasive appointments impossible. All tertiary surgical dental care plans should include preventive recommendations.

Tools to Delay Treatment Under Sedation or General Anesthesia

- Basic and advanced behavior guidance techniques are generally effective for tertiary treatment of dental caries in typically developing children. On the other hand, CSHCN can present behavioral and physical challenges that complicate providing definitive restorative treatment. In these situations, it may be desirable to avoid pharmacological interventions that are necessary to facilitate patient cooperation due to medical fragility. Alternately, logistical concerns such as hospital OR waitlists, parent concerns with pharmacologic techniques, and desire to delay treatment until a later date (for eruption of a full component of primary or permanent teeth, extraction of third molars, etc.) can drive the choice to defer definitive treatments. This chapter discusses a number of minimally invasive strategies to treat or defer treatment of caries.

Hall Crowns

Preformed metal crowns have been a part of the dental providers' restorative arsenal since 1950 [5]. Often made of stainless steel, these full-coverage restorations outperform class II amalgam and resin restorations in primary teeth both in durability and longevity. They are ideal for restoring large, multi-surface cavitated lesions in primary teeth with or without pulpal involvement and should strongly be considered for use in children being treated under general anesthesia [6]. The traditional method of preparation involves administration of local anesthesia, occlusal and interproximal reduction of the primary tooth surfaces with caries removal, and fitting and crimping of the stainless steel crown (SSC) before cementation with a glass ionomer cement. Given the technique-sensitive nature of this process, some dental providers have asked whether the same treatment could be provided in a less invasive but equally effective method.

In the 1990s, an audit of Scottish general dentist Dr. Norna Hall's dental records challenged the traditional approach to SSC placement. Instead of using the standard SSC technique, she selected an appropriately sized SSC, filled it with glass ionomer cement, and placed the crown using finger pressure or the child's own occlusal forces without any caries removal or local anesthesia [7]. This novel method is now known as the Hall technique. An initial retrospective audit of her dental records showed a clinical success rate that was similar to the traditional SSC placement [7]. Biologically this may occur because of the full-coverage nature of the SSC. Once it is placed, it seals off the decay process from nutritive substrates, stopping the decay process. Additionally, the glass ionomer cement seals the margins of the SSC and provides fluoride release, further preventing the growth of caries.

Multiple follow-up studies and randomized controlled trials performed in general dental office settings have supported the use of the Hall technique as a viable alternative for dental practitioners [8–12]. A 2015 Cochrane review concluded that in addition to a moderate quality of evidence that crowns placed with the Hall technique were less likely to cause pain and abscesses than fillings, the Hall technique may also reduce discomfort at the time of treatment [13]. Another benefit is that the use of this method may also increase the use and acceptability of preformed metal crowns by general dentists. A survey of British undergraduate dental students suggests that instruction in the Hall technique increased the use of SSCs as a treatment modality over other noninvasive techniques such as glass ionomer cement [8].

The Hall technique may be a beneficial option for the dental practitioner to use in children with special health care needs. This is especially true in cases where there are minimal treatment needs that could be restored without the need for sedation or general anesthesia. As for all children, case selection using clinical, and preferably also radiographic data, for diagnosis is key. In cases where pulpal involvement is questionable, traditional crown preparation and pulpal therapy are preferable. When the underlying medical condition or behavior contraindicates pulpal therapy, extraction is likely the treatment of choice [14]. Given that the Hall technique requires no tooth preparation and a larger-sized SSC than the traditional method, it is not possible to place multiple SSCs in the same quadrant in the same visit. Children who require treatment of multiple adjacent teeth must be appointed several weeks apart to allow for tightness of interproximal contacts to relax. Therefore, for logistical reasons, the Hall technique may not be appropriate for children with extensive dental needs requiring adjacent SSCs in multiple quadrants. Additionally, space loss due to multiple carious lesions in a quadrant can cause challenges in fitting crowns. It may be possible to place one and, then after a period of days to weeks, place an adjacent one once the periodontal ligament has had a chance to adjust. Second primary molars that are treated using the Hall technique will need additional monitoring to ensure that the chance of ectopic eruption of the permanent first molars is minimized.

It is important to note that all randomized control trials used to analyze the Hall technique excluded children with "significant health problems" and "systemic disease requiring special considerations during their dental treatment" from their study population [9, 15]. The inclusion of children with special health-care needs in retrospective studies is unknown [7, 11]. There are however few contraindications for using traditionally placed or Hall technique-placed SSCs as a restorative option for individuals with special health-care needs. They may be in fact the preferred restorative option over intracoronal fillings due to their durable and definitive nature [6]. Perhaps the biggest contraindication to placement may be the child's ability to safely tolerate the procedure. While patients have rated the Hall technique as less painful than traditional restorative care, it is still uncomfortable and requires cooperation from the patient. Another concern is that Hall crowns are delivered without a rubber dam in place to protect the airway. It is imperative that the clinician establish a baseline of cooperation and confirm that the patient can remain still for the procedure. This will help ensure that a SSC is not inadvertently swallowed or aspirated due to sudden movements or a slip of the provider's finger.

Hall Crown Protocol (Box 1)

This technique can be initiated the same day as diagnosis but may benefit from a two-appointment approach. Initially, the tooth should have an appropriate diagnosis using patient and caregiver report of symptoms, clinical, and ideally radiographic data. Case selection is critical, and teeth with pulpal involvement should not be considered for this approach.

A documented informed consent from the parent or guardian for the procedure should be included in the patient chart. If a two-appointment approach is used, the clinician can place rubber orthodontic separators or spacers interproximally to gain space for the crown delivery (Fig 2a). Patients and caregivers should be advised not to pick at or floss the interproximal areas where these have been placed. This minimizes the chance that separators will fall out. Regular toothbrushing should still be encouraged.

If spacers were placed, as when placing orthodontic bands, the second appointment should be scheduled at least 3–5 days after the initial appointment but less than 2 weeks later. This maximizes the effectiveness of the separators' orthodontic movement (Fig. 2b). At the delivery appointment, any remaining spacers should be removed. An appropriately sized, precontoured stainless steel crown (e.g., Ni-Chro

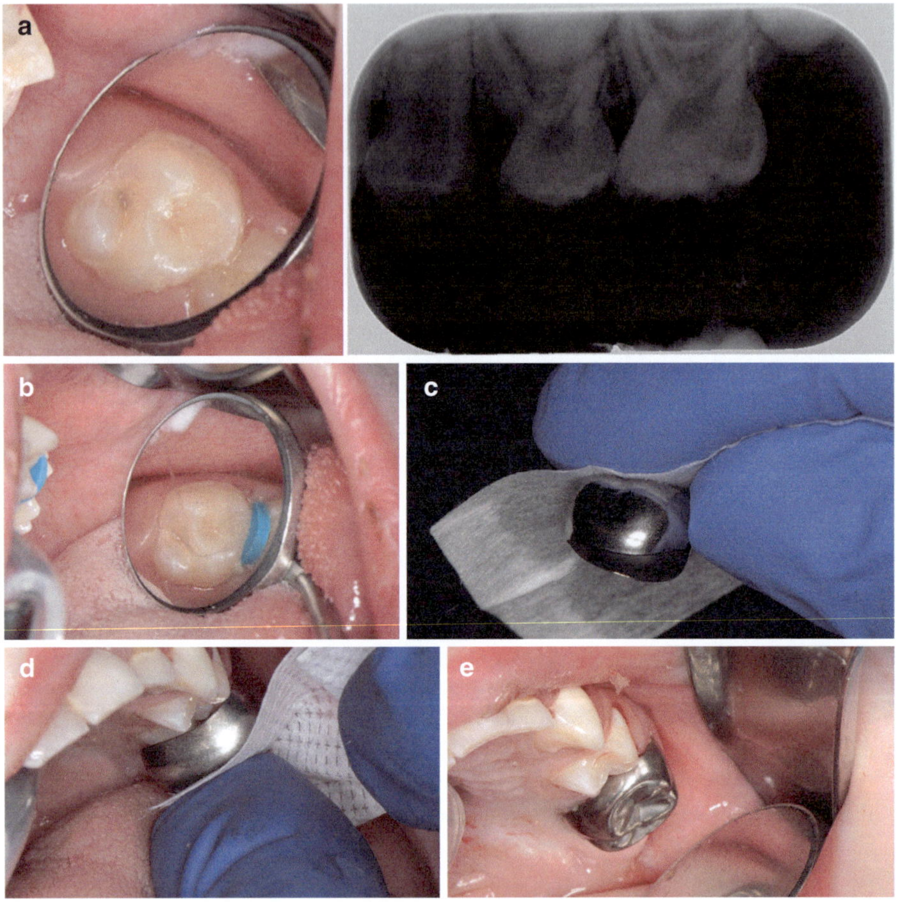

Fig. 2 (**a**) Tooth #J with carious occlusal lesion. (**b**) Orthodontic separator placed interproximally prior to Hall crown try-in. (**c**) Occlusal surface with surgical tape to secure crown. (**d**) Try-on of Hall crown. (**e**) Fully seated Hall crown with excess cement removed

Ion Crowns, Unitek Stainless Steel Crowns—3M, Saint Paul, MN) should be selected. A precontoured crown works best as it requires minimal trimming, crimping, and contouring prior to placement. The size of the crown should be based on the interproximal width of the tooth's occlusal plane and the availability of space between the adjacent teeth. A periodontal probe may be helpful in measuring this space and selecting an appropriate crown size.

To protect the patient's airway, a gauze throat shield should be placed posterior to the tooth, and the high-speed suction should be readily available. Some clinicians also find it helpful to stabilize the crown by placing a piece of tape (e.g., surgical cloth or masking tape) on the dried occlusal surface for increased security (Fig. 2c). The crown is then fitting on top of the occlusal surface of the tooth, up to halfway into the interproximal contacts, but not fully seated. The clinician should judge if the crown is appropriately sized for the interproximal dimensions of the tooth and assess if it has adequate clearance to seat over the buccal bulge with pressure. Usually the selected crown is one to two sizes larger than a crown used in a traditional preparation to achieve this goal.

Once the appropriate size is selected, the tooth should be dried, and the patient's airway should be checked once again to ensure it is protected. The crown is then filled three-quarters full with glass ionomer cement and placed on the tooth (Fig. 2d). Using finger pressure, the crown is seated below the interproximal contacts and is further seated by the clinician using either a crown-seating instrument such as a bite stick or the child's own occlusal forces by having her bite down on a cotton roll. Pressure should be maintained until the crown is fully seated to the gingival margin. Excess cement is removed with the air and water syringe and hand instruments and by bringing knotted dental floss through the interproximal contacts (Fig. 2e).

The patient's occlusion should be checked and noted in the dental record. Often because the crown selected is larger than used in a traditional preparation, it may come into premature contact with the opposing arch. This typically resolves in 1 to 2 weeks, as the primary tooth intrudes and the periodontal ligament adjusts. Observe any changes to the occlusal relationship at follow-up appointments. This procedure will cause minor discomfort similar to the pain that children experience after braces are adjusted. To improve patient postoperative comfort, advise caregivers to administer acetaminophen and/or ibuprofen for a day or two.

Box 1	
Appointment 1	1. Diagnosis of tooth to be restored using clinical and (ideally) radiographic data 2. Caries risk assessment and behavioral analysis 3. Informed verbal and written consent 4. Placement of orthodontic separators to open proximal contacts if possible
Appointment 2	1. Remove orthodontic separators if previously placed 2. Select appropriately sized SSC based on interproximal width of occlusal plane 3. Dry tooth with air or gauze 4. Place throat shield 5. Fill SSC with glass ionomer cement 6. Place SSC on occlusal surface of tooth 7. Seat the crown below the interproximal contacts using finger pressure and/or have the child bite down on a cotton roll 8. Remove excess cement with air/water syringe, dental instruments, and floss 9. Check occlusion 10. Suggest acetaminophen or ibuprofen for postoperative comfort

ART/ITR

The alternative or atraumatic restorative treatment (ART) was one of the first tools developed to control caries using a minimally invasive approach. Originally used in the developing world and reported on in 1985, it has been endorsed by the World

Health Organization for use in populations without access to traditional dental care [16]. This technique was intended for treatment without the use of adjunctive pharmacologic management (e.g., oral conscious sedation, general anesthesia), so it holds promise for caries control in CSHCN and other behaviorally challenging patients.

The original ART technique involves removal of the carious lesion using hand instruments without local anesthetic or power-driven equipment. Caries removal using this method is usually incomplete and can be prone to pulpal exposure. The tooth is then restored with an adhesive material such as glass ionomer, glass ionomer cement (GIC), resin-modified glass ionomer, composite resin, or compomer [17]. Modified ART techniques have since been introduced. These modified techniques include opening the enamel to access the dentin with a high-speed handpiece, using alternative materials such as amalgam, or first applying silver diamine fluoride (SDF) to arrest decay as in the silver-modified atraumatic restorative treatment (SMART) technique [18, 19].

ART has two goals: (1) to restore teeth with cavitated carious lesions and (2) to seal pits and fissure to prevent future decay [20]. To achieve both of these aims, the current material of choice is high-viscosity GIC due to its survival and fluoride-releasing properties [21]. GIC is relatively inexpensive and readily available in the dental practitioner's arsenal. It easily flows into class I preparations and covers pits and fissures by pressing a gloved finger onto the surface of teeth. ART is not typically meant to be a definitive restoration, but because the circumstances of where and how it is placed do not generally allow for follow-up care, it often becomes the final restoration. Another minimally invasive technique called interim therapeutic restoration (ITR) uses similar methods as ART but has different therapeutic goals. The main difference between ITR and ART is that ITR requires active monitoring of a tooth's condition after this minimally invasive treatment until a definite restoration can be placed. The ITR technique more accurately describes the dental professional's approach to care in the developed world where conditions allow for patient follow-up.

The American Academy of Pediatric Dentistry states that ITR "may be used to restore, arrest or prevent the progression of carious lesions in young patients, uncooperative patients, or patients with special health care needs or when traditional cavity preparation and/or placement of traditional dental restorations are not feasible and need to be postponed" [22]. ITR may also be used for stepwise caries excavation when the carious lesion is deep and/or approximates the pulp chamber.

ITR Protocol

The technique for ITR is similar to ART: caries removal is completed with hand or rotary instruments. This is usually done without anesthetic unless the lesion is deep. The clinician should take care to ensure that the margins of the preparation are as caries-free as possible to allow for proper chemical bonding along the dentin-enamel junction (DEJ). Optimal bonding at this site ensures that any remaining bacteria are sealed off from nutrients in the oral cavity, thereby increasing the success rate of these restorations.

If possible, the tooth should be isolated and acid etched with polyacrylic acid. The lesion is rinsed and air-dried. It is important not to over dry the dentin, as the glass ionomer will draw in moisture during its setting phase. If the preparation is too dry, the material will draw moisture through the dentin tubules and may cause post-operative sensitivity in large preparations. Glass ionomer cement is then placed in the lesion and shaped with finger pressure or hand instruments. Excess cement is removed and smoothed to final contour. A curing light can be used to speed the chemical reaction by applying heat, but is not necessary.

Modified ITR Technique for Anterior Teeth

Some clinicians have combined the full-coverage benefits of the Hall technique with the advantages of using ART/ITR materials. Nelson first described how durable, esthetic anterior restorations could be delivered using celluloid strip crowns and resin-modified glass ionomer (RMGI) [23]. Young pre-cooperative children and individuals with behavior-modifying special health-care needs are often not candidates for traditional anterior esthetic restorations of composite or full-coverage zirconia. These restorations are extremely technique and moisture sensitive and must be done on a cooperative or sedated patient. The option for strong, tooth-colored anterior restorations where traditional methods are unfeasible is also important for minimizing inequities in care for CSHCN. Non-esthetic anterior restorations like stainless steel crowns or untreated caries may negatively affect the individual's self-esteem and/or highlight their health differences to the non-dental public [24]. This modified technique can be especially beneficial when a patient who is minimally cooperative presents with early childhood caries affecting the maxillary incisors because it can be done in the knee-to-knee position with no local anesthesia. Additionally it can be used as a more durable interim restoration on permanent teeth for a patient with special health-care needs until the child finishes growing and is a candidate for full-coverage adult crowns.

Modified ITR Technique Protocol

Tooth preparation is contingent on the natural spacing of the teeth. If there are interproximal contacts, interproximal reduction may be performed ("sliced") with a carbide or tapered diamond bur so that there is adequate clearance for the strip crown form or forms to be placed. If there is adequate interproximal spacing to place the strip crowns, this step can be skipped (Fig. 3a). Carious tissue may be removed with hand or slow-speed rotary instruments. Complete caries removal is not necessary. Care must be taken with both the slicing and caries removal procedures so as not to damage the adjacent gingiva to minimize bleeding and prevent moisture contamination of the restorative material. The most conservative approach should be used when behavior or patient positioning threatens to compromise the surgical field. If bleeding does occur, gauze pressure should be held over the area to encourage hemostasis. Incisal reduction is not performed.

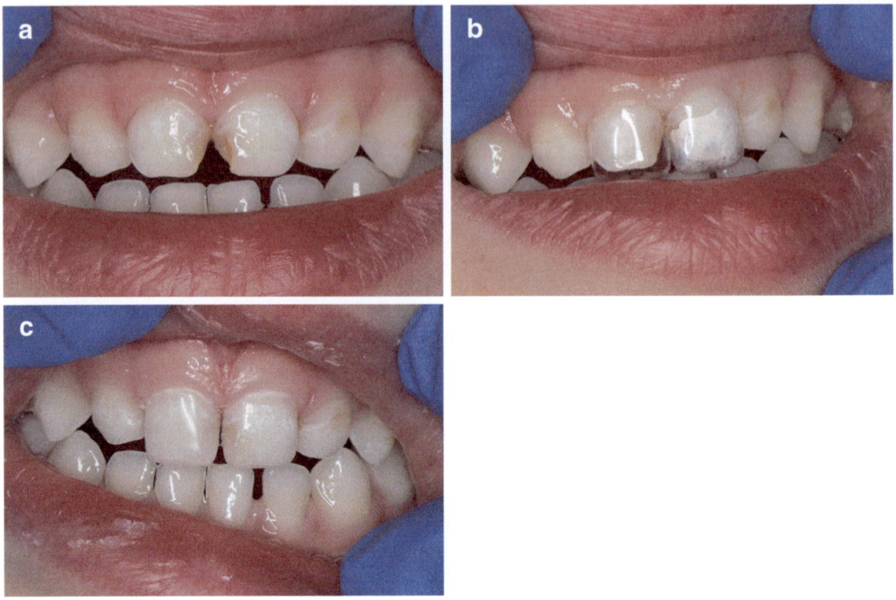

Fig. 3 (**a**) Mesial caries on #E and F on 2-year and 1-month-old female. Lesions previously treated with RMGI, but restoration has fractured. (**b**) Fitting strip crown forms to #E and F. Selected crown forms should allow for closed gingival margins and ideally have interproximal clearance for cleansibility. (**c**) After removal of crown forms, RMGI can be smoothed using soft flex discs and finishing burs. It is important that the crowns are not in occlusion to prevent wear and breakage

Appropriately sized crown forms should be selected (e.g., 3M, Success Essentials, Space Maintainers Lab) (Fig. 3b). Depending on the brand, the gingival collar of the crown may need to be removed with scissors. Crown forms are typically one size larger than with traditional strip crown methods and will be longer than the natural tooth as incisal reduction is not performed [23]. To set realistic expectations, caregivers should be made aware of this during the informed consent process. Crown forms should extend to the gingival margin and should approximate the circumference of the gingival collar but may be larger than traditionally placed strip crowns. If the crown form seats firmly to the gingival margin, it may be necessary to cut vent holes along the lingual surface to allow excess restorative material to escape. This step is not necessary if there is spacing around the gingival margin, as any excess material will vent gingivally.

The crown forms are removed and filled three-quarters full with RMGI. They are then immediately placed on the tooth or teeth and seated with gentle finger pressure. The curing light should be used to tack cure on the facial and lingual for 3 s each. This will allow sufficient polymerization of the excess material around the gingival margin to allow for easier removal with a hand instrument like the Hollenbeck carver. Once this is removed, the restorations should be cured on the facial and lingual for 20 s each.

Place a gauze throat shield, and have the high-speed suction ready to protect the patient's airway during crown form removal. Remove the crown form or forms with a hand instrument such as the Hollenbeck or discoid-cleoid carver by lifting from the gingival margin towards the incisal edge. The restorations should require minimal finishing (Fig. 3c). If a vent hole was necessary, remove excess lingual material with a football-shaped finishing bur. Sandpaper discs can be used to smooth or reduce overly long incisal edges.

This technique may be modified for adult anterior teeth by using permanent celluloid crown forms. More interproximal tooth reduction may be necessary due to less natural spacing in the permanent dentition. Patients in both dentitions should be cautioned to not use these restored teeth to bite or tear hard foods as this may compromise the durability of these crowns. They should be encouraged to cut hard foods into bite-sized pieces and counseled to chew with their posterior teeth instead.

Silver Diamine Fluoride (SDF)

History of Silver Compounds in Dentistry

Silver has been valued for its antimicrobial properties for thousands of years, even before the germ theory of disease was fully conceptualized. Alexander the Great stored water in silver containers on his long military campaigns, and ancient Romans describe packing wounds with silver foil in their first book of medicine [25]. Healthcare inventors adopted silver to produce safer medical devices as the microbial origin of disease became better understood. The advent of silver sutures, catheter parts, and other surgical devices paved the way for successful medical breakthroughs [26].

Silver was first used in dentistry as early as the 1840s in the form of the salt "nitrate of silver" (known today as silver nitrate; $AgNO_3$). Early dentists observed that some carious lesions that turned dark would signal a stop in the disease process, while ones that remained light in color would progress. They endeavored to find a medicament that would instantly cauterize these lesions and create the dark, hard surface that some lesions seemed to fortuitously develop [27]. Silver nitrate's extremely caustic properties created this effect quickly and safely. It continued to be a popular treatment through the era of G.V. Black and his modernization of operative dentistry. In 1917, Percy Howe introduced an updated version of this medicament in an ammoniacal silver nitrate mixture ($AgNH_3NO_3$). Known eponymously as Howe's solution, it was marketed as an antimicrobial product that could penetrate deeper into dentin. Until the 1950s it was used to sterilize carious lesions after preparation and was even promoted as a disinfectant in early root canal therapy [28].

The developments of dental medicaments are advantageous for providers in settings with low resource areas because they offer a quick, economical solution to populations with heavy disease burdens. Dental providers at the Western Australia School Dental Service first used silver fluoride (AgF) as the initial part of a minimally invasive treatment process for a cohort of disadvantaged young children in

New South Wales in the 1970s [29]. Faced with a backlog of dental cases in a rural location, silver fluoride was first applied to inhibit the growth of existing lesions. Next, a coat of stannous fluoride (SnF_2) was applied to act both as a reducing agent for AgF and to prevent new lesions from occurring. This two-step "metal fluoride" approach resulted in arrest of three-quarters of the existing lesions. Only one-third of the original lesions required additional surgical treatment after the initial application [28]. Despite the success of this protocol, few studies continued to investigate this method after the 1990s.

SDF in Dentistry

Around the same time as researchers were combining silver and fluoride in Australia, a similar, but chemically different, medicament was being investigated in Japan. Dr. Mizuho Nishino sought to combine the powerful antimicrobial properties of silver with the benefits of a high dose of fluoride as part of her master's thesis in cariology at Osaka University in 1969 [30]. The difference between this solution and the two-step process was that this formulation also created a dark precipitate which could block dentinal tubules and reduce sensitivity associated with hydrostatic pressure [31]. Soon, "diammine silver fluoride" was granted approval by the Central Pharmaceutical Council of the Ministry of Health and Welfare of Japan as a caries-arresting or cariostatic agent and marketed under the name "Saforide." This compound, $AgF(NH_3)_2$, is commonly misspelled or misinterpreted as silver diamine fluoride. The proper chemical nomenclature is silver diammine fluoride as it contains two a*mm*ine groups (NH_3), not two a*m*ine groups (NH_2) [28]. The use of the term "diamine" is so ubiquitous; however, it has become the accepted form both in the current scientific and marketing literature.

Researchers in the developing world quickly adopted Dr. Nishino's medicament to treat populations where access to traditional dental care is or was extremely limited. In vivo and in vitro studies using SDF were conducted with great success in Argentina, Brazil, China, Cuba, Japan, and Nepal in the 1990s and early 2000s [32, 33]. Comparing the outcome of this geographically diverse research is challenging however, owing to the different methodologies used and study populations examined. Despite the inconsistencies, several key themes emerged. First, the most effective concentration of SDF to arrest dental caries was 38% when compared to lower concentrations of 10–12% [34]. Second, the addition of reducing agents such as potassium iodide or tannic acid (found in local teas) to mitigate the color change of the lesion did not change the efficacy of 38% SDF [35, 36]. Third, SDF was more effective at arresting existing caries and preventing new lesions than previously used methods such as interim therapeutic restorations with fluoride-releasing glass ionomer cement, fluoride varnish application, frequent chlorhexidine rinses, and oral hygiene instruction [32, 37, 38]. SDF has been found to work best when applied in multiple intervals than a one-time placement. Since the protocols in these population studies varied considerably, consistent evidence on the optimal frequency and interval between applications does not exist, but most recommend an application every 6–12 months [32, 39].

SDF has been found to be up to 80% effective for arresting carious lesions after a one-time application [28]. Most research to date has focused on SDF's effect on buccal, lingual, and occlusal surfaces where the medicament can be easily applied and monitored for its distinctive color change. Like other fluoride formulations, SDF is most beneficial on smooth surface lesions. Its effect is enhanced when these lesions are shallow and self-cleansing and do not trap additional plaque and food particles. When comparing SDF to dental sealants as treatment for pit and fissure caries, resin and glass ionomer cement sealants were both more effective at preventing and arresting early enamel decay [35, 40]. There are no observed differences in success rates between primary and permanent teeth [28].

The two main components of SDF, silver and fluoride, are made dissolvable in water by the addition of ammonia. Silver acts as a broad-spectrum antimicrobial, with a high biocompatibility and low toxicity in humans. Its ions act as tiny "silver bullets" that damage and degrade bacterial cell walls, disrupt bacterial DNA synthesis and replication, and disrupt intracellular metabolic activity, eventually leading to cell death [41]. The remaining silver ions can also accumulate in the hulls of dead bacteria, and these reservoirs kill other living bacteria in a process known as the "zombie effect" [42]. Fluoride preferentially forms fluorohydroxyapatite crystals and strengthens surface enamel. It both promotes remineralization and protects against demineralization. The 5% SDF solution contains 44,800 fluoride parts per million (ppm), almost twice that of 5% sodium fluoride varnish containing 22,600 ppm; to date it is the medicament with the highest concentration of fluoride ions available on the market.

SDF Protocol

Due to the significant and permanent discoloration of a tooth after SDF application, a separate informed consent document form should be considered. Ideally, this would also include photos of the black staining that indicates caries arrest (see Fig. 4). To apply SDF, a tooth should first be as isolated as possible to prevent contamination of the saliva and ensure ideal contact between the medicament and the lesion. A cotton roll or gauze isolation with a saliva ejector in place may be helpful. To protect surrounding mucous tissues, a thin layer of petroleum jelly can be applied as a barrier. SDF is a clear or color-tinted liquid, but once the free silver ions are reduced with environmental oxygen, it will turn black and irreversibly stain the carious lesion, any physical harbors (e.g., craze lines, demineralized crevices), and mucosa (Fig. 5). Care should be taken to protect the patient's skin, clothing, and other clinical surfaces that may come in contact with the SDF during the procedure. A thin layer of petroleum jelly can be applied to surrounding soft tissues to prevent SDF from staining. If SDF does contact the mucosa or skin, a dark stain will result but will disappear in a few days to weeks after the epithelium exfoliates. Air-drying of the intended target area is thought to be helpful in placement. Food debris and plaque should be removed from the lesion to allow for optimal contact of the medicament.

Date: ________________

Informed Consent for Silver Diamine Fluoride

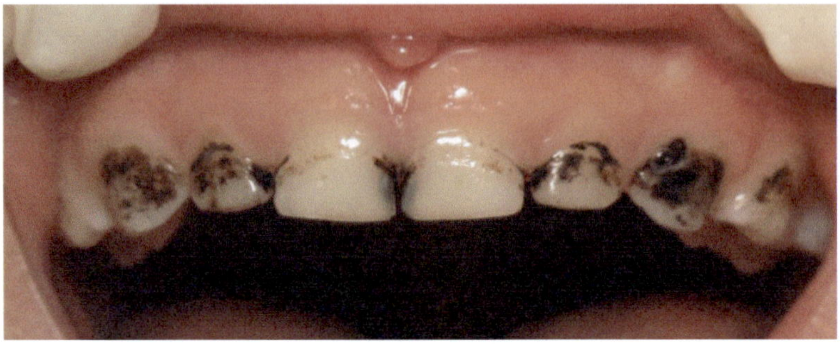

Advantages

- Can help stop tooth decay
- Can help reduce dental sensitivity

Disadvantages

- Will turn the cavity on the tooth **permanently dark in color.**
- May stain other areas. This includes gums, skin, other teeth, or clothing. Areas where tooth -colored restorations meet the tooth surface may also stain.
- May not stop all decay. Some cavities may require more than one application of SDF or other dental treatment such as a filling, crown, root canal therapy, or extraction may be needed.
- May leave a metallic taste in the mouth. This usually dissipates quickly.
- Cannot be used for patients with a metal allergy or open mouth sores.

Alternatives

- No treatment of the cavity is an option. However, progression of the cavity may occur and cause it to become worse.
- Traditional dental treatment is an option. This includes fillings or crowns.

Signature of patient or authorize representative: ______________________________

Signature of clinician: ____

Fig. 4 Sample informed consent form

Once the tooth is isolated, a small drop of SDF is applied to the carious lesion using a microbrush or cotton pellet. Again, care should be taken to restrict application to the intended target. If conditions allow, the SDF should be allowed to be absorbed by the lesion for up to 1 min and any excess blotted off with a clean microbrush, cotton pellet, or other sponge [43]. Multiple teeth may be treated during one appointment. Once applied, a physical barrier precipitates out of the clear solution onto the carious lesion. Two major products form: silver phosphate (Ag_3PO_4), which acts a reservoir of phosphate ions, and calcium fluoride (CaF_2), which is a pH-regulated fluoride supply available during cariogenic challenge [28, 30]. Minor products such as silver-protein complexes form, but their role is poorly understood. It is hypothesized that silver fills the microtubules, further sealing the tooth from disease [44].

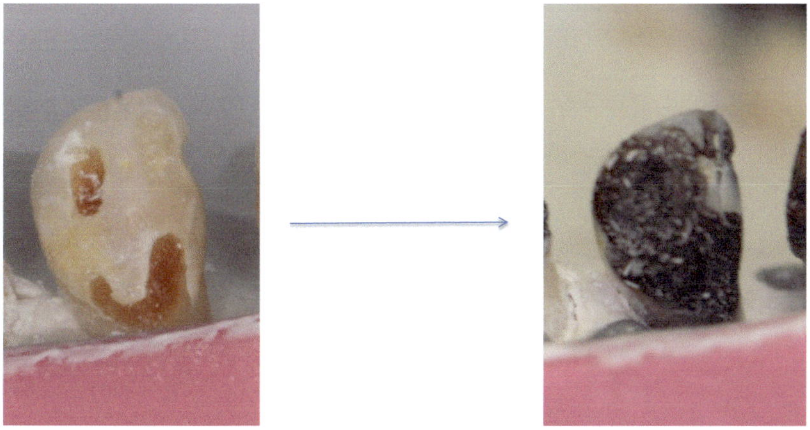

Fig. 5 Color change 24 h after SDF application

A one-time application of SDF is approximately 80–85% effective in arresting decay. This makes follow-up a crucial part of the SDF application process. Lesions should be checked within 1–2 weeks to ensure that the physical barrier has precipitated which will lead to caries arrest. Carious areas should be dark and hard to explorer touch. Leathery lesions, soft lesions, or lesions that have not turned the characteristically dark color will need a reapplication of SDF. This is common if the lesion was not adequately cleared of plaque and debris prior to SDF placement and the medicament could not penetrate to the level of the caries. Patient cooperation can also determine the success of an SDF application. A cooperative child where the medicament can be carefully brushed into the lesion may be a more successful candidate than an uncooperative patient seen in a medical immobilization/protective stabilization device. After caries arrest has been clinically achieved, the lesion will need to be monitored every 3–6 months and SDF applied periodically until the tooth is restored or exfoliates.

SDF's major side effect, the dark staining, can be off-putting to some parents. Some caregivers are more accepting of SDF on posterior teeth than for anterior teeth. It should be noted however that silver particles from an application to posterior teeth might travel through the saliva and stain anterior sites inadvertently. Silver particles may also lodge in enamel defects or craze lines on teeth that are not targeted for therapy and stain them black. Parental acceptance can also rise if the use of SDF may prevent the use of more invasive, traditional treatment modalities. A study of caregiver perception of SDF staining in anterior teeth found that parental acceptance of this treatment modality rose from 29.7 to 60.3% if it meant that treatment under general anesthesia could be avoided [45].

Silver-Modified Atraumatic Restorative Technique Protocol

SDF application alone does not restore the form and function of teeth, and space loss in the dental arch could occur as a result. For large carious lesions, other minimally invasive techniques should be considered as an adjunct to SDF. Placement of

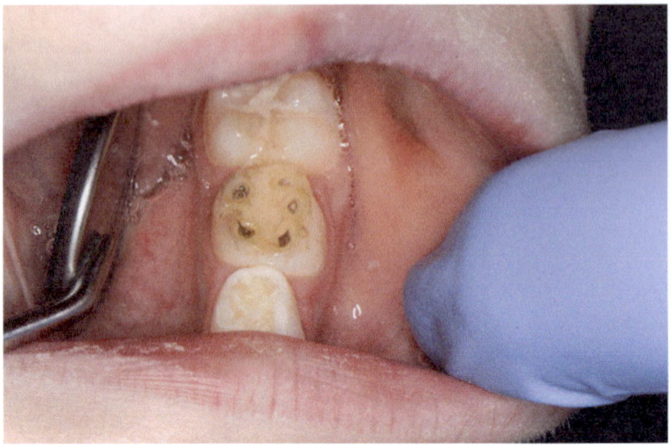

Fig. 6 SMART with immediate GIC over SDF placement—note discoloration

glass ionomer cement over an SDF-treated lesion using the silver-modified atraumatic restorative technique (SMART) is an option [19]. This restoration should be done several hours or days after initial SDF placement, as the ammonia in the wet medicament can be corrosive to glass per the manufacturer's instructions. By delaying placement, the clinician can also ensure that caries arrest has taken place for a favorable outcome. This achieves a better esthetic result as the silver ions will mix less with the glass ionomer cement and not discolor the restoration (Fig. 6).

It should be noted that because there is a plan for follow-up and continuous monitoring of the lesion, this technique more resembles interim therapeutic restorations (ITR) than ART.

Case Scenario

Rachel is a 2-year and 9-month-old female who presents to your clinic for a consult request by her medical oncology team. Her medical history is significant for acute lymphoblastic leukemia that was diagnosed 3 weeks ago. Rachel lives with her mother, father, and older brother who are all healthy. Her medical team noted in their referral that she has caries on her anterior teeth.

On clinical exam you note that Rachel has all primary teeth present with open molar contacts and adequate spacing in her primary dentition. All soft tissues are pink, firm, and healthy. You confirm that Rachel has caries in all anterior teeth as well as the occlusal surfaces of her first primary molars. This is consistent with severe early childhood caries as classified by the American Academy of Pediatric Dentistry [46]. There are no abscesses or fistulas present. On speaking with her parents, you learn that Rachel was breastfed ad libitum until a few months ago. Her parents brush occasionally with a non-fluoridated "training" toothpaste, but use has been infrequent because they report she did not like it. She eats a varied diet with frequent snacks of crackers, cheese, and fruit.

You consult with Rachel's medical oncology team, and they would like to begin chemotherapy this week. This will necessitate delaying dental treatment for 3–4 months. While none of her carious lesions are approximating the pulp chamber, she does have significant dental decay that compromises form and function. You discuss options with her team and her parents.

First, you give Rachel's parents primary preventive recommendations that are focused on care during chemotherapy. This includes appropriate use of fluoridated toothpaste twice a day. You also discuss healthy diet options that limit carbohydrates and processed sugars. Rachel may also take oral medications during chemotherapy that are high in sucrose, and you discuss the cariogenic potential of these elixirs.

To address Rachel's current dental disease, you want to arrest the decay currently present until it can be addressed once her medical condition is stable. Since there are no large lesions with risk for pulpal involvement, you feel comfortable delaying her dental treatment per the recommendation of her medical team. SDF can arrest the current lesions and prevent new lesions from occurring during the course of chemotherapy treatment. The downside, the dark discoloration, is discussed with the parents. This side effect is also discussed with the medical team, as physicians may not recognize that these dark lesions are arrested caries. The parents provide written and verbal consent to SDF application, and you place the medicament in your office the same day. You reappoint Rachel for a return visit 1 month later. At that appointment you determine that most, but not all, the lesions have arrested. You reapply SDF at that visit.

Rachel begins chemotherapy and you are unable to follow up with her for 6 months. After the course of her oncology treatment, you see Rachel for a recare visit at your clinic. You discover that all of the anterior teeth have arrested and that one of the most caries-compromised incisors has fractured. You discuss treatment options with Rachel's care team and her family. Her parents find the cosmetic appearance of the teeth objectionable, and her oncologist clears her for comprehensive oral rehabilitation in the operating room. You finalize the plan to see Rachel for comprehensive dental care and rehabilitation under general anesthesia. In the operating room, you note that all smooth surface and cavitated pit-and-fissure lesions are arrested and hard to explorer touch. Operatively you remove the most superficial layer of the dark hardened crust and restore the anterior teeth with zirconia crowns and posterior molars with stainless steel crowns. These full-coverage restorations completely mask the dark staining. Rachel's parents are pleased with the esthetic and restorative results.

Conclusion

- Modern dentistry is undergoing a paradigm shift from surgical management of caries to a medical management approach.
- In addition to primary prevention and tertiary surgical treatment, minimally invasive treatment techniques are emerging as secondary treatment options.
- Minimally invasive treatment options include Hall crowns, interim therapeutic restorations, medicaments such as silver diamine fluoride, and combinations of these.

- Children with special health-care needs can greatly benefit from these minimally invasive options as they may prevent the need for dental treatment under sedation or general anesthesia.

References

1. AAPD. Guideline on caries-risk assessment and management for infants, children, and adolescents. Pediatr Dent. 2016;38(6):142–9.
2. ADA. American Dental Association Caries Risk Assessment Form. http://www.ada.org/~/media/ADA/Science%20and%20Research/Files/topic_caries_over6.ashx. Published 2011. Accessed 1 Jan 2017.
3. Jenson L, Budenz AW, Featherstone JDB, Ramos-Gomez FJ, Spolsky VW, Young DA. Clinical protocols for caries management by risk assessment. J Calif Dent Assoc. 2007;35(10):714–23.
4. Sarvas EW, Schwantes SA, Karp JM. Preparing the pediatric dentist for palliative and end-of-life care. Pediatr Dent. 2016;38(4):295–9.
5. Humphrey W. Use of chrome steel in children's dentistry. Dent Surv. 1950;26:945–9.
6. Seale N, Randall R. The use of stainless steel crowns: a systematic literature review. Pediatr Dent. 2015;37(2):147–62.
7. Innes NPT, Stirrups DR, Evans DJP, Hall N, Leggate M. A novel technique using preformed metal crowns for managing carious primary molars in general practice—a retrospective analysis. Br Dent J. 2006;200(8):451–4.
8. Gilchrist F, Morgan AG, Farman M, Rodd HD. Impact of the Hall technique for preformed metal crown placement on undergraduate paediatric dentistry experience. Eur J Dent Educ. 2013;17(1):e10–5.
9. Innes NP, Evans DJP, Stirrups DR. The Hall Technique; a randomized controlled clinical trial of a novel method of managing carious primary molars in general dental practice: acceptability of the technique and outcomes at 23 months. BMC Oral Health. 2007;7:1–21.
10. Innes N, Stewart M, Souster G, Evans D. The Hall Technique; retrospective case-note follow-up of 5-year RCT. Br Dent J. 2015;219(8):395–400.
11. Ludwig KH, Fontana M, Vinson LQA, Platt JA, Dean JA. The success of stainless steel crowns placed with the Hall Technique: a retrospective study. J Am Dent Assoc. 2014;145(12):1248–53.
12. Schwendicke F, Stolpe M, Innes N. Conventional treatment, Hall Technique or immediate pulpotomy for carious primary molars: a cost-effectiveness analysis. Int Endod J. 2015;49:1–10.
13. Innes NPT, Ricketts D, Chong LY e, Keightley AJ, Lamont T, Santamaria RM. Preformed crowns for decayed primary molar teeth. Cochrane Database Syst Rev. 2015;12(12):CD005512. https://doi.org/10.1002/14651858.CD005512.pub3.
14. Garrocho-Rangel A, Echavarria-Garcia A, Rosales-Berber M, Flores-Velazquez J, Pozos-Guillen A. Dental management of pediatric patients affected by pulmonary atresia with ventricular septal defect: a scoping review. Med Oral Patol Oral Cir Bucal. 2017;22(4):e458–66.
15. Santamaria RM, Innes NPT, Machiulskiene V, Evans DJP, Alkilzy M, Splieth CH. Acceptability of different caries management methods for primary molars in a RCT. Int J Paediatr Dent. 2015;25(1):9–17.
16. Frencken JE. The ART approach using glass-ionomers in relation to global oral health care. Dent Mater. 2010;26(1):1–6.
17. Tyas MJ, Anusavice KJ, Frencken JE, Mount GJ. Minimal intervention dentistry—a review: FDI Commission Project 1-97. Int Dent J. 2000;50:1):1–12.
18. Monse-Schneider B, Heinrich-Weltzien R, Schug D, Sheiham A, Borutta A. Assessment of manual restorative treatment (MRT) with amalgam in high-caries Filipino children: results after 2 years. Community Dent Oral Epidemiol. 2003;31(2):129–35.
19. Alvear Fa B, Arron J, Wong A, Young D. Silver modified atraumatic restorative technique (SMART). Stoma EDU J. 2016;3(2):18–24.

20. Frencken JE, Holmgren CJ. Caries management through the Atraumatic Restorative treatment (ART) approach and glass-ionomers: update 2013. Braz Oral Res. 2014;28(1):1–4.
21. Hesse D, Bonifacio CC, Bonecker M, et al. Survival rate of Atraumatic Restorative Treatment (ART) restorations using a glass ionomer bilayer technique with a nanofilled coating: a bi-center randomized clinical trial. Pediatr Dent. 2016;38(1):18–24.
22. The American Academy of Pediatric Dentistry. Policy on interim therapeutic restorations (ITR). Pediatr Dent. 2017;39(6 Suppl):57–8.
23. Nelson T. An improved interim therapeutic restoration technique for management of anterior early childhood caries: report of two cases. Pediatr Dent. 2004;35(4):124–8.
24. Soares FC, Cardoso M, Bolan M. Altered esthetics in primary central incisors: the child's perception. Pediatr Dent. 2015;37(5):29–34.
25. Barillo DJ, Marx DE. Silver in medicine: a brief history BC 335 to present. Burns. 2014;40(Suppl 1):S3–8.
26. Lansdown ABG. Silver in health care: antimicrobial effects and safety in use. Curr Probl Dermatol. 2006;33:17–34.
27. Stebbens E. What value has argenti nitras as a therapeutic in dentistry? Int Dent J. 1891;12(10):661–71.
28. Peng JJ-Y, Botelho MG, Matinlinna JP. Silver compounds used in dentistry for caries management: a review. J Dent. 2012;40(7):531–41.
29. Craig GG, Powell KR, Cooper MH. Caries progression in primary molars: 24-month results from a minimal treatment programme. Community Dent Oral Epidemiol. 1981;9(6):260–5.
30. Nishino M, Yoshida S, Sobue S, Kato J, Nishida M. Effect of topically applied ammoniacal silver fluoride on dental caries in children. J Osaka Univ Dent Sch. 1969;9:149–55.
31. Yamaga R, Nishino M, Yoshida S, Yokomizo I. Diammine silver fluoride and its clinical application. J Osaka Univ Dent Sch. 1972;12:1–20.
32. Gao SS, Zhang S, Mei ML, Lo EC-M, Chu C-H. Caries remineralisation and arresting effect in children by professionally applied fluoride treatment—a systematic review. BMC Oral Health. 2016;16(1):12.
33. Llodra JC, Rodriguez A, Ferrer B, Menardia V, Ramos T, Morato M. Efficacy of silver diamine fluoride for caries reduction in primary teeth and first permanent molars of schoolchildren: 36-Month clinical trial. Practitioner. 2005;249(1675):721–4.
34. Dos Santos VE, De Vasconcelos FMN, Ribeiro AG, Rosenblatt A. Paradigm shift in the effective treatment of caries in schoolchildren at risk. Int Dent J. 2012;62(1):47–51.
35. Monse B, Heinrich-Weltzien R, Mulder J, Holmgren C, van Palenstein Helderman WH. Caries preventive efficacy of silver diammine fluoride (SDF) and ART sealants in a school-based daily fluoride toothbrushing program in the Philippines. BMC Oral Health. 2012;12(1):52.
36. Yee R, Holmgren C, Mulder J, Lama D, Walker D, van Palenstein Helderman W. Efficacy of silver diamine fluoride for arresting caries treatment. J Dent Res. 2009;88(7):644–7.
37. Tan HP, Lo ECM, Dyson JE, Luo Y, Corbet EF. A randomized trial on root caries prevention in elders. J Dent Res. 2010;89(10):1086–90.
38. Nantanee R, Santiwong B, Trairatvorakul C, Hamba H, Tagami J. Silver diamine fluoride and glass ionomer differentially remineralize early caries lesions, in situ. Clin Oral Investig. 2016;20(6):1151–7.
39. Zhi QH, Lo ECM, Lin HC. Randomized clinical trial on effectiveness of silver diamine fluoride and glass ionomer in arresting dentine caries in preschool children. J Dent. 2012;40(11):962–7.
40. Liu BY, Lo ECM, Chu CH, Lin HC. Randomized trial on fluorides and sealants for fissure caries prevention. J Dent Res. 2012;91(8):753–8.
41. Jung WK, Koo HC, Kim KW, Shin S, Kim SH, Park YH. Antibacterial activity and mechanism of action of the silver ion in Staphylococcus aureus and Escherichia coli. Appl Environ Microbiol. 2008;74(7):2171–8.
42. Wakshlak RB-K, Pedahzur R, Avnir D. Antibacterial activity of silver-killed bacteria: the "zombies" effect. Sci Rep. 2015;5(1):9555.
43. Horst JA, Ellenikiotis H, Milgrom PL. UCSF protocol for caries arrest using silver diamine fluoride: rationale, indications and consent. J Calif Dent Assoc. 2016;44(1):16–28.

44. Seto J, Horst JA, Parkinson DY, Frachella JC, DeRisi JL. Silver microwires from treating tooth decay with silver diamine fluoride. bioRxiv. 2017. doi: https://doi.org/10.1101/152199.
45. Crystal YO, Janal MN, Hamilton DS, Niederman R. Parental perceptions and acceptance of silver diamine fluoride staining. J Am Dent Assoc. 2017;148(7):510–518.e4.
46. American Academy of Pediatric Dentistry. Policy on early childhood caries (ECC): classification, consequences, and preventive strategies. Oral Health Policies. 2017;37(6):50–2.

Pharmacologic Management of the Pediatric Patient with Special Healthcare Needs

James W. Tom

Introduction

Numerous non-pharmacologic strategies exist to effectively render dental and surgical care to children with special healthcare needs. Desensitization, tell-show-do, and hypnosis remain common considerations, while directed strategies focusing upon environmental and situational modifications are discussed elsewhere in this text. Certain dental procedures and surgeries combined with the particular concerns of the child with special healthcare needs may exceed the utility of some of these methods, and pharmacologic strategies must be considered as possible alternatives when such situations arise.

From a 2016 US Census report, the population of children aged 17 years and younger with severe disabilities stands at approximately 6.2% [1]. Within this population, a portion of children with medical complexities exists with severe chronic illness and some with the use of various life-sustaining technologies [2]. These children, by virtue of their condition alone, may require treatment in hospital settings and may require advanced anesthesia and perioperative care. For those who may not require extensive perioperative care for dental treatment, it is prudent to first explore methods and strategies of basic behavior support techniques in traditional settings in an effort to provide ready access for comprehensive oral healthcare. According to the American Academy of Pediatric Dentistry (AAPD) Guideline on Behavior Guidance for the Pediatric Patient [3], six concepts should be approached first when attempting behavior support:

- Voice control
- Nonverbal communication

J. W. Tom, DDS, MS (✉)
Herman Ostrow School of Dentistry, University of Southern California,
Los Angeles, CA, USA
e-mail: jtom@usc.edu

T. M. Nelson, J. R. Webb (eds.), *Dental Care for Children with Special Needs*,
https://doi.org/10.1007/978-3-030-10483-2_10

- "Tell-show-do"
- Positive reinforcement
- Distraction
- Parental presence or absence during treatment

Other chapters in this text address modalities such as desensitization, occupational therapy approaches, and protective stabilization. Hypnosis, repetitive tasking, contingent/non-contingent escape, and escape extinction have also been described in the literature [4]. Yet when these and additional strategies fail to provide a safe, predictable, and minimally traumatic environment for Children with Special Healthcare Needs (CSHCN), the use of pharmacologic means to render treatment becomes a viable treatment option.

When Non-pharmacologic Strategies Are Not Enough

Providing safe and high-quality dental care demands that patients be relatively immobile to produce clear diagnostic imaging, atraumatic local anesthesia delivery, safe operative dentistry and surgical conditions with high- and slow-speed rotary instruments, and accurate dental impressions and occlusal registrations. Children that have difficulty in communication, sensory perception, or behavior are certainly put at risk when preventative and restorative dentistry or surgery is performed. Non-pharmacologic treatment modalities to reduce movement and increase patient safety may be unreliable from appointment to appointment, and factors outside of the control of the operative team and caretakers can be highly unpredictable.

Additionally, the course of time needed for caretakers and the operative team to adapt to a child's behavioral patterns and routines, sensory and psychological sensitivities, and ongoing therapies may be impractical in timely treatment of pressing or immediate oral healthcare conditions. Limitations to cognitive and developmental age, assessment of the efficacy of therapeutic medications for daily living, and nonpharmacologic interventions may also hinder timely delivery of needed care.

Various methods ranging from inhalation sedation with nitrous oxide and oxygen to general anesthesia exist for these particular circumstances. Yet particular attention must be directed toward preoperative preparation, health history gathering, and specific postoperative care considerations when treating CSHCN.

Equally important are the preoperative, perioperative, and postoperative concerns and needs of the parents or caretakers. The myriad of pharmacologic treatment options coupled with the dental treatment options must be clearly delineated for individuals involved in long-term care of the CSCHN. This enables them to make informed and appropriate decisions regarding safe care. Parents and caretakers also play vitally important roles in gathering needed information from other healthcare providers for preoperative assessment, postoperative management, and follow-up care.

The Sedation and Anesthesia Continuum

Current understanding of the wide range of pharmaceutically induced depression of the central nervous system is best described as a continuum. Because of the myriad of patient presentations and types of procedures performed in dentistry, no one level or plane of anesthesia may be suitable for every patient. For some CSCHN, each appointment or scheduled visit may require different sedation and anesthesia demands due to a variety of factors that may include ongoing development or growth, changing medical or psychological therapies, or the dental procedure or planned surgery. Likewise, within a single procedure, different levels of central nervous system depression may be needed to assist the patient through surgically stimulating or invasive procedures, while at other times, periods of minimal operative stimulation or manipulation may require lighter levels of sedation or anesthesia.

The American Dental Association (ADA), American Academy of Pediatrics (AAP), American Academy of Pediatric Dentistry (AAPD), American Society of Dentist Anesthesiologists (ASDA), and the American Society of Anesthesiologists (ASA) have all agreed upon and adopted standard terminology to describe the continuum of sedation and anesthesia [5–7]. Being a continuum, levels of consciousness, respiratory drive and patency, and cardiovascular function can vary depending on the medical complexity of the child and the medications administered. The standard definitions are as follows:

Minimal Sedation (anxiolysis) is a drug-induced state during which patients respond normally to verbal commands. Although cognitive function and physical coordination may be impaired, airway reflexes and ventilatory and cardiovascular functions are unaffected.

Moderate Sedation/Analgesia ("conscious sedation") is a drug-induced depression of consciousness during which patients respond purposefully (Note: reflex withdrawal from painful stimulus is *not* considered a purposeful response) to verbal commands, either alone or accompanied by light tactile stimulation. No interventions are required to maintain a patent airway, and spontaneous ventilation is adequate. Cardiovascular function is usually maintained.

Deep Sedation/Analgesia is a drug-induced depression of consciousness during which patients cannot be easily aroused but respond purposefully following repeated or painful stimulation. The ability to independently maintain ventilatory function may be impaired. Patients may require assistance in maintaining a patent airway, and spontaneous ventilation may be inadequate. Cardiovascular function is usually maintained.

General Anesthesia is a drug-induced loss of consciousness during which patients are not arousable, even by painful stimulation. The ability to independently maintain ventilatory function is often impaired. Patients often require assistance in maintaining a patent airway, and positive pressure ventilation may be required because of depressed ventilation or drug-induced depression of neuromuscular function. Cardiovascular function may be impaired.

Although the definitions seemingly present distinct levels of central nervous depression, the continuum of sedation and anesthesia in the context of treating children may not have such well-defined parameters. An important concept undergirding these definitions when treating CSHCN with sedatives or general anesthesia medications is careful consideration of the overall initial presentation of the patient. Children often present with anatomical, medical, and behavioral complexity that may already impair neurologic, respiratory, and/or cardiovascular functioning. The administration of drugs may further suppress these physiologic systems. Accordingly, there exists a high potential for exceeding the intended level of sedation when usual behavioral and physiologic indicators of depth of sedation are obscured or absent. Without question, a comprehensive and thorough preoperative evaluation and medical history are paramount before undertaking any procedure involving pharmacologic sedation and/or general anesthesia.

Routes of Administration

Enteral Administration

Introducing sedative medications into the body may prove challenging for providers caring for CSHCN. With children in general, the enteral, or oral, route is typically preferred by many dental practitioners for its relative ease of acceptance by patients, painless administration to children, and achievement of acceptable levels of moderate sedation. This is also a convenient route for some patients who are administered medications through a gastronomy tube. Pediatric absorption of medications via the enteric system differs from that of adult absorption. Generally, drug uptake and delivery to target organs by the oral route occurs much more slowly in pediatrics than adults. Gastric pH, emptying time, immaturity of secretions, and activity of bile and pancreatic fluids all account for a slower uptake when compared to adult oral absorption [8].

Advantages Enteral administration of sedative medications is generally well-tolerated by children who are able to take medications via the oral route. Those children unable to accept medications in pill or tablet forms may have medications made into powder form using pill crushers and then mixed into a liquid or familiar food (apple sauce, syrup, etc.). Many sedative medications are available in oral suspension or liquid form. Additionally, permitting requirements for dental practitioners employing oral moderate sedation and, in particular, oral sedation for pediatrics are generally easier to obtain but vary from state to state [9]. Deep sedation and general anesthesia employed by dental practitioners require extensive residency training and more stringent permitting requirements.

Disadvantages Enteral administration is subject to first-pass hepatic metabolism, where the orally or gastronomy tube administered drug undergoes metabolism via portal circulation before ever reaching systemic circulation. Because of this first-pass hepatic metabolism, pharmacologic effects of sedative medications can be highly variable and unpredictable. Intended levels of sedation may never be achieved or, more dangerously, may be exceeded, and a child may enter levels of deep sedation/general anesthesia when lighter levels were intended. Additionally, pediatric patients with hepatic dysfunction or genetic dispositions in hepatic enzyme production may exhibit even greater unpredictability than is typical for this inherently unpredictable route of administration. Re-dosing of oral medications in a single appointment is not advised. "Stacking" of doses can lead to oversedation, and achieving ideal levels of moderate sedation with a singular dose may be difficult when using weight-based dosing regimens.

Parenteral Administration

Techniques of drug administration that circumvent first-pass hepatic metabolism lead to predictable blood serum levels of sedative medications. Parenteral administration of sedative medications can range from the minimally invasive, such as inhaled nitrous oxide/oxygen sedation, to those requiring advanced training in performing venipuncture and vein catheterization. In the United States, the permitting process for dentists to provide parenteral moderate sedation has been a more rigorous and intensive educational process, generally requiring both a didactic and clinical component. Parenteral moderate sedatives are commonly administered intravenously in dental settings, with intramuscular and even intranasal routes being employed occasionally. General anesthesia, in most common forms, is also delivered via various parental routes that include inhalation, intravenous, and intramuscular injections.

Advantages Parenteral administration, because of its direct route into the venous circulation, bypasses first-pass hepatic metabolism and delivers a reliable concentration of drug into the bloodstream. Parenteral administration allows titration, the incremental dosing to effect, with forms such as intravenous or inhalational routes. Because of less albumin and protein present in the pediatric bloodstream, there are more active molecules of drug than in adult administration. Induction into moderate sedation, deep sedation, or general anesthesia is often rapid and ideal for children who present with apprehension and an inability to tolerate dental treatment. Short-acting sedative medications with rapid onset of action can allow for more rapid and complete recovery from sedation and anesthesia than sedatives that are administered enterally.

Disadvantages Accessibility to providers who offer parenteral moderate sedation or deep sedation/general anesthesia in dental office-based settings can be limited due to heightened training requirements and state licensing restrictions. Parenteral moderate sedation via the intravenous route may be difficult to achieve in a young child who is unable to tolerate invasive procedures such as intravenous cannulation. Furthermore, relatively few deep sedation and general anesthesia practitioners in dentistry, namely, dentist anesthesiologists and oral and maxillofacial surgeons, are readily available to treat CSHCN and those with complex medical conditions. Delivery of parenteral deep sedation and general anesthesia demands proper equipment specific to pediatric care, monitoring during the perioperative phase, and trained personnel involved in all aspects of patient care. This can be challenging outside of hospital-based settings. For medically and behaviorally complex CSHCN, an office-based or ambulatory setting for parenteral administration of sedative medications may be wholly inappropriate, and hospital care may be the only option.

Note: *Deeper than intended levels of sedation can be achieved by any route of administration (enteral, sublingual, intramuscular, intranasal, etc.).*

Minimal Sedation or Anxiolysis

For some CSHCN, a minimal level of central nervous depression, or anxiolysis, may be adequate for dental treatment. Also, minimal sedation may be used as an introductory phase of an overall anesthetic strategy to reduce preoperative anxiety prior to deep sedation or general anesthesia. Minimal sedation may also be the primary mode of pharmacologic management when CSHCN present in the dental setting for minor procedures or procedures of relatively short duration.

Nitrous Oxide

A popular and classic agent used in many pediatric dental office settings is nitrous oxide inhalation sedation. Used alone, or in combination with an enteral sedative, nitrous oxide/oxygen inhalation minimal sedation has a rapid onset of action, can be titrated, and allows for almost complete recovery from any sedative effect once it is discontinued. Specifically, nitrous oxide's low solubility in both blood and fat allows for its quick clinical effect and short duration of action once administration of the gas is terminated. Its actions have been described as an anxiolytic, an analgesic, and a weak anesthetic. It acts via inhibition of the *N*-methyl-D-aspartate (NMDA) of the excitatory glutamate receptor. The additional effects of nitrous oxide upon the γ-aminobutyric acid (GABA) and α-amino-3-hydroxyl-5-methyl-4-isoxazole-propionate receptors have also been implicated in its sedative and analgesic effects [10].

Commonly, rapid induction into minimal sedation or anxiolysis involves the administration of nitrous oxide at a concentration of 50–70% for a brief period followed by careful titration of the inhaled mixture to below 50% nitrous oxide concentrations. Prolonged exposure to concentrations above 50% may lead to increased risks of nausea and vomiting, oversedation, or an inability of the patient to follow verbal commands.

Limitations CSHCN presenting with respiratory conditions that preclude breathing through a nasal hood generally will not be candidates for nitrous oxide/oxygen sedation. Upper respiratory infections, partial or complete choanal atresia, cleft lip and/or palate, or any situation where placement of the typical nitrous oxide nasal hood and effective nasal breathing will compromise delivery of effective minimal sedation are relative contraindications.

Lower respiratory conditions, although not absolute contraindications, may also impede gas exchange and restrict effective sedation attempts. Children with significant respiratory conditions, such as incapacitating cystic fibrosis, pulmonary sequestrations (blebs), closed air spaces, bronchogenic or adenomatoid cysts, congenital lung disorders, or severe inflammatory disease, should generally be treated in the hospital setting. Care of these children in office-based settings is only appropriate after close consultation with pediatric pulmonology specialists and possibly pediatric anesthesia specialists familiar with outpatient and office-based settings.

The American Academy of Pediatric Dentistry (AAPD) describes other contraindications for nitrous oxide administration. Along with the aforementioned respiratory considerations, the AAPD lists avoiding the use or exposure of nitrous oxide for those individuals in the first trimester of pregnancy, concurrent treatment with bleomycin sulfate for malignancies, methylenetetrahydrofolate reductase (MTHFR) deficiency, and cobalamin (vitamin B12) deficiency [11].

Children presenting with MTHFR deficiency, an autosomal recessive disorder that implicates gene mutation at C677T and A1298C locations, have increased risk factors for heart disease, stroke, hypertension, glaucoma, psychiatric disorders, and neural tube birth defects. MTHFR is responsible for folate metabolism and homocysteine regulation, and nitrous oxide inhibits the transformation of homocysteine to methionine and subsequently leads to an accumulation of unconverted homocysteine in affected children. Homocysteine levels can also stem from deficiencies in vitamin B12, folic acid, and vitamin B6. As a result of increased homocysteine levels, increased prothrombotic activity and platelet adhesiveness (clotting) have been observed [12]. Nitrous oxide exposure in children with known MTHFR deficiency must be avoided.

Moderate or Procedural Sedation

Moderate sedation provides a deeper plane of central nervous system depression that may allow for more invasive or lengthier procedures that would otherwise be poorly tolerated or painful without this modality. With proper licensing, facilities, training, personnel, and monitoring, it can occur in dental office-based settings, ambulatory surgical centers, and hospital-based settings. A multitude of agents can be employed to provide moderate sedation for CSHCN. This may include enteral or parenteral routes of administration or a combination of both. For all children with complex medical conditions, it is critical to conduct a thorough evaluation and consultation with members of the healthcare team and engage in shared decision-making regarding the use of moderate sedation among parents, caretakers, practitioners, and consultants.

While often itself the intended goal of procedural sedation, moderate sedation can also be employed as a premedication prior to the induction of general anesthesia. It can provide an effective means of alleviating significant anxiety and reducing difficult behavior prior to mask inhalation induction, intramuscular induction, or intravenous attempts in general anesthesia. The following additional benefits can also be accomplished [13]:

- Reduction in autonomic (vagal) reflexes
- Reduction in airway secretions
- Anterograde amnesia
- Prophylaxis against pulmonary aspiration of gastric contents
- Provide analgesia

Patient Evaluation for Moderate Sedation

Particular emphasis must be placed upon the evaluation of a CSHCN's ability to maintain a patent airway for oxygenation and ventilation. In extreme situations, a "difficult airway" is described by the ASA as "the clinical situation in which a trained anesthesiologist experiences difficulty with facemask ventilation of the upper airway" (Table 1). In dental office-based situations where immediate management from experienced and trained anesthesia providers may not be possible, avoidance of such situation is paramount. Patients presenting with conditions that involve narrowed or inflamed airways, limited mouth opening, limitations to head and neck movement and extension, anatomic obstruction, and limited neurologic control of respiration are particularly at risk for adverse moderate sedation outcomes. Cardiovascular conditions also play an important role in patient evaluation for

Table 1 Difficult airways in congenital syndromes based on anatomical site [14]

Anatomical site	Common related syndromes
Nasopharynx	Mucopolysaccharidoses
Oral cavity/oropharynx	Trisomy 21 Beckwith-Wiedemann syndrome Mucopolysaccharidoses
Mandible/maxilla	Pierre Robin sequence Treacher Collins syndrome Goldenhar syndrome Apert syndrome
Pharynx/larynx	Trisomy 21
Trachea	Trisomy 21 Mucopolysaccharidoses
Cervical spine	Trisomy 21 Klippel-Feil syndrome Goldenhar syndrome Mucopolysaccharidoses

moderate sedation. Parenteral administration via the intravenous route may affect circulation and cardiac output. Certain agents used in moderate sedation may precipitate untoward increases or decreases in heart rate or inotropy.

Shared decision-making involves bidirectional, or two-way, exchange of information between providers, patients, and caregivers to reach treatment plan agreement [15]. The treatment plan should allow for multiple preoperative evaluation appointments to gather needed information from consultants. For CSHCN with complex medical conditions, it is not uncommon to involve physician consultants far outside the range of the usual pediatrician and cardiologist. Previous anesthesiologists, surgeons, pulmonologists, endocrinologists, psychiatrists and psychologists, or neurologists can be welcome contributors to the overall dental care plan.

Monitoring in Moderate Sedation

As of this writing, the ADA, the AAPD, the AAP, and the ASA [16] recommend the following monitoring and personnel in their published guidelines concerning the use of moderate sedation in dental settings (Table 2). Boards of Dentistry also mandate specific practice parameters for each state.

Capnography, the measurement of exhaled carbon dioxide during respiration, is an extremely valuable monitoring parameter during moderate sedation. It is also extremely useful in resuscitation efforts and rescue. Dentistry, however, poses a unique problem in the use of capnography since the airway is relatively open, and exhaled carbon dioxide oftentimes exits the oral cavity rather than the nose. Typical nasal cannulas depend on exhaled carbon dioxide gases via the nasal route for accurate measurement. Also, in pediatric dental moderate sedation, supplemental oxygen is delivered via nasal hood versus a nasal cannula, so adaption of current

Table 2 Monitoring and personnel requirements for moderate sedation

	ADA	AAP/AAPD	ASA
Pulse oximetry	Yes	Yes	Yes
Noninvasive blood pressure measurement	Yes	Yes, 15 min increments	Yes
Capnography	Capnography or pre-tracheal stethoscope	Capnography (preferred) or pre-tracheal stethoscope + bidirectional communication	Yes, unless precluded by the nature of the patient, procedure, or equipment. Institute capnography after moderate sedation has been achieved
Personnel with requisite permitting and training	Two individuals: operating dentist with ACLS and BLS-HCP, dental assistant with BLS-HCP	Two individuals: operating dentist (PALS certification recommended), assistant (trained in advanced airway management)	Two individuals: operating dentist and assistant trained in recognition of apnea and airway obstruction

monitoring technologies to the pediatric dental setting is often required. Figure 1 is an example of adapting a common Luer lock-type connector to a nitrous oxide nasal hood, and Fig. 2 is the resultant capnograph waveform displayed on a typical vital signs monitor.

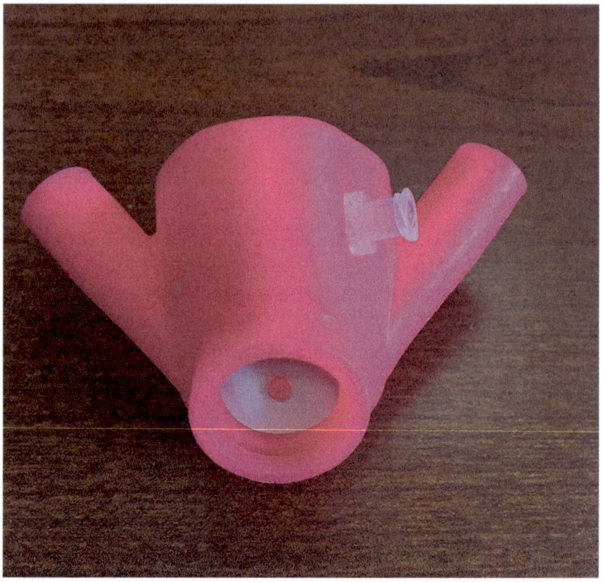

Fig. 1 Nitrous oxide nasal hood adapted to receive capnography line

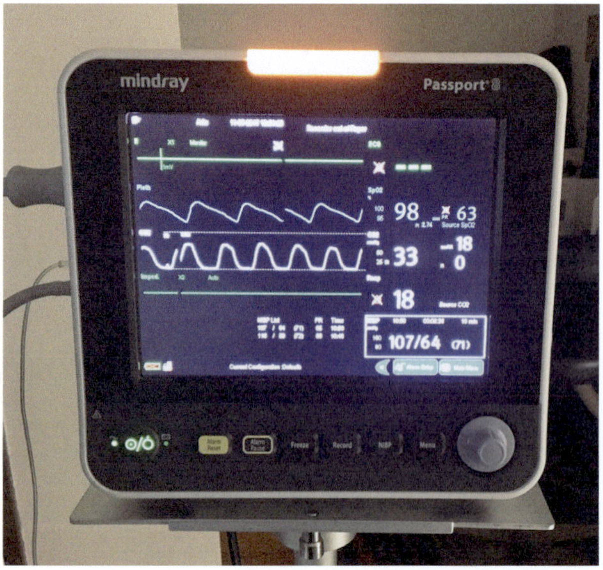

Fig. 2 End-tidal CO2 being displayed at 33 mm/Hg measured via nasal hood

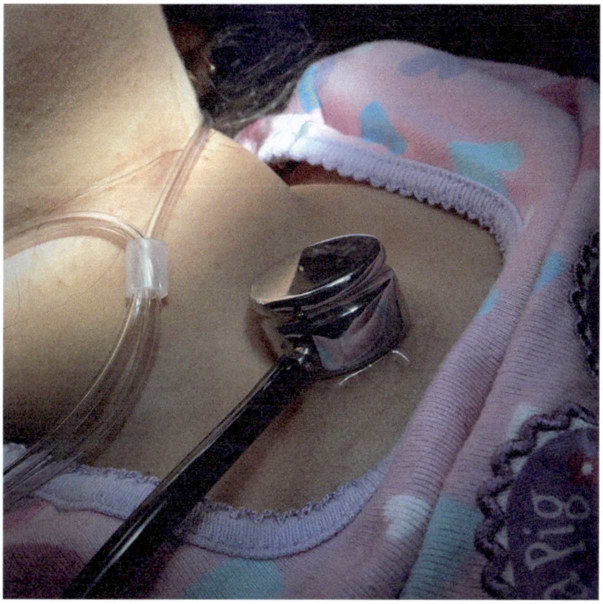

Fig. 3 Pre-tracheal stethoscopy on a pediatric patient during moderate sedation

Alternatively, pre-tracheal or tracheal stethoscopy can be an immediate, real-time auditory monitor of patient respiration (Fig. 3). This method is not subject to mouth breathing artifacts. Pre-tracheal stethoscopes, placed above the sternal notch and midline on or around the thyroid cartilage with double-sided adhesive tape, can transmit the sounds of respiration, the "gurgling" of fluids in the airway, and even the heart rate from adjacent carotid arteries through direct auscultation or electronic amplification.

Personnel

Because moderate sedation relies on purposeful response from the patient, at least two individuals are required for patient monitoring. The operating dentist or surgeon in office-based settings usually orders and administers the sedative agents, while a dental assistant, termed "support personnel" by the AAPD, may monitor or contribute in "supportive or resuscitative" measures. Dental assistants, while monitoring, may be engaged in interruptible patient-related tasks of short duration (suctioning, light curing, retraction, irrigation, etc.) or even be troubleshooting equipment. The practitioner should be trained in recognizing and rescuing a pediatric patient from unintended deep sedation and managing the airway in an unconscious patient.

Very often, moderate sedation techniques are accompanied by protective stabilization. This may cause typical methods of observing patient stability—chest excursion upon respiration, patient movement, and skin/mucosal color—to be obscured. Other protective measures used in pediatric dentistry such as patient eye protection

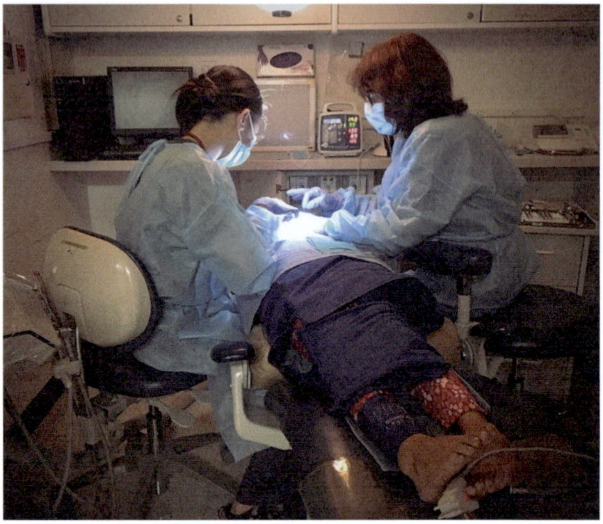

Fig. 4 Typical pediatric dentistry "quiet room" where direct observation and monitoring can be obscured by protective stabilization, lack of light, and auditory distractions

(sometimes tinted) and rubber dams or pharyngeal isolation devices can cause more indicators of patient ventilation, sedation level, and patient oxygenation to be obfuscated. Pediatric treatment rooms where moderate sedation is performed are often isolated and dark to calm patients and provide a less distracting environment. The lack of operatory lighting may hinder direct visualization of mucous membranes and patient response. Lastly, auditory cues are often masked by dental high-volume suction and dental high-speed handpieces. Figure 4 shows a typical pediatric treatment "quiet room."

Common Agents Used in Moderate Sedation

Antihistamines

In pediatric moderate sedation, antihistamines are often administered for both sedative and antiemetic effects. H_1 receptor inhibition decreases the amount of histamine released and has utility for patients with chronic inflammatory conditions such as asthma or allergic rhinitis. Additionally, a decrease in mucous secretions and the antisialogogue action of antihistamines also is an added benefit in pediatric dentistry.

Of the antihistamines used for sedation, both hydroxyzine and diphenhydramine have been popular agents used alone or in combination with another sedative or inhaled nitrous oxide. Both diphenhydramine and hydroxyzine are available in oral formulations and provide antisialogogue and sedative effects. Both agents readily cross the blood-brain barrier and also provide antimuscarinic anticholinergic effects that can raise heart rate and cardiac output. However, paradoxical reactions, where the central nervous system becomes stimulated instead of depressed, occur

Table 3 Antihistamines used in sedation

Antihistamines	Dose	Duration of action	Notes
Diphenhydramine	0.5–1.25 mg/kg PO Maximum daily dose: 300 mg [17]	3–6 h	Paradoxical reaction possible, anticholinergic properties, may potentiate other sedative medications
Hydroxyzine	0.6–2.5 mg/kg PO Maximum daily dose: Under 6 years—50 mg, over 6 years—100 mg [18]	4–6 h	Paradoxical reaction possible, anticholinergic properties, may potentiate other sedative medications

commonly with the use of antihistamines alone. Extrapyramidal symptoms, where motor restlessness and agitation occur with antihistamine administration, are also unwanted side effects (Table 3).

Other non-sedating antihistamines include cimetidine and ranitidine. These are used for reducing gastric acidity prior to general anesthesia. Cimetidine is well known to inhibit liver enzymes used in the metabolism of many drugs and can prolong their half-lives.

Benzodiazepines

Benzodiazepines have been the cornerstone of moderate sedation practice and are often used in combination with other sedatives. By acting as an agonist to the GABA receptor, benzodiazepines depress central nervous system activity and reduce anxiety. Benzodiazepines offer versatile routes of administration that include oral, intravenous, intramuscular, intranasal, sublingual, or rectal routes. Not only do benzodiazepines impart sedative properties, they also provide variable degrees anterograde amnesia. Benzodiazepines do not provide analgesia, and other agents (opioids, local anesthesia, nitrous oxide) must be employed if adequate pain control is needed for the dental or surgical procedure. Additionally, benzodiazepines have been described as relatively safe drugs when used at therapeutically appropriate doses for moderate sedation [19].

Perhaps the most significant safety aspect attributed to benzodiazepines is the ability to be reversed or competitively inhibited, by flumazenil. If a patient experiences respiratory depression that is significant enough to cause a precipitous decline in oxyhemoglobin saturation or becomes unconscious when moderate sedation was intended, a dose of 0.01–0.02 mg/kg of flumazenil given parenterally may reverse the sedative effects of a benzodiazepine, while basic life support measures are simultaneously administered (Table 4).

Benzodiazepines also have antiepileptic properties that make them ideal for the management and sedation of children with seizure activity. Used as both rescue medications for seizure activity and status epilepticus in CSHCN, administration of benzodiazepines for moderate sedation and preoperative sedation raises seizure threshold levels (Table 5).

Table 4 Benzodiazepine antagonist flumazenil

Benzodiazepine antagonist	Parenteral dose	Notes
Flumazenil	0.01–0.02 mg/kg [20] Maximum recommended dose: 3 mg	May precipitate seizure activity in patients with seizure history or on long-term benzodiazepine therapy

Table 5 Benzodiazepines commonly used for sedation

Benzodiazepine	Route	Usual dose
Diazepam	Oral	0.1–0.3 mg/kg Maximum recommended dose: 10 mg [21]
Midazolam	Oral Intranasal Intramuscular Intravenous	0.25–0.75 mg/kg 0.2 mg/kg 0.1–0.15 mg/kg 0.05–0.6 mg/kg (<6 years) 0.025–0.4 mg/kg (6–12 years) Maximum recommended dose: 20 mg oral dose, 10 mg IV dose [22]
Triazolam	Oral (crushed tablets)	0.02 mg/kg Maximum recommended dose: 0.5 mg [23]

Midazolam

Midazolam has long been utilized as a versatile and effective moderate sedation agent that can be administered in a variety of routes. This water-soluble benzodiazepine has a beta elimination half-life of approximately 3–7 h in children and a clinical duration of action anywhere between 1 and 6 h depending on dose. The oral administration of midazolam has been well described in the literature alone or with various combinations of other sedatives. Onset of action is described as being 10–15 min. Doses ranging from 0.5 to 0.75 mg/kg were demonstrated to enhance sedation and cooperation with a concomitant lowering of heart rate and blood pressure [24]. Depending on state regulations and practitioner licensing, parenteral intranasal (IN) administration and atomized intranasal (AIN) administration have found popularity for children not receptive to oral administration. Because of the circumvention of first-pass hepatic metabolism via IN/AIN administration, the dosing of midazolam is reduced to 0.35–0.5 mg/kg, and onset of action is more rapid than in the oral route. If the dental practitioner is permitted to administer sedative medications via the intravenous or intramuscular route, dosing and onset of action are similar to that of IN/AIN administration.

Diazepam

Historically, oral and intravenous diazepam has been popular in pediatric dental moderate sedation regimens. Although diazepam use in infants and CSHCN with hepatic insufficiency is discouraged, many regimens that employ oral diazepam along with antihistamines and opioids have been described for preschool-aged children and older. Pisalchaiyong et al. demonstrated that oral midazolam had slight advantages over oral diazepam in reducing movement and crying behaviors in children with autism [25]. Parenteral diazepam is not water soluble, and intramuscular injections can be painful and absorption unpredictable. Diazepam has a half-life of up to 43 ± 13 h in adults, and its active metabolite (desmethyldiazepam) has a half-life of up to 9 days. Diazepam undergoes enterohepatic circulation where its active metabolite from the liver is stored in bile and is released back into enteric circulation repeatedly [26]. Rectal administration in office-based settings is uncommon but can be used for CSHCN unable to intake medications via the oral route. Gastronomy tube administration and dosing are equivalent to oral dosing, and anywhere from 0.1 to 0.3 mg/kg has been shown to be effective for moderate sedation. At 60 min however, onset of action of diazepam is slower compared to that of midazolam [27].

Triazolam

Triazolam has been gaining popularity within adult dentistry as an "off-label" moderate sedation agent despite its primary indication for the short-term treatment of insomnia. Pediatric efficacy and safety have not been established, and the use is off-label in children under 12 years old. However one small study ($n = 20$) by Meyer et al. demonstrated that no statistical differences were measured in comparing 0.02 mg/kg triazolam versus 40 mg/kg chloral hydrate + 25 mg hydroxyzine in patients ranging in age from 21 to 74 months [28]. Triazolam has a short plasma half-life of 1.5–5.5 h in adults and reaches peak plasma levels at 2 h after oral administration. It is a potent amnestic and is currently available in tablet form.

Limitations The benzodiazepines may cause respiratory depression, central nervous system disturbances and depression, unconsciousness in moderate to high doses, or when combined with other sedative medications. As stated above, the benzodiazepines impart no analgesic qualities, and operative dentistry procedures or dental surgery must factor in the use of local anesthesia or other analgesics to control pain. Additionally, unwanted reactions have been reported with the administration of midazolam to children where paradoxical excitement or "angry child syndrome," occurs [29]. Irritation and discomfort are associated with intranasal administration of midazolam with parenteral formulations, and a potential for neurotoxicity is present with the close proximity of nasal mucosa to the central nervous system through the cribriform plate.

Chloral Hydrate

Chloral hydrate, an oral sedative in common use for pediatric moderate sedation in dental office-based settings, was discontinued from commercial manufacture in 2012 (oral solution by Pharmaceutical Associates, oral capsules by Breckenridge) for business reasons. Compounding pharmacies, in both outpatient and hospital settings, have continued to manufacture oral solutions from crystals or powder; however no FDA-approved formulations exist today that contain chloral hydrate [30]. When compounded, practitioners must ensure proper dosing is followed, as standard commercially available concentrations are no longer commonplace.

Table 6 Chloral hydrate

Chloral hydrate (compounded)		
Chloral hydrate	Oral	10–100 mg/kg (up to 2500 mg) [32]

Chloral hydrate, when administered enterally, is metabolized to trichloroethanol by alcohol dehydrogenase and has significant central nervous system depressant effects. High doses of chloral hydrate, 50–100 mg/kg, may lead to clinically significant respiratory depression, cardiac dysrhythmias, and hypoxemia. Onset of action occurs within 15 min with sleep-like effects occurring within 60 min of oral administration. Chloral hydrate has a plasma half-life of 8–12 h. Residual motor impairment and lethargy may persist for up to a day after administration in healthy individuals [31] (Table 6).

Nausea and vomiting have been reported as the most frequent side effects regarding oral administration of chloral hydrate because of gastric and mucous membrane irritation. Chloral hydrate may also exacerbate acute intermittent porphyria, as its metabolite is an ethanol derivative.

Limitations Because of its long clinical duration of action and plasma half-life, chloral hydrate has been implicated in adverse outcomes related to pediatric sedation [33]. The inability of chloral hydrate to be reversed also becomes problematic when overdose or toxicity is encountered. High-dose chloral hydrate in animal studies has demonstrated genotoxicity and carcinogenicity, but human studies are inconclusive [34].

Opioids

Of all of the moderate sedatives described here, only opioids impart a significant degree of analgesia along with euphoria, sedation, and central nervous system depression. Like the antihistamines and benzodiazepines described above, oral opioids are frequently used in combination with other agents by pediatric dentists with experience in oral sedation. Opioids can also blunt gag reflexes and have been described as providing a "quiet" surgical field with less patient movement.

Opioids are agonists of the μ, κ, and δ receptors located in the periphery, dorsal root ganglion, spinal cord, and brain. Transient side effects are well known in clinical settings, and among them, respiratory depression, sedation, and nausea and vomiting are expected from administration. Persistent side effects, including opioid-induced constipation, biliary tract spasm, and urinary retention, can be problematic in CSHCN.

Like benzodiazepines, the transient side effects can be reversed by administration of an opioid receptor antagonist—naloxone. When life-threatening respiratory depression occurs with the administration of an opioid analgesic, either alone or in combination with other oral sedatives, a rescue dose of naloxone should be administered. Naloxone is typically administered via injection but has also been shown to be effective when administered via intranasal route. When administered, a patient must be closely monitored for at least 2 h after administration for possible re-sedation and respiratory depression (Table 7).

Limitations Opioids used alone do not have anterograde amnestic properties, nor is the degree of sedation as reliable as with benzodiazepines or other sedative-hypnotics. Opioid use must be closely monitored, and its use is cautioned in CSHCN that present with respiratory compromise, obstructive or central sleep apnea, obesity, and anatomical restrictions in ventilation and respiration during the perioperative and recovery period (Table 8).

Codeine

Codeine not recommended for pediatric use (under 12 years of age) and has been removed from many hospital formularies. Codeine is a prodrug that relies on hepatic isoenzyme CYP2D6 for metabolism into its active form of morphine. It has been implicated in adverse outcomes where children with specific "ultrafast metabolizer" genotypes may be subject to overdose [37]. Adverse events reported to the FDA included fatal respiratory depression. Once common formulations of acetaminophen with various codeine concentrations are not recommended for sedation or postoperative analgesia in children.

Meperidine

Meperidine has been commonly used in combination with antihistamines, benzodiazepines, chloral hydrate, and nitrous oxide for various pediatric oral sedation regimens. It is well absorbed through the gastrointestinal tract and makes for an ideal

Table 7 Opioid antagonist naloxone

Opioid antagonist (naloxone)	Intravenous (IV) dose	Intramuscular (IM) dose
1 month–5 year and <20 kg	0.1 mg/kg q2–3min	0.1 mg/kg q3–8 min
>5 year and >20kg	2.0 mg q2–3min	2.0 mg q3–8 min

Table 8 Common narcotics used for sedation

	Oral dose	Duration of action	Notes
Meperidine	1.0–2.2 mg/kg Maximum recommended oral dose: 50 mg [35]	2–4 h	Respiratory depressant, may trigger seizures, use with caution with antidepressants and serotonergic drugs, histamine release, mild to moderate tachycardia
Morphine	0.5–0.7 mg/kg A maximum recommended dosage for oral morphine solution has not been established for pediatric patients [36]	4 h	Respiratory depressant, histamine release

oral analgesic adjunct to other oral sedatives. Meperidine has been shown to cause less histamine release than morphine in recent observational studies and has a plasma half-life after intravenous injection of 3.7 ± 1.6 h. Meperidine has anticholinergic properties and has some antisialogogue effects. Along with the reduction in salivary flow, slight increases in heart rate can also be observed.

Meperidine has a potency described to be approximately one-tenth of morphine with a dose-dependent duration of action of 2–4 h. Efficacy studies demonstrate oral dosing above 1.7 mg/kg as being "high dose" and did not correlate into greater effectiveness when co-administered with hydroxyzine [38]. Sedation, euphoria, and potential for nausea and vomiting are equal to morphine when given in equal analgesic doses. Meperidine has found utility in postoperative settings to reduce shivering associated with general anesthesia administration. Meperidine's active metabolite, normeperidine, has a plasma half-life of 14–21 h and can accumulate with repeated oral dosing. Because of the significant first-pass metabolism when administered via the enteral route, meperidine and meperidine-containing oral sedation regimens must be used with caution in CSHCN that have pre-existing seizure disorders [39]. Additionally, meperidine must be used with caution in patients concurrently prescribed selective serotonin reuptake inhibitors (SSRI), serotonin-norepinephrine reuptake inhibitors, St. John's Wort, tricyclic antidepressants, and other medications affecting the serotonergic and serotonin metabolism. Along with possible serotonin syndrome complications, meperidine administration may also potentiate seizures in susceptible patients.

Morphine

Although historically regarded as the prototypical opioid in which all opioids are compared against, the popularity of oral morphine utilized in pediatric oral sedation is low. Morphine produces analgesia, euphoria, sedation, and a decreased ability to concentrate. Morphine absorption through the gastrointestinal tract is not as reliable as oral meperidine, and peak effects of the drug are observed in 45–90 min after administration [40]. Oral morphine sulfate is available in an immediate-release liquid form that is easily combined with other oral sedative medications.

Morphine sulfate also causes histamine release from circulating mast cells, and its use in CSHCN sensitive to increases in inflammatory mediators (e.g., patients with asthma, allergic rhinitis, eczema) is discouraged. Morphine use in combination with other oral sedatives, such as midazolam, diazepam, hydroxyzine, and nitrous oxide, was shown to be effective in a small study by Chen and Tanbonliong [41]. Adverse events in this retrospective study included transient oxyhemoglobin desaturations below 95% that resolved with repositioning of the head and airway and one report of wheezing after administration.

α-2 Adrenergic Agonists

α-2 adrenergic agonists include both clonidine and dexmedetomidine. The activation of α-2A and α-2C subtype receptors, which are located primarily in the central nervous system, is responsible for the sedative, analgesic, and sympatholytic effects seen with the administration of oral clonidine and parenteral dexmedetomidine

[42]. Suppression of neuronal firing within the central nervous system inhibits release of the neurotransmitter norepinephrine that results in hypnosis and sedation.

A major advantage of the α-2 agonists when used in the context of sedation is the lack of respiratory depressant effects typically seen with benzodiazepines and opioids. Although both clonidine and dexmedetomidine can induce hypotensive episodes, the effects on mean arterial pressure and cardiac output are generally dose dependent. Dexmedetomidine also finds utility in decreasing the incidence of emergence delirium or an acute phase of impaired cognitive functioning that includes agitation and combativeness, which can occur after general anesthesia administration. Many CSHCN may already be on therapeutic levels of α-2 adrenergic agonists, such as tizanidine, for control of spasticity associated with cerebral palsy or off-label use for the treatment of attention deficit hyperactivity disorder or autism [43] (Table 9).

Limitations Both α-2 adrenergic agonists discussed in this chapter lack the ability to provide anterograde amnesia that benzodiazepines provide during sedation. Because of this, it may be necessary to introduce a benzodiazepine into the moderate sedation regimen if amnesia is needed. The analgesic effects α-2 adrenergic agonists may not be as profound as that of opioids, and augmentation with local anesthesia or other analgesics may be considered. Additionally, with the minor to moderate decrease in cardiac output that both clonidine and dexmedetomidine can induce, it is prudent for the healthcare team to assess the suitability of such medications in the treatment of CSHCN with significant cardiovascular issues.

Clonidine

Orally administered clonidine has a long history as an antihypertensive, antimigraine, and treatment for menopausal flushing in adults. Other applications of clonidine include the treatment of attention deficit hyperactivity disorder, chronic pain, and substance abuse withdrawal symptoms [46]. It has a slow onset of action in pediatric moderate sedation, with peak blood levels occurring at 60–90 min after administration. Oral clonidine is available in both tablet and liquid forms, and because of clonidine's lipophilicity, transmucosal (buccal oral rinses) routes have been described for patients able to perform oral rinsing [47]. Intranasal administration significantly accelerated onset of action to approximately 30 min, although uptake of the drug can be unpredictable.

Table 9 α-adrenergic agonists used for sedation

α-agonist	Dose	Onset of action
Clonidine	2–4 μg/kg oral Not to exceed 5μg/kg orally [44]	60–90 min
Dexmedetomidine	1–4.5 μg/kg (IM, IN, oral) Not to exceed 4.5 μg/kg [45]	20 min

Dexmedetomidine

A relatively new agent to be used in pediatric enteral and parenteral sedation in office-based settings is dexmedetomidine. With a greater affinity for the α-2 adrenergic receptor site, dexmedetomidine exhibits a unique biphasic effect on cardiac output where lower intravenous infusion rates produce a lower cardiac output while higher infusion rates or bolus dosing will produce hypertension for a brief period [48]. When used orally or transmucosally (as in an oral rinse), absorption is predictable and effective enough to facilitate intravenous cannulation on otherwise uncooperative children [45].

Combination Oral Moderate Sedation Regimens

Benzodiazepines used in conjunction with inhaled nitrous oxide have historically been the most popular approach to procedural sedation in pediatric dentistry. Today this regimen continues to be commonly utilized by pediatric dentists [49]. However, because of the procedural and surgical demands of pediatric dentistry, a combination of sedation, analgesia, and amnesia is often required to render humane and effective care. It is not uncommon for practitioners to employ oral sedation regimens that include a combination of two or even three sedatives.

When developing anesthesia and moderate sedation treatment plans for CSHCN that include multiple agents, it is particularly important to conduct an expanded evaluation of medical history, current and past medications, and postoperative pain management strategies.

Deep Sedation and General Anesthesia

The provision of deep sedation and general anesthesia (GA) in dental settings is limited to dentist or physician practitioners with permits and training to offer this modality. Current recommendations from the ASA, the AAP/AAPD, and the ASDA state that a separate and independent anesthesia provider must be present whenever deep sedation or general anesthesia is planned in dental settings for the pediatric dental patient [50, 51]. Deep sedation or general anesthesia may be provided in private dental clinics, accredited ambulatory surgical centers (ASCs), or hospital-based operating rooms. CSHCN may have more airway or physical complexities than healthy peers. Therefore, for deep sedation and GA cases, it is critical to engage in shared decision-making with the anesthesia provider and facility in which treatment will be rendered.

Of all of the pharmacologic modalities employed in the treatment of CSHCN, general anesthesia is considered the most effective in ensuring that dental practitioners will be able to complete dental procedures. However, as the Special Care in Dentistry Association (SCDA) also warns, general anesthesia is the most complex to arrange, can be the most expensive to the patient in some circumstances (especially in office-based settings), and may entail the greatest risk [52]. An additional challenge when considering general anesthesia for CSHCN is the manner in which anesthesia is induced. Parental separation and intravenous access in anesthesia induction can be challenging for typically developing children, due to apprehension, fear, limited patient cooperation, or limited understanding. The additional complexities of neurologic, anatomic, and physiologic conditions seen in CSHCN must be addressed well in advance of the treatment day by an experienced general anesthesia provider. Further, those CSHCN with medical complexities, with severe chronic illness, and with technology dependence may require extensive medical support care to circumvent complications [2].

The techniques and methods of delivering deep sedation and general anesthesia care exceed the scope of this chapter, yet it is beneficial for the practitioner to familiarize themselves with names and properties of pharmaceuticals that are used with frequency (Table 10). The following list of general anesthesia medications are commonly used in isolation or in combination with previously mentioned sedatives for induction and maintenance of deep sedation and general anesthesia. Drugs intended for deep sedation and general anesthesia have a particularly narrow therapeutic range. With propofol, for instance, there is a very small difference in dosing between moderate sedation and unconsciousness. Ketamine can also be described as a general anesthetic medication with a similarly narrow therapeutic range, making it unsuitable for moderate sedation providers. Most medications intended for deep sedation or general anesthesia do not have reversal agents, and experience in managing the apneic patient with airway support and advanced airway instrumentation is critical when caring for CSHCN using these drugs.

Table 10 Drugs used commonly to administer general anesthesia

Deep sedation/ general anesthesia agent	Type and typical route of administration	Malignant hyperthermia triggering agent?	Details
Ketamine	Intramuscular, Intravenous, intranasal, oral	No	Versatile induction agent, sympathomimetic, does not cause respiratory depression
Propofol	Intravenous	No	Sedative-hypnotic agent
Sevoflurane	Inhalational	Yes	Inhaled induction agent, patient must be able to tolerate facemask
Desflurane	Inhalational	Yes	Used for general anesthesia maintenance only via endotracheal intubation
Succinylcholine	Intravenous, intramuscular	Yes	Depolarizing muscle relaxant, may cause fasciculations, short duration of action
Rocuronium	Intravenous	No	Non-depolarizing muscle relaxant, intermediate duration of action

Ketamine

Ketamine, a derivative of phencyclidine, is a versatile *N*-methyl-D-aspartate (NMDA) antagonist that provides amnesia, analgesia, and dissociative anesthesia. In higher doses, it can cause cerebral excitation and increases sympathetic output. Various routes of administration are available, including oral, intramuscular, intranasal, and intravenous routes. Ketamine is particularly useful in the treatment of CSHCN, because it can be injected intramuscularly on uncooperative patients, providing a rapid induction into general anesthesia, facilitate intravenous cannulation, and ease transport into the operatory while maintaining protective reflexes. Intranasal single-dose administration at a relatively high dose of 5 mg/kg results in onset of action of approximately 11–30 min and a duration of action of approximately 50 min [53].

Ketamine may stimulate secretion of saliva, and salivary excess can precipitate laryngospasm. Because of this, anticholinergics such as glycopyrrolate or atropine may be co-administered. The increases in heart rate and cardiac output are dose dependent, and ketamine should be used with caution in patients unable to tolerate increases in sympathetic tone.

Limitations Ketamine causes increases in both intracranial and intraocular pressure. Ketamine administration should be carefully considered in CSHCN with intracranial hypertension and those presenting with a ventriculoperitoneal (VP) shunt. Because of the inherent increase in cerebral excitation, caution should be exercised for patients with seizure disorders. Ketamine may also exacerbate secretions associated with common upper respiratory tract infections and precipitate airway compromise.

Propofol

Propofol, or 2,6-diisopropylphenol, is a common agent used in intravenous moderate-to-deep sedation maintenance, general anesthesia induction, and general anesthesia maintenance. Reductions in cardiac output and respiratory depression are dose dependent, and this milk white drug can provide unconsciousness and general anesthesia in low doses. Propofol imparts no analgesic effects, and amnesia is unreliable in doses that do not produce general anesthesia. The main advantage of propofol is its rapid onset of action (3–5 min) and short duration of action. Infusions using propofol in total intravenous anesthesia (TIVA) techniques often allow for rapid, complete recovery and facilitate a safer discharge in outpatient settings [54]. Propofol also has an antiemetic effect that is effective in reducing the nausea and vomiting associated with both anesthesia exposure and dental or oral surgery.

Limitations Propofol is only effective via the parenteral route, and practitioners trained in managing the pediatric airway must be present during its use. CSHCN may pose even greater risks for airway obstruction and apnea than healthy peers.

Although propofol is formulated with egg product (egg lecithin lipids without egg white proteins) and soy products (soybean oil), pediatric patients with anaphylaxis to both rarely have demonstrated allergy to propofol formulations [55]. Longer infusions of propofol have been associated with propofol infusion syndrome which is a potentially fatal condition characterized by metabolic acidosis, hyperlipidemia, bradycardia, and possible rhabdomyolysis [56]. CSHCN presenting with complex medical needs may be more at risk for complications with propofol induction or maintenance infusions.

Sevoflurane

Sevoflurane is a popular inhalational general anesthetic agent that has a minimally irritating odor and can be inhaled with limited rejection by many pediatric patients. Upon administration, sevoflurane is a potent bronchodilator and has a rapid onset. That makes it an ideal agent for pediatric mask induction for CSHCN that can tolerate inhalational methods. Used alone or in conjunction with nitrous oxide, mask inhalation induction with sevoflurane has been popular since the discontinuation of the production of halothane. Sevoflurane can trigger a malignant hyperthermia crisis in susceptible patients (see below) (Fig. 5).

Desflurane

Desflurane is another inhaled anesthetic that, unlike sevoflurane, is unsuitable for mask inhalation induction. Desflurane is pungent and extremely irritating to pediatric airways, and its use should be considered carefully in patients with reactive airway diseases, such as asthma. Additionally, desflurane may cause transient

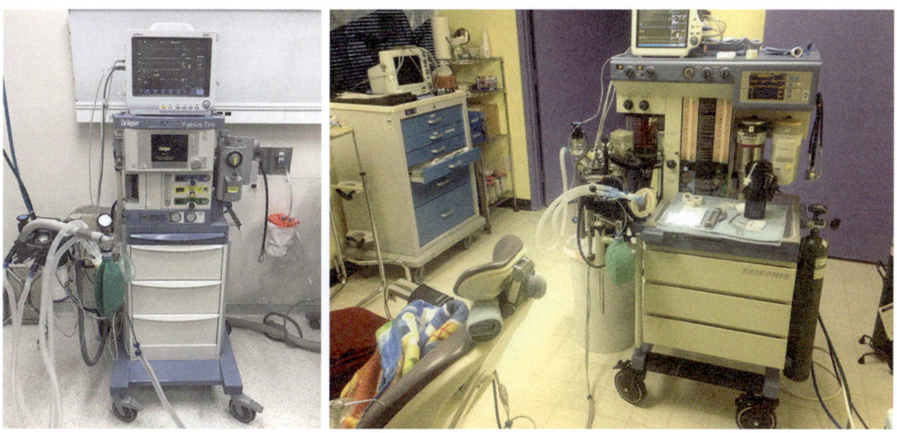

Fig. 5 Examples of compact anesthesia machines and monitors used in dental settings

tachycardia and increased cardiac output due to stimulation of the sympathetic nervous system. This can be problematic for CSHCN that cannot tolerate increases in heart rate or blood pressure. The main advantage of using desflurane in inhaled general anesthesia regimens is its low blood gas solubility. This allows for rapid recovery from general anesthesia without the residual effects of accumulated inhaled drug. Desflurane can also trigger a malignant hyperthermia crisis in susceptible patients (see below).

Succinylcholine

Succinylcholine is a depolarizing skeletal muscle relaxant that is used to facilitate tracheal intubation on patients undergoing dental procedures with intubated general anesthesia. It is also used as a rescue medication for laryngospasm by general anesthesia trained and permitted providers. With a bolus dose, succinylcholine's duration of action is approximately 5–10 min depending on dose and activity of the patient's own cholinesterase activity. Because of its depolarizing action at the neuromuscular junction, an initial and brief period of skeletal muscle contraction followed by relaxation, or fasciculations, is often seen upon intravenous administration. Succinylcholine may increase serum potassium and is a triggering agent for malignant hyperthermia in susceptible patients. For CSHCN that may not be able to tolerate disorganized and sometimes vigorous muscle contractions, succinylcholine use should be considered carefully. For CSHCN with cholinesterase deficiency, the action of succinylcholine may be prolonged for several hours.

Rocuronium

Rocuronium is a non-depolarizing muscle relaxant with a longer duration of action than succinylcholine. Rocuronium administration results in flaccid muscle paralysis that facilitates tracheal intubation and muscle relaxation needed for some surgeries. Although dental surgery rarely requires the degree of skeletal muscle flaccidity needed in abdominal or orthopedic surgery, its use in intubated general anesthesia for dental procedures is relatively common and requires mechanical ventilation throughout the duration of the procedure. It, as well as other non-depolarizing neuromuscular blockers, can be reversed with the administration of an anticholinesterase, such as neostigmine or edrophonium, or by a newer γ-cyclodextrin agent, sugammadex [57]. Rocuronium is not a triggering agent for malignant hyperthermia, but it can precipitate allergic reactions. Non-depolarizing neuromuscular blockade can also be prolonged in patients presenting with muscular dystrophies [58].

Malignant Hyperthermia

Malignant hyperthermia (MH) is a rare and emergent (1:14,000 to 1:200,000 prevalence) autosomal dominant genetic condition that is triggered by the use of inhaled

Table 11 Conditions associated with malignant hyperthermia

Malignant hyperthermia-associated conditions
Duchenne muscular dystrophy
Central core disease
King-Denborough syndrome
Multiminicore disease

volatile general anesthetics, depolarizing neuromuscular blockers (succinylcholine), or other factors. It can be fatal if interventions are not delivered early, and nearly 1% of all general anesthesia-related fatalities can be attributed to malignant hyperthermia. This condition has a pediatric male predilection, and nearly half of all cases occur in children. Mutations in two genes related to skeletal muscle calcium regulation have been identified: ryanodine receptor type 1 (RYR1) and voltage-dependent L-type calcium channel 1S subunit (CACNA1S) gene. Recent investigations into STAC3, a protein involved in Native American myopathy, have been implicated in MH susceptibility [59] (Table 11).

Clinical manifestations will include increased end-tidal carbon dioxide, tachycardia, cardiac dysrhythmias, elevated temperature, muscle rigidity, masseter spasm, cola-colored urine, eventual rhabdomyolysis, elevation in creatine kinase, cardiovascular collapse, and death if not treated [60]. Definitive treatment of an MH episode includes the administration of dantrolene 2.5–3.0 mg intravenously as soon as possible, discontinuation of triggering agents, cooling, aggressive management of electrolyte imbalances, and transport to a pediatric intensive care unit [2].

The Malignant Hyperthermia Association of the United States (MHAUS) is an important resource for patients diagnosed or suspected of being autosomal dominant for malignant hyperthermia. Whenever general anesthesia is planned for a CSHCN and a risk for MH is identified, additional information and a crisis emergency hotline are available at http://www.mhaus.org or 800-644-9737.

Setting Reasonable Expectations

Depending on patient presentation and treatment goals, a wide variety of pharmacologic options exist for CSHCN. Prior to developing a pharmacologic treatment plan for minimal or moderate sedation and/or deep sedation and general anesthesia, it is of prime importance to perform a thorough and extensive evaluation of:

- Medical history
- Psychological and social development
- Ritualistic and repetitive behaviors
- Sensory management
- Intellectual disability
- Sleep patterns [61]

Without question, the most predictable method of delivering effective dental care and surgery is with pharmacologically induced general anesthesia, but this modality can carry significant risk to CSHCN with complex medical conditions. General anesthesia, in most states, requires properly trained and credentialed providers with expertise in both pediatrics and patients with special needs. The drug-drug interaction with commonly prescribed medications may also increase the risk for intraoperative complications related to various organ systems and physiologic processes. Arrhythmias and cardiac conduction abnormalities, agranulocytosis, increased anesthetic medication demand or marked reduction in dose, and other potential disturbances have been reported with popular medications used for the treatment of autism spectrum disorder, attention deficit hyperactivity disorder, cerebral palsy, or depression and mania.

Moderate sedation by any route is less predictable in providing optimal conditions for delivery of dental care and surgery, but the advantages of lower cost, greater accessibility to credentialed and trained providers, and performance in a familiar dental office-based setting may favor its use. Limitations of moderate sedation include a an abbreviated working time due to both the duration of action of sedative medications and a route of administration that may only allow for singular doses of drugs. Additionally, any method short of general anesthesia depends on effective local anesthesia for stimulating or invasive dental treatment. CSHCN who cannot tolerate commercial formulations of dental local anesthetics may have a limited range of treatment options with minimal, moderate, or even deep sedation techniques that rely on local anesthesia administration [62].

Appropriate Dental Treatment Planning

Advanced pharmacologic sedation and general anesthesia modalities often require an unusually large amount of effort to coordinate. This requires the involvement of practitioners, allied healthcare professionals, parents and caregivers, and the patient themselves. Because follow-up appointments that involve dental treatment may be impractical and may involve more pharmacologic interventions, dental treatment planning must include realistic and long-term goals. CSHCN may not be candidates for removable or fixed dental appliances, orthodontic hardware, extensive cosmetic dental restorations, or invasive procedures because of inabilities to maintain regular oral hygiene, limited motor control, overwhelming sensory sensibilities, or complex medical conditions. Exposure to minimal and moderate sedation or general anesthesia should be kept to an absolute minimum to complete dental procedures because of undetermined risks to neurological development. The impact and association of sedation and general anesthesia agents on neuronal apoptosis and future neurocognitive impairment are currently being studied, and some investigations suggest children under the age of 4 years are at-risk populations [63, 64]. Because CSHCN present greater medical risk than healthy peers, careful consideration of the risks of sedation and general anesthesia must be weighed against the benefits. This involves a thoughtful consideration of the nature of the procedure, urgency, and potential for deferral.

Case-Based Scenario

After receiving an urgent call from a patient's parent regarding possible dental trauma to their 5-year-old son, the dentist reviews the patient record and notes that his child has been previously diagnosed with autism and a seizure disorder. Previous appointments have been marked with difficulty because the patient was unable to tolerate longer procedures without significant physical restraint from parents. Further questioning from the dentist reveals that this patient sustained a fall, and two maxillary primary central incisors have palatal luxation that interferes with occlusion.

The patient arrives later today with his parents to the dentist, and a thorough medical history is conducted. Before arrival, the patient was instructed to fast in order to keep a treatment option of sedation available. He is currently 20 kg and stands at 110 cm tall. He generally has generalized tonic-clonic seizures once or twice a month that are self-limiting to about 3 min in duration. He currently takes oral levetiracetam (Keppra) twice a day for the management of seizure disorder and, before today's appointment, has been taking oral acetaminophen to control pain from the injury. His previous medical history is significant for extreme preterm birth (delivery at 27 weeks) and strabismus surgery at 2 years of age with no complications. As expected, the patient is anxious and apprehensive, but with assistance from parents, an occlusal and periapical radiographs are obtained. He can respond verbally but often requires a repetition of questions or statements. It is determined that the ideal treatment for the traumatized primary incisors is extraction.

Consultation with the patient's primary care physician and neurologist include the following topics:

1. Description of the current dental trauma and plan to extract the traumatized primary teeth
2. Therapies for autism spectrum disorder and seizures
3. Proposed plan of using therapeutic doses of midazolam and nitrous oxide as an adjunct for safe and predictable dental care
4. Discussions regarding risks and benefits for using a method of pharmocosedation, use of local anesthesia for the extractions, and alternatives to treatment that include general anesthesia or nontreatment
5. Consensus agreement to provide oral moderate sedation with appropriate monitoring and recovery care

Further discussion with the patient's parents confirms that oral moderate sedation would be the most appropriate treatment option to allay anxiety, provide safe and reasonably predictable operating conditions for local anesthesia and surgery, and ensure a degree of amnesia to an otherwise traumatic event. Because the patient had been nil per os (NPO) for over 6 h for solid foods, and he only had less than 2 ounces of water prior to arrival; all ASA guidelines for preoperative fasting prior to sedation had been satisfied. The patient has already taken his morning dose of Keppra and has not had a seizure in about 2 weeks.

The dentist and dental assistant conduct a thorough airway evaluation that includes noting a full range of motion of the head and neck, oral opening greater than 30 mm, a thyromental distance of greater than 6 cm, and an ability to breathe easily through the nose. The dentist also notes a normal occlusion, and the parents report no snoring at night. With a brief glimpse of the oropharyngeal area, the dentist sees that the airway is a Mallampati Grade I designation—uvula and both tonsillar pillars could easily be seen. Baseline blood pressure, room air pulse oximetry, and heart rate were measured, and the patient is accompanied to the restroom to void prior to beginning sedation. An ASA Physical Status II designation is assigned to this patient as he has autism and a well-controlled seizure disorder.

An oral solution of midazolam is administered in the waiting area to minimize a lengthy waiting time in the dental chair, and the patient readily accepts since he is hungry and thirsty. The dose administered is calculated to 10 mg (approximately 0.5 mg/kg). Within 15 min, he shows some signs of sedation, and the patient is carefully guided into a wheelchair and brought back with his parents into the treatment area. With assistance from his parents and the dentist, the patient is helped into the dental chair, and a vital signs monitor is placed onto the patient. Baseline vital signs (blood pressure, oxygen saturation, and heart rate) are measured as the beginning stages of moderate sedation are seen. The dentist recognizes that it may be an opportune time to place a nasal hood and begin to administer approximately 4 L/min of oxygen. Because the vital signs monitor also records end-tidal (exhaled) carbon dioxide through a small attachment, a waveform on the monitor appears and corresponds with the ventilation of the patient. The patient breathes through his nose and closes his mouth upon verbal command, and he also verbally mentions that he is comfortable.

At this point, the dentist begins titrating the administration of nitrous oxide inhalation sedation to 50% over a period of 10 min. After each minute, the dentist regular checks the patient's response by asking him to open his mouth as wide as he can. The dentist notices that at 50% nitrous oxide concentration, the patient is somewhat sluggish and has a 1–2 s delay in response. At this point the dentist places a rubber bite block with a piece of floss attached to it in the patients mouth, and she also places a large 4″ × 4″ piece of cotton gauze, also with an attached piece of floss for retrieval, in the posterior portion of the patients mouth. A regular and consistent capnograph waveform is noted on the vital signs monitor.

With parents holding the patient's hands and the dental assistant providing adequate suction and immobilizing the patient's head with a light hold, an intraoral infiltration of local anesthesia with 2% lidocaine and 1:100,000 epinephrine is administered in the buccal vestibule. The patient remains calm and does not complain of pain. Another injection is administered to the palatal aspect, in the nasopalatine region, and both the dentist and the assistant notice a slight wince from the patient. After a few minutes with a distractive story, the dentist begins elevation and extraction of the luxated incisors.

Within 10 min, the incisors are extracted, and the nitrous oxide is titrated to a level of 0%. The patient remains on 100% oxygen for approximately 10 min and allowed to recover completely for another 30 min upright in the chair. A large cotton gauze with long pieces of floss are used to tamponade the surgical area, and bleeding is ascertained to be quite minimal. After approximately an hour in total treatment time with vital signs recorded every 5 min, the patient displays no delays in verbal response. Because of present limitations to ambulation and coordination, the patient is carefully wheeled to the car with his parents. Parents also receive a very thorough postoperative written instruction sheet for both sedation and postoperative surgical care, and they are instructed to administer his usual evening dose of Keppra with soft foods.

Later this evening, the dentist gives the parents a call for a postoperative care check. The parents report that the local anesthesia has worn off and he is now eating soft foods and drinking liquids with no problems. He is walking steadily and is asking when his new front teeth are going to grow in.

Conclusion

- Pharmacologic strategies to enable safe and effective dental treatment for CSHCN should be integrated into treatment plans early and discussed with relevant caregivers as treatment options.
- In some cases and for some procedures, non-pharmacologic strategies may not be able to accommodate safe and predictable dental treatment.
- The provision of pharmacologic therapies for dental treatment falls into a dynamic continuum of sedation and anesthesia.
- Dental providers must be cognizant of particular regional limitations to provide sedation and anesthesia that includes training, choice of drugs, settings, personnel, and required monitoring.
- Many medications with long histories of effective sedation and a wide margin of safety exist for office-based settings. Newer agents should be considered in particular situations, and a working knowledge of agents used in general anesthesia is helpful in developing treatment options.
- Dental practitioners opting to provide pharmacologic management must be able to prevent and recognize common complications associated with sedation and anesthesia.
- For CSHCN minimal to moderate sedation modalities may not prove to be effective in all situations. Reasonable expectations must be discussed with all individuals involved in dental care when minimal to moderate sedation is considered.

References

1. Waldman BH, Perlman SP, Wong A. The largest minority population in the U.S. without adequate dental care. Spec Care Dentist. 2017;37(4):159–63.
2. Graham RJ, Wachendorf MT, Burns JP, Mancuso TJ. Successful and safe delivery of anesthesia and perioperative care for children with complex special health care needs. J Clin Anesth. 2009;21:165–72.

3. American Academy of Pediatric Dentistry. Clinical guideline on behavior guidance for the pediatric patient. Pediatr Dent. 2018;39(6):246–59.
4. Lyons RA. Understanding basic behavioral support techniques as an alternative to sedation and anesthesia. Spec Care Dentist. 2009;29(1):39–50.
5. American Dental Association. Guidelines for the use of sedation and general anesthesia by dentists. Adopted by the ADA House of Delegates. 2016 Oct.
6. American Society of Anesthesiologists. Continuum of depth of sedation: definition of general anesthesia and levels of sedation/analgesia. Approved by the ASA House of Delegates. 2014 Oct.
7. American Academy of Pediatric Dentistry and American Academy of Pediatrics. Guideline for monitoring and management of pediatric patients before, during, and after sedation for diagnostic and therapeutic procedures: update 2016. Am Acad Pediatr Dent Ref Manual. 2016; 38(6).
8. Edginton AN, Fotaki N. Oral drug absorption in pediatric populations. In: Dressman J, Reppas C, editors. Oral drug absorption: predication and assessment. 2nd ed. New York: Informa Healthcare; 2010. p. 108–26.
9. LaPointe L, Guelmann M, Primosch R. State regulations governing oral sedation in dental practice. Pediatr Dent. 2012;34(7):489–92.
10. Tobias JD. Applications of nitrous oxide for procedural sedation in the pediatric population. Pediatr Emerg Care. 2013;29(2):245–65.
11. American Academy of Pediatric Dentistry. Use of nitrous oxide for pediatric dental patients. Am Acad Pediatr Dent Ref Manual. 2013;39(6):273–7.
12. Orhon ZN, Koltka EN, Tüfekçi S, Buldag C, Kisa A, Durakbasa U, Çelik M. Methylene tetrahydrofolate reductase deficiency: the hidden risk in pediatric anesthesia. Turk J Anaesthesiol Reanim. 2017;45(5):277–81.
13. Cote CJ, Todres ID, Ryan JF, Goudsouzian NG. A practice of anesthesia for infants and children. 3rd ed. Philadelphia: WB Saunders Company; 2001. p. 172.
14. Raj D, Luginbuehl I. Managing the difficult airway in the syndromic child. Contin Educ Anesth Crit Care Pain. 2015;15(1):7–13.
15. Lin JL, Cohen EC, Sanders LM. Shared decision making among children with medical complexity: results from a population-based survey. J Pediatr. 2018;192:216–22.
16. American Society of Anesthesiologists. Practice guidelines for moderate procedural sedation and analgesia 2018: a report by the American Society of Anesthesiologists Task Force on Moderate Procedural Sedation and Analgesia, the American Association of Oral and Maxillofacial Surgeons, American College of Radiology, American Dental Association, American Society of Dentist Anesthesiologists, and Society of Interventional Radiology. Anesthesiology. 2018;128(3):437–79.
17. Diphenhydramine [FDA package insert] Franklin Lakes NJ. BD Simplist. 2012 Dec.
18. Atarax [FDA package insert] Roerig. 2006 Jun.
19. Lourenço-Matharu L, Ashley PF, Furness S. Sedation of children undergoing dental treatment. Cochrane Database Syst Rev. 2012;3:CD003877.
20. Romazicon [FDA package insert] Nutly NJ. Roche. 2007 Feb.
21. Valium [FDA package insert] Nutley NJ. Roche. 2008 Jan.
22. Midazolam [FDA package insert] Lake Zurich IL. Fresenius Kabi. 2017 Mar.
23. Triazolam [FDA package insert] New York NY. Pfizer. 2008 Feb.
24. Gentz R, Casamassimo P, Amini H, Claman D, Smiley M. Safety and efficacy of 3 pediatric midazolam moderate sedation regimens. Anesth Prog. 2017;64:66–72.
25. Pisalchaiyong T, Trairatvorakul C, Jirakija J, Yuktarnonda W. Comparison of the effectiveness of oral diazepam and midazolam for the sedation of autistic patients during dental treatment. Pediatr Dent. 2005;27(3):198–206.
26. Mandelli M, Tognoni G, Garattini S. Clinical pharmacokinetics of diazepam. Clin Pharmacokinet. 1978;3:72–91.
27. Wilson S. Management of child patient behavior: quality of care, fear and anxiety, and the child patient. Pediatr Dent. 2013;35(2):170–4.

28. Meyer ML, Mourino AP, Farrington FH. Comparison of triazolam to a chloral hydrate/hydroxyzine combination in the sedation of pediatric dental patients. Pediatr Dent. 1990;12(5):283–7.
29. Uldum B, Hallonsten AL, Poulsen S. Midazolam conscious sedation in a large Danish municipal dental service for children and adolescents. Int J Paediatr Dent. 2008;18(4):256–61.
30. Institute for Safe Medication Practices. Chloral hydrate: is it still being used? Are there safer alternatives? 2016: November. Accessed via the World Wide Web at: http://www.ismp.org/newsletters/acutecare/showarticle.aspx?id=1152 on 20 Feb 2018.
31. Pershad J, Palmisano P, Nichols M. Chloral hydrate: the good and the bad. Pediatr Emerg Care. 1999;15(6):432–5.
32. Greenberg SB, Faerber EN, Aspinall CL, Adams RC. High-dose chloral hydrate sedation for children undergoing mr imaging: safety and efficacy in relation to age. Am J Roentgenol. 1993;161:639–41.
33. Cote CJ, Karl HW, Notterman DA, Weinberg JA, McCloskey C. Adverse sedation events in pediatrics: analysis of medications used for sedation. Pediatrics. 2000;106(4):633–44.
34. HaselKorn T, Whittemore AS, Udaltsova N, Friedman GD. Short-term chloral hydrate administration and cancer in humans. Drug Saf. 2006;29(1):67–77.
35. Demerol [FDA package insert] Parsippany NJ. Validus Pharmaceuticals LLC. 2017 Aug.
36. Morphine Sulfate (oral) [FDA package insert]. Accessed online at: https://www.accessdata.fda.gov/drugsatfda_docs/label/2010/022195s002lbl.pdf on Dec 2009.
37. United States Food and Drug Administration. FDA drug safety communication: FDA restricts use of prescription codeine pain and cough medicines and tramadol pain medicines in children; recommends against use in breastfeeding women. 2018. Accessed via World Wide Web at https://www.fda.gov/Drugs/DrugSafety/ucm549679.htm on 20 Feb 2018.
38. Lenahan M, Wells M, Scarbecz M. A retrospective study of 248 pediatric oral sedations utilizing the combination of meperidine and hydroxyzine for dental treatment. J Clin Pediatr Dent. 2015;39(5):481–7.
39. Modica PA, Tempelhoff R, White PF. Pro- and anticonvulsant effects of anesthetics (part I). Anesth Analg. 1990;70:303–15.
40. Stoelting RK. Opioid agonists and antagonists, chapter 3. In: Stoelting RK, editor. Pharmacology and physiology in anesthetic practice. 3rd ed. Philadelphia: Lippincott-Raven; 1999. p. 77–112.
41. Chen N, Tanbonliong T. Comparison of two morphine-benzodiazepine-hydroxyzine combinations for the oral sedation of pediatric dental patients: a restrospective study. Pediatr Dent. 2018;40(1):43–8.
42. Giovannitti JA, Thoms SM, Crawford JJ. Alpha-2 adrenergic receptor agonists: a review of current clinical applications. Anesth Prog. 2015;62:31–8.
43. Henney HR, Chez M. Pediatric safety of tizanidine: clinical adverse event database and retrospective chart assessment. Paediatr Drugs. 2009;11(6):397–406.
44. Almenrader N, Passariello M, Coccetti B, Haiberger R, Pietropaoli P. Premedication in children: a comparison of oral midazolam and oral clonidine. Paediatr Anaesth. 2007;17:1143–9.
45. Zub D, Berkenbosch J, Tobias J. Preliminary experience with oral dexmedetomidine for procedural and anesthetic premedication. Paediatr Anaesth. 2005;15:932–8.
46. Owens JA. The practice of pediatric sleep medicine: results of a community survey. Pediatrics. 2001;108:E51.cc.
47. Hanning SM, Gul MO, Toni I, Neubert A, Tuleu C. A mini-review of non-parenteral clonidine preparations for paediatric sedation. J Pharm Pharmacol. 2017;69:398–405.
48. Dyck JB, Maze M, Haack C, et al. The pharmacokinetics and hemodynamic effects of intravenous and intramuscular dexmedetomidine hydrochloride in adult human volunteers. Anesthesiology. 1993;78:813–20.
49. Wilson S, Houpt M. Project USAP 2010: use of sedative agents in pediatric dentistry-a 25-year follow-up survey. Pediatr Dent. 2016;38(2):127–33.
50. American Society of Dentist Anesthesiologists. Parameters of care. Approved by ASDA General Assembly. 2018 May 4. Accessed via: https://www.asdahq.org/sites/default/files/ASDA%20Parameters%20of%20Care.pdf

51. American Society of Anesthesiologists. ASA statement on sedation & anesthesia administration in dental office-based settings. Approved by the ASA House of Delegates. 2017 Oct 25.
52. Glassmand P, Caputo A, Dougherty N, Lyons R, Messhieha Z, Miller C, Peltier B, Romer M. Special Care Dentistry Association consensus statement on sedation, anesthesia, and alternative techniques for people with special needs. Spec Care Dentist. 2008;29(1):2–8.
53. Surendar M, Pandey R, Saksena A, Kumar A, Chandra G. A Comparative evaluation of intranasal dexmedetomidine, midazolam and ketamine for their sedative and analgesic properties: a triple blind ranomized study. J Clin Pediatr Dent. 2014;38(3):255–62.
54. Pershad J, Godambe SA. Propofol for procedural sedation in the pediatric emergency department. J Emerg Med. 2004;27(1):11–4.
55. Murphy A, Campbell DE, Baines D, Mehr S. Allergic reactions to propofol in egg allergic children. Anesth Analg. 2011 Jul;113(1):140–4.
56. Okamoto MP, Kawaguchi DL, Amin AN. Evaluation of propofol infusion syndrome in pediatric intensive care. Am J Health-Syst Pharm. 2003;60:2007–14.
57. Won YJ, Lim BG, Lee DK, Kim H, Kong MH. Suggamadex for reversal of Rocuronium-induced neuromuscular blockade in pediatric patients: a systematic review and meta-analysis. Medicine. 2016;95(34):e4678.
58. Wick S, Muenster T, Schmidt J, et al. Onset and duration of rocuronium-induced neuromuscular blockade in patients with Duchenne muscular dystrophy. Anesthesiology. 2005;102:915–9.
59. Bamaga AK, Riazi S, Amburgey K, Ong S, Halliday W, Diamandis P, Guerguerian A, Dowling JJ, Yoon G. Neuromuscular conditions associated with malignant hyperthermia in paediatric patients: a 25-year retrospective study. Neuromuscul Disord. 2016;26:201–6.
60. Larach MG, Gronert GA, Allen GC, Brandom BW, Lehman EB. Clinical presentation, treatment, and complications of malignant hyperthermia in North America from 1987 to 2006. Anesth Analg. 2010;110:498–507.
61. Taghizadeh N, Davidson A, Williams K, Story D. Autism spectrum disorder (ASD) and its perioperative management. Pediatr Anesth. 2015;25:1076–84.
62. Wang Y, Lin I, Huang C, Fan S. Dental anesthesia for patients with special needs. Acta Anaesthesiol Taiwanica. 2012;50:122–5.
63. Glatz P, Sandin RH, Pederson NL. Association of anesthesia and surgery during childhood with long-term academic performance. JAMA Pediatr. 2017;17(1):e163470. https://doi.org/10.1001/jamapediatrics.2016.3470.
64. Sun L, Li G, Miller TLK, Salorio C, Byrne MW, Bellinger DC, Ing C, Park R, Radcliffe J, Hays SR, DiMaggio CJ, Cooper TJ, Rauh W, Maxwell LG, Youn A, McGowan FX. Association between a single general anesthesia exposure before age 36 months and neurocognitive outcomes in later childhood. JAMA. 2016;315(21):2312–20.

Protective Stabilization in the Dental Setting

Janice A. Townsend

Introduction

Children with special healthcare needs (CSHCN) are more prone to caries, periodontal disease, inadequate oral hygiene, and decreased access to daily preventive care and routine dental visits [1–3]. To compound this problem, delivery of dental care for these patients, especially those with intellectual difficulties, can be challenging. A combination of sensory-stimulating activities, an unfamiliar environment, possible discomfort, and loss of control are typically inherent to a dental visit [4]. Dental visits, and even daily preventive care, can be distressing and may prompt resistant or aggressive behavior [1]. Restrictive behavior guidance techniques may, therefore, be needed to ensure patients receive necessary preventive care [1, 5]. These techniques are referred to as "protective stabilization" or "medical immobilization." This differentiates temporary immobilization needed for a specific procedure from general behavior restraints. Restraint for CSHCN, especially those with intellectual disability, has been inappropriately used for general behavior management and may have a negative connotation [2]. This is a highly controversial topic and dentists must be aware of the perceptions, legal implications, and practical concerns of protective stabilization for CSHCN.

Ethical Implications

All patients have a right to adequate dental care and to be free of the outcomes associated with dental neglect such as pain, infection, poor nutritional status, and low self-esteem [2]. People with intellectual disabilities also have the same rights to

J. A. Townsend (✉)
The Ohio State University, Columbus, OH, USA

Nationwide Children's Hospital, Columbus, OH, USA
e-mail: Janice.Townsend@nationwidechildrens.org

T. M. Nelson, J. R. Webb (eds.), *Dental Care for Children with Special Needs*,
https://doi.org/10.1007/978-3-030-10483-2_11

bodily integrity and respect as individuals as any other person. It can put the clinician in a challenging position to honor these rights simultaneously. The balance of autonomy, patient safety, and quality of life is central to the issue of protective stabilization for patients with CSHCN [2, 5]. In 2000 the US Surgeon General's Report specifically acknowledged that individuals "who have disabilities are at greater risk for oral diseases, and in turn, oral diseases further jeopardize their health" [3]. Failure to employ proper prevention, examination, and treatment services can be interpreted as passive neglect or a failure to provide the patient's constitutionally guaranteed right to adequate medical care [2, 5]. However, the need for dental care must be balanced with the dentist's duty to respect the patient's right to self-determination [6]. When a person does not have the capacity to consent, issues of autonomy are complex [2]. The negative history of the use of restraint in the intellectual disability and psychiatric community further complicates this issue.

Historical Perspective

Challenging behaviors such as self-injury, aggression, and stereotypies are prevalent in persons with intellectual disability [7]. Historically these individuals have been subjected to restrictive behavioral practices to limit their movement or restrict their liberties [8]. Physical or mechanical restraint originated in French psychiatric hospitals during the eighteenth century as a way of preventing physical injury. These practices were a source of controversy almost from the beginning [7]. Since that time, the following methods have been used in with CSHCN:

- *General behavioral restraint* can take a number of forms including environmental barriers such as locked doors or the use of furniture to prevent movement. These may be referred to as "calming rooms" or "time-out rooms" [8].
- *Protective stabilization* methods have included mechanical restraints such as straightjackets; boards; ties to chairs, wheelchairs, beds, or other furniture; gloves used to manage self-biting or pica; and clothing worn to restrict movement such as reversed jumpsuits [8].
- *Psychotropic medications* are intended to limit movement or make a person drowsy all of the time. They restrict free movement and are a form of chemical restraint [8].

These interventions are used to prevent children or adults from harming others or themselves through aggressive or self-injurious behavior, but they carry their own risks [9]. Behavioral restraints may result in reduced socialization and autonomy of the individual. They are a form of seclusion that limits access [8]. Physical restraints can be invasive, and the process of applying restraint can injure the person being restrained and the people responsible for implementation [10, 11]. The use of restraint can also provoke additional behavior problems or aggression [11, 12]. Finally, psychotropic restraints present major issues of autonomy plus the additional concern of medication safety.

The harmful use of restraint in long-term care facilities has been reported widely in the last few decades. Restraint should only be used when all other techniques have failed, but studies have shown the frequency of use was consistent with routine rather than last resort use [9]. Service users, or patients who have required restraint, have differing view of its efficacy and purpose and report observing abuse [12]. They also reported poor staff training resulting in injury to the staff member or patient [12]. One example of objectionable use of restraint was in a school setting where a child was tied to a toilet seat for 2 h [7]. A 1999 US government report found conclusively that CSHCN are especially targeted by facility staff for unsafe restraint practices and are at greater risk of injury and death [13]. A 1998 *Hartford Courant* investigation reported on 142 deaths in the prior decade in mental health settings connected to the use of physical restraint. Those who died were disproportionally children [14]. This investigation suggested that failure of government oversight contributed to these incidents [14]. Typically severe physical injuries or death caused by restraints result from dehydration, choking, circulatory and skin problems, loss of strength and mobility, incontinence, and injury from other patients [15].

Despite concerns about improper use, many feel there is still a place for properly executed restraint in general behavioral therapy. For example, restraint to prevent harm, such as preventing a child from running into traffic or the use of seatbelts, is pervasive in our society. Failure to employ such controls would be deemed negligent or malicious [8]. In the context of healthcare, patients are entitled to effective treatment. Failure to use restraint when other measures are not as likely to be effective is unethical, particularly when the possibility of harm is high [7, 16, 17]. As a reflection of this responsibility, the Society for the Advancement of Behavioral Analysis advocates for strict and limited criteria for use of restraint, with careful weighing of risk and benefits [7, 16, 17].

A contemporary goal of behavior management for CSHCN is to build a repertoire of adaptive skills that reduces the need for patients to resort to aggression or self-injury [7, 18, 19]. However, these behaviors remain powerful ways to communicate and control one's environment and can be difficult to extinguish [7]. While ideally we work with patients to decrease the need for restraint, these methods continue to be employed due to the serious and possible harmful nature of these behaviors [7, 15, 19]. To prevent improper use, organizations have attempted to reduce physical restraint by making the criteria for implementation more stringent, requiring more accurate documentation, instituting performance improvement projects, and setting criterion-referenced standards [10].

Criticism of restraint has typically focused on use in behavioral environments. However, detractors have suggested it is overutilized in dentistry in the United States. Since the system of payment for dentists is based upon fees for treatment performed, there is financial incentive to complete as many procedures as possible [1]. Behavioral techniques such as desensitization are not always predictable or reimbursable and involve more visits and time compared to the rapid effect of chemical or physical restraints [1]. Thus the current reimbursement model in dentistry incentivizes the use of protective stabilization over potentially effective, but lengthy, behavioral therapies [1]. Parents of children with CSHCN may have concerns about any type of restrictive behavior guidance due to this history. They may benefit from education on the difference between protective stabilization and general restraints and the justification for use in dentistry.

Nomenclature and Regulatory Perspectives

Throughout the world the use of protective stabilization is governed by a wide variety of authorities. We focus here on the United States, providing a few examples of regulation that occurs at local and regional levels. The US Department of Health and Human Services Center for Medicare and Medicaid Services (CMS) glossary states that:

> Physical restraints are any manual method or physical or mechanical device, material, or equipment attached to or adjacent to the resident's body that the individual cannot remove easily which restricts movement or normal access to one's body. Chemical restraints are any drug used for discipline or convenience and not required to treat medical symptoms. [20]

However, this definition is geared toward residential care facilities for behavior purposes. The Joint Commission that accredits US healthcare organizations and programs differentiates between restraints of patients for medical/surgical procedures and for behavioral health. It states that standards that limit movement for general behavioral reasons do not apply to "limitation of mobility or temporary immobilization related to medical, dental, diagnostic, or surgical procedures" [2].

The New York State Office for People with Developmental Disabilities defines medical immobilization/protective stabilization (MIPS) as "the partial or complete control of an individual's arms, legs, head or torso which is necessary to protect the individual or others from injury for the duration of a medical or dental appointment. It may include manual and mechanical immobilization/stabilization and use of a papoose board" [21] and is acceptable when used in accordance with specific procedural rules for consent and documentation (Administrative Memorandum 2010-02) [21]. The use of protective stabilization must be part of an individual-specific plan (except in an emergency) and must be in accordance with the orders of a dentist [21, 22]. Brief holds of short duration needed for routine activities such as toothbrushing does not require the same level of consent or documentation [21]. For example, the use of mouth prop to facilitate toothbrushing is not considered a type of protective stabilization and does not require informed consent but should be documented in the individuals' service plan [21].

Policies, Guidelines, and an International Perspective

The acceptability of protective stabilization varies widely in different parts of the world, and this is reflected in the differing guidelines of professional groups.

The American Academy of Pediatric Dentistry (AAPD) does acknowledge that "Protective stabilization can be helpful in patients for whom traditional behavior guidance techniques are not adequate" [23]. The AAPD has a specific guideline dedicated to protective stabilization with practice recommendations which will be discussed in greater depth later in the chapter [24].

The European Academy of Paediatric Dentistry (EAPD) does not have a specific guideline on protective stabilization. The EAPD guideline on sedation states "The use of restraint in dentistry (including such restraining devices as the papoose board) is practiced to a varying extent in European countries, but in some countries, as the Nordic, forbidden to use by law. A mouth prop may be used to help a child support the lower jaw and thus assist it in holding the mouth open. It may not be used to forcefully get a child to hold the mouth open, which may also make it more difficult to assess the level of sedation" [25].

British guidelines emphasize that any physical restraint of children must be carried out with regard for the Human Rights Act (15) and the European Convention "On the Rights of the Child," Consent and Capacity Assessment (1989) [26]. From this perspective, the use of physical intervention is forcibly providing treatment for a patient that has withheld their permission [27]. This is viewed as a major infringement on an individual's right to liberty [27]. It is only justified if the individual lacks capacity, the intervention is necessary to protect that individual from harm, and the intervention is proportionate to the likelihood and seriousness of the potential harm [27]. Therefore one could argue that according to these guidelines, the use of the papoose board for a preventive visit would not be appropriate.

The British Society for Disability and Oral Health permits "clinical holding" for patients unable to comply with routine oral healthcare [28]. The group places emphasis on the determination of mental capacity, informed consent, and use of the least restrictive intervention [28]. British guidelines also focus on the difference in capacity rules between England, Wales, and Scotland with the Scotland rules being more complex [28]. Perhaps the most restrictive guideline on this topic is the Scottish Intercollegiate Guideline Network Document on Safe Sedation of Children Undergoing Diagnostic and Therapeutic Procedures that states "physical restraints and HOM(E) have no place in dental treatment of children and should not be used" [29]. The hand-over-mouth exercise (HOME) behavior guidance technique is also no longer included in the AAPD guidelines.

Protective Stabilization in the Dental Office

Before using any restrictive physical intervention, an individual assessment should be carried out to consider the underlying condition and treatment, environment, the child/young person's behavior, age, and mental capacity [24, 26].

Indications

Protective stabilization for dentistry is primarily distinguished from general behavioral restraints by its temporary nature [19]. The goal of protective stabilization is to safely complete an exam or procedure versus accomplishing generalized behavior management. The duration should only be long enough to complete the dental procedure, and the extent of immobilization is determined by specific needs of the patient [19]. Protective stabilization should be reserved for only the most serious problem behavior, and it should only be used after less restrictive procedures are shown to be ineffective and in conjunction with other proactive therapies [1, 10, 19, 21, 22, 24, 26, 27]. Various behavior modification approaches such as distraction, play, shaping, modeling, sensory integration, desensitization, and repetitive task performance have been shown success in children with CSHCN and are discussed in more detail throughout this book [16, 24, 26, 27, 30]. After considering a variety of options, the least restrictive method of stabilization should be used [5].

According to the AAPD, protective stabilization is indicated under the following circumstances:

1. A patient requires immediate diagnosis and/or urgent limited treatment and is unable to cooperate, and uncontrolled movements pose a safety risk.
2. A previously cooperative patient becomes uncooperative, and the appointment needs to come to a safe end.
3. An uncooperative patient requires limited treatment and is not a candidate for sedation or treatment under general anesthesia.
4. A sedated patient requires stabilization to control movements.
5. A patient with CSHCN exhibits uncontrolled movements that are potentially harmful or interfere with care [24].

Protective stabilization should only be used when necessary to protect the individual and others during a dental appointment and should not be used for coercion, convenience, or punishment [5, 7, 19, 21, 22, 27, 31].

Most patients with CSHCN can undergo dental treatment without protective stabilization [5]. However, anticipating its potential need is necessary because planned protective stabilization is safer than unplanned [11, 24]. Unplanned stabilization is generally used reactively to address a behavior that may cause harm to the individual or others [7, 11]. This reactionary approach is more likely to result in injuries to the person exhibiting challenging behavior and the person implementing the restraint [7, 24].

Observation of behavior in the waiting room is helpful, as patients displaying hyperactivity and aggression may exhibit these same behaviors in the treatment area [19]. Patients who cannot cooperate for physical examination, blood draws, or nail care likely will not be able to cooperate for dental appointments [19]. Marshall et al. found the following factors predicted uncooperative behavior in children with autism: nonverbal/minimal or echolalic language, inability to understand language appropriate for age, inability to follow multistep instructions, parents providing almost all toothbrushing, incomplete toilet training by age 4, inability to cooperate for a haircut, attending special education, and inability to read at age 6 [32]. This does not mean a child with these characteristics will always require protective stabilization, but they are good areas of inquiry during the parent interview. Discussing patient strengths and limitations may be useful in making the determination of whether he will require protective stabilization.

Medical Considerations

A full review of the patient's medical history should be completed before use of protective stabilization, as some medical or physical conditions impact its use [10, 18, 21, 24]. Consultation may be needed to determine the impact of stabilization and associated elevated levels of distress on the patient's medical conditions. For example:

- In a patient with respiratory disease such as *asthma*, *cystic fibrosis*, or complications of *obesity*, restriction of the chest or full supine positioning may be contraindicated [18, 24].
- Patients with severe *cardiac* or *sickle cell disease* may not be able to compensate physiologically if they are distressed by restraint.
- The potential for atlantoaxial instability should be ruled out in predisposing conditions such as *Down syndrome*, *Goldenhar syndrome*, *spondyloepiphyseal dysplasia*, *Morquio syndrome*, and *rheumatoid arthritis* [18, 33].
- Any form of medical immobilization should be used with extreme caution or avoided entirely in patients with recent fractures, a history of dislocated joints, *osteogenesis imperfecta*, *severe osteoporosis*, and *osteopetrosis* [18, 24].
- Stabilization with a papoose board or blanket should be used with caution in patients prone to overheating such as *anhidrotic ectodermal dysplasia* and *uncontrolled hyperthyroidism*.
- Patients with a history of abuse may be psychologically impacted by use of protective stabilization.

Environment

Protective stabilization should be used in an environment of family and caregiver involvement, and most parents feel they should be present to increase the child's stability and comfort [4, 34]. While parental presence and involvement should be encouraged, parents should not be made to feel guilty if they do not want to be present [26]. If they choose to be absent, it should be documented [24, 26]. If parents are denied access, they must be informed of the reason, and the rationale must be documented in the patient's chart [24]. It is helpful to attempt and create an environment that is based on the child's specific coping mechanisms and preferred level of stimuli [4]. When possible, continuity of dentist, staff, location, and order of dental procedures also facilitates a minimally restrictive environment [4].

Informed Consent

The process of informed consent is an ethical obligation and a legal requirement that goes beyond a signature on a consent form [2, 24]. In the case of protective stabilization, it is advisable to obtain specific, written informed consent [2, 19, 21, 24]. Failure to obtain informed consent may result in a criminal charge of battery (unwanted touching) or a claim of negligence (malpractice) for failure to fully "inform" the patient about a treatment or procedure [2, 35].

First, it is critical to ascertain who can consent for care for the patient, including the patient's ability to give consent. Laws concerning the age of consent vary widely, so to ensure compliance, the dental provider should become familiar with the regulations in their region [2, 24, 27]. Sfikas advises getting a copy of the court order appointing any guardian and inspecting it to ensure they are authorized to consent to treatment on behalf of the patient [35]. For example, some guardians are authorized to handle financial decisions but cannot make healthcare decisions [35]. For children who reside in a group home, it may not be possible for the practitioner to meet the guardian face-to-face [2]. The residence manager or nurse can help communicate with the guardian and help ensure consent is obtained and documented [2]. It is also advisable to have the practitioner's information on the form so the guardian can contact the dental clinic [2]. When a patient does not have the capacity to give consent, an explanation should still be given at his level of understanding, and the provider should obtain his assent if possible [1, 24, 27].

The informed consent process should begin with a conversation regarding the possible need for protective stabilization, what type is recommended and why, possible risks and benefits, likely outcomes, and alternatives [24]. Involvement of parents in the informed consent process is crucial because they frequently will ultimately authorize treatment and they are a wealth of information about the child. Marshall et al. found that parents of children with autism were able to predict cooperation for examination and radiographs [4]. Parents often know which appointment structure and coping strategies yield the best results and should be part of the behavior guidance planning process [4]. If at all possible, this should take place on a day prior to treatment so parents or caregivers have time to reflect on options and ask questions [24]. If past behavior suggests immobilization may be necessary, it is advisable to obtain consent in advance and have any devices needed in place with the goal of managing behavior with other modalities as shown in Fig. 1.

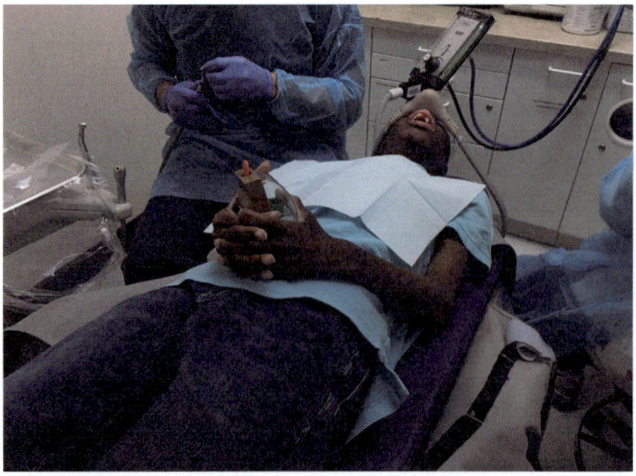

Fig. 1 Teenage male with autism is having a tooth restored with a board passive stabilization device in place due to a previous history of uncooperative behavior. The patient was successfully treated using communicative behavior guidance techniques and nitrous oxide sedation without protective stabilization. Note the patient was allowed to hold his toy to provide distraction for the appointment

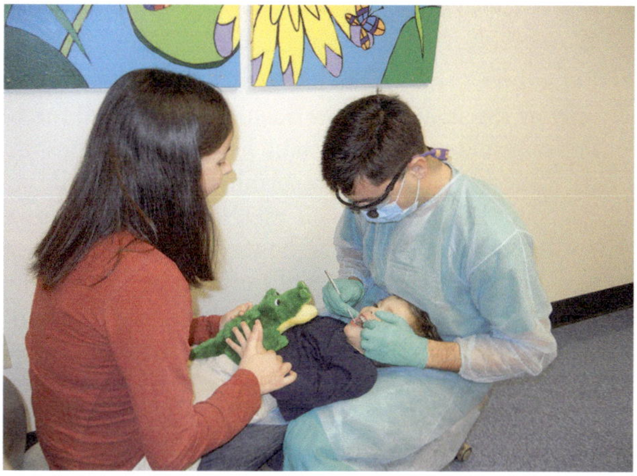

Fig. 2 An infant is examined in the knee-to-knee position. Note that the dentist is using his non-dominant hand to keep the patient from closing and injuring himself on the mirror

Knee-to-Knee Exam

The purpose of protective stabilization is to support the child patient. This value is most apparent in the knee-to-knee exam or knee-lap exam. This patient positioning technique allows the child to remain in the parent's lap and for the child's head to be placed into the dentist's lap. The child's legs are controlled by straddling the parent's lap, the parent gently restrains the arms and hands, and the dentist stabilizes the child's head as shown in Fig. 2. Special foam support mats are manufactured to support infants and young children in this position but are not necessary. This exam is primarily used for very young children unable to cooperate for examination in the dental chair, but it may be used for older CSHCN when patient size permits safe positioning.

During these examinations it is important to protect the child from injuring himself by closing on dental instruments such as the mirror or explorer. For very young children with few teeth, the dentist can place a finger on the alveolar ridge posterior to the most erupted tooth to prevent the child from closing. Older children with more teeth erupted may benefit from the use of a foam or child-sized mouth prop if both the mirror and explorer are needed. Knee-to-knee positioning is almost universally acceptable to parents, and even critics that oppose any type of restraint generally agree that some type of physical contact and steadying is acceptable in pediatric dentistry [36].

Active Stabilization

Active stabilization involves restraint by another person such as the dentist or dental auxiliary. Active stabilization or "holding" must avoid the use of unnecessary force, which could cause pain or put pressure on joints [37]. This may also be referred to as physical or personal restraint [19].

A number of specific techniques are included in active stabilization:

- Sometimes parts of the patient's body are gently held, and pressure is intended only as resistance to slow down the speed and force of movement [18].
- For minimal restriction, some have suggested a staff member form an "arc" over the patient's body, which permits the individual to move more freely since limited contact is made with their body [18]. More extensive movements of the patient's body are restricted by contact with the person's arcing arm [18].
- Hand guarding is employed for most pediatric dental patients during injections to prevent unexpected movements and injury and is accepted by critics of restraint [19, 38]. In this technique the dental assistant proactively places her arms over the hands of the child to block them if they are raised to the mouth [19].
- Head holding is a method of controlling movement, often side to side, of the patient [19]. Mild movement may be employed by the operator by cradling the patient's head between the operator's forearm and chest of the non-dominant arm [19]. This can provide stabilization for patients with poor head control, and the dentist can sense impending movement through patient tensing. This allows her to compensate by removing instruments or stopping the handpiece for patient safety [19]. More rigorous movement may require an additional staff member to support the head through sitting or kneeling behind the patient to firmly secure the head [19]. Care must be taken to keep the hands out of the operating field and avoid injury to the patient's ears [19].
- Therapeutic holds are utilized to control large movements by patients and require two or three additional assistants [19]. The arms may be crossed across the chest and held firmly by the patient's hips [19]. An alternative to this is the leg over method where the patient's arms drape off of the chair and are secured between the legs of the dentist and dental assistant. Therapeutic holds can be applied to the legs by crossing the ankles and holding them firmly [19]. This technique is usually accompanied by some form of passive immobilization above the knees [19].

Full immobilization by active stabilization for more than a few seconds is almost impossible. For lengthier procedures or procedures that risk harm to the patient, such as prolonged use of a high-speed handpiece, alternatives are needed. During active immobilization patients may detect a heightened sense of stress or anxiety from the staff which may promote more distress [2]. Patients may also feel threatened by being overpowered by the staff [2].

The use of parents or caregivers to provide active stabilization should be regarded with caution [28]. While caregivers provide ideal assistance and emotional support by holding the patient's hand [28], they are not trained to provide active protective stabilization. They may inadvertently harm the patient through improper stabilization or provide inadequate stabilization resulting in patient injury from treatment [28]. Involvement of parents or caregivers remains an individual decision for each provider, but ultimately the safety of the patient is the responsibility of the dentist.

Passive Immobilization

Passive immobilization involves the use of mechanical devices which assist the patient in remaining properly positioned [19, 24]. Examples include Papoose Boards®, Pedi-Wraps®, sheets, straps, seat belts, towels, wrist bracelets, and vests [19]. Typically the use of passive immobilization is accompanied by active immobilization to apply the mechanical device or to immobilize portions of the body that are not restrained by the device, so consent for both methods is prudent [19].

Sheets have long been used as stabilizing devices [19, 38, 39]. A bedsheet wrapped around the patient can effectively limit extremity movement in a non-threatening way [19]. These blankets can be used to "swaddle" the patient which affords protection and security [18]. The sheet can be secured with durable tape that can be cut or with large safety pins [19, 38]. The patient can also participate in application of the sheet. This technique is typically well accepted and can provide a sense of security [19].

A board-type device (Papoose Board®, Olympic Medical Corp., Seattle, Washington, USA) is perhaps the most commonly used form of passive protective stabilization (Fig. 3). Typically this device consists of a rigid but cushioned board covered in vinyl with Velcro® straps for the wrists and three heavy canvas wraps that go over the arms and torso, shoulders, and knees. A removable rigid head stabilizer may also be used, but many feel it is bulky and ineffective [19]. With proper patient selection and application, these devices can enable safe diagnosis and treatment in large, uncooperative patients and can be invaluable for emergency care [19, 38]. However, the use of canvas fabric can be very hot in a resisting patient which increases the risk of overheating [38].

Other commercially available devices have a similar design but use a wrap made of an open weave nylon material that reduces the risk of overheating (Rainbow® Stabilizing Products, Hampton, New Hampshire, USA) (Fig. 4) [5, 19]. They are also nonrigid, so patients may be treated upright or semireclined [19]. Children may

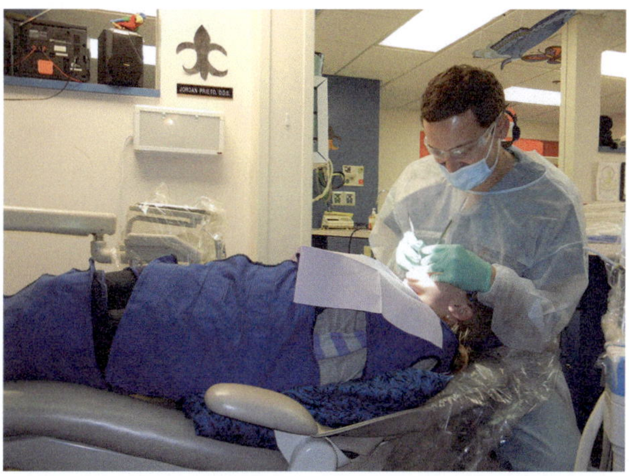

Fig. 3 Protective stabilization utilizing a Papoose Board (Olympic Medical Corp., Seattle, Washington, USA)

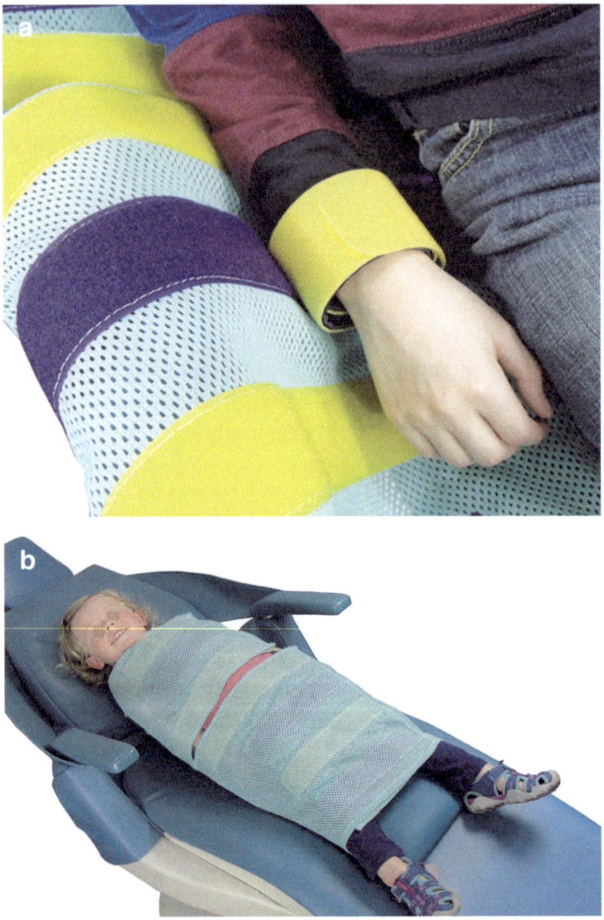

Fig. 4 (**a**)Wrist straps and (**b**) nylon fabric wrap used in an alternative protective stabilization device (Rainbow® Stabilizing Products, Specialized Care Company, Inc., Hampton, New Hampshire, USA, image courtesy of http://specializedcare.com/)

associate this device with a security blanket and feel it is less restrictive [19]. However, the, nonrigid design, difference in wrap material, and smaller size can make this device inadequate for larger, more combative patients [19, 38].

Most board-type devices are made from fabric that presents infection control challenges. A newer device has no fabric (Joey Board, Queen Creek, AZ, USA) and can be cleaned with disinfectants, without laundering. This device also has a recessed area in the board for the patient's head which permits different positions for sedation procedures.

Regardless of the type of immobilization board, wrist straps must be carefully placed and monitored periodically to ensure adequate circulation and correct positioning. Patients with muscle contractures should not have limbs stretched or straightened for wrist holders or knee wraps. Stabilization devices for these children should be secured in the patient's natural condition as shown in Fig. 5. Application of full-body stabilization should be accomplished in a sequential manner, and if a head stabilizer is used, it should be applied last [24]. The torso must be supported actively at all times while wrist straps are in place. This helps to ensure proper positioning of the hands and limits the potential for injury due to improper flexion [24]. All devices should be positioned to permit monitoring of vital signs, chest movement, and color, especially for sedation procedures [24]. Devices with a flat board design may not adapt to the dental chair and may need pillows and beanbags under the board to promote stability. Alternately, the board can be secured to the chair with straps or belts [19].

Although a board type device can be perceived as objectionable by critics, it also has advocates. These devices have been proposed as a tactile stimulus therapy device as part of a sensory adapted dental environment (SADE). Shapiro et al. found a "friendly butterfly" stabilization device that "hugged" the child tightly as part of a SADE intervention to be more effective at decreasing anxious behaviors than a loosely wrapped stabilization device in CSHCN [40]. Others agree the protective stabilization can serve as a source of deep pressure during dental procedures [41]. Weighted blankets have been shown to facilitate the ability to feel safe, comforted, and "grounded in the world," and stabilization boards may provide a similar

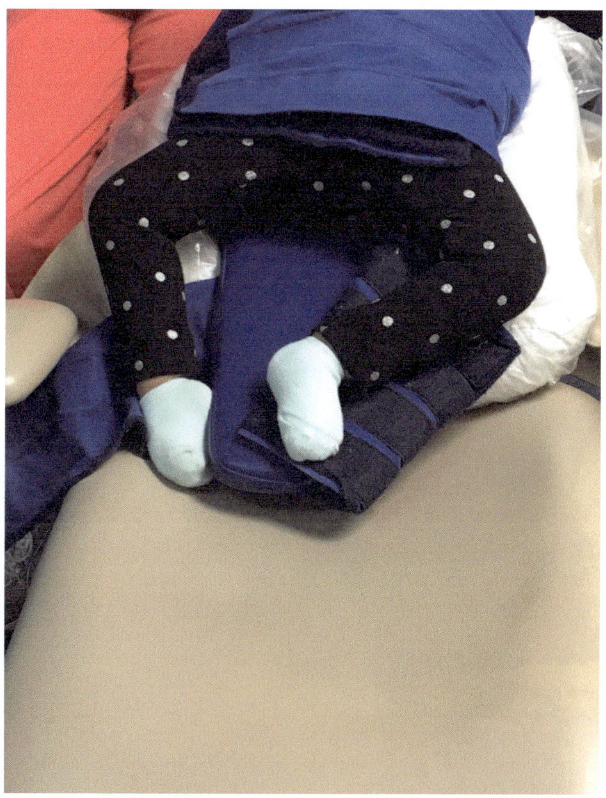

Fig. 5 Note that the legs are allowed to stay in a natural position in this patient with limb contracture associated with spina bifida

sensation [2, 42]. Deep pressure stimulation is a form of touch pressure applied to the body providing the feeling of a firm hug, holding, swaddling, or massage [42]. Aside from the benefit of deep touch pressure, passive stabilization may be less stressful to patients than active stabilization due to lack of physical contact with others, less of a sense of being overpowered, and reduced anxiety on the part of the staff [2]. Passive stabilization is associated with fewer injuries than active stabilization [11, 24].

Positioning Devices or Stabilizers

Adjunct devices can be used to enable positioning and support but are not necessarily forms of protective stabilization. For example, many patients with specialized wheelchairs can receive high-quality dental procedures while remaining in their chairs [19]. Wheelchair head supports may already be present on the chairs of patients with muscular instability disorders. These can be used to provide familiarity and support during dental procedures (Fig. 6a) [19]. The use of chairlifts can securely place the chair in an ergonomically acceptable position for the dental provider during lengthier procedures.

For patients who are transferred to the dental chair, additional means of support should be used to ensure patient comfort and stability [19]. Bean bag pillows or chairs may be placed into the reclined dental chair to stabilize the patient's body as shown in Fig. 6b [19]. Commercially available devices combine bean bags with a vacuum source to create a customized, molded form around the patient for stability and security [19].

Mouth Props

Mouth props can be used provide support or comfort to any patient. They may be especially helpful in patients with cerebral palsy, where they can be used to stabilize

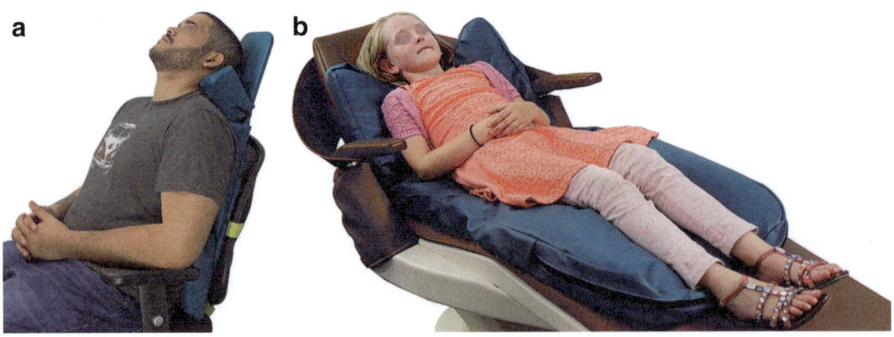

Fig. 6 Stabilization devices can be utilized to enable positioning and support such as (**a**) head support for wheelchair and (**b**) chair cushion (Specialized Care Company, Inc., Hampton, New Hampshire, USA, image courtesy of http://specializedcare.com/)

reflexive closing movements the patient cannot voluntary control. There are many different types of mouth props available—each with specific indications and contraindications. Prior to the use of any mouth prop, the teeth should be assessed for previous injury and mobility. The use of exfoliating primary teeth or previously traumatized teeth risks avulsion and subsequent aspiration.

- Molt®-style mouth props (Hu-Friedy Manufacturing Company, Chicago, IL, USA) have an adjustable, scissor-type design and are available in adult, child, and infant sizes as shown in Fig. 7a [19]. A soft material, such as rubber tubing, is placed over the metal blades [19]. Care must be taken to ensure overly large tubing does not slip off the blades and become an aspiration risk. The advantages of these mouth props are their ability to adjust to accommodate the opening potential of the patient and the ability to be stabilized extraorally [19, 38]. However, there is potential for these mouth props to become anteriorly positioned and fracture, luxate, or avulse teeth—including permanent incisors [19, 38]. These mouth props can leave an extraoral imprint which can be

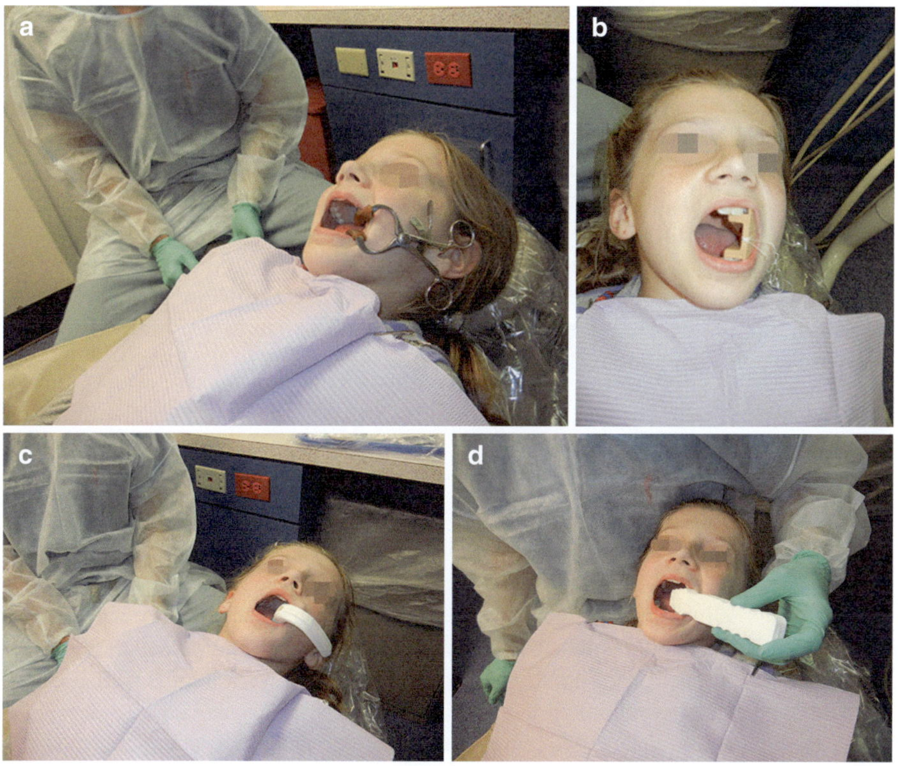

Fig. 7 A variety of different mouth props are available including (**a**) Molt® adjustable mouth prop, (**b**) block-style mouth prop, (**c**) Open Wide® Reusable Mouth Prop (Specialized Care Company, Inc., Hampton, New Hampshire, USA), and (**d**) Open Wide® Mouth Rests (Specialized Care Company, Inc., Hampton, New Hampshire, USA)

prevented by securing a 4 × 4 inch gauze between the cheek and the mouth prop [19]. They can also impinge on the intraoral soft tissues, so care must be taken in their placement [19]. These mouth props can be used to gently increase opening if they are positioned correctly on the posterior teeth but should not be used to forcibly open the mouth or open beyond patient comfort [19].

- Dental bite blocks (e.g., McKesson®) are wedge shaped and made out of a firm rubber block and come in a variety of sizes as shown in Fig. 7b [19]. These blocks provide comfort and support and pose less risk of injury to hard and soft tissue [19]. However these mouth props are more easily dislodged from an uncooperative patient, are not adjustable, and may provoke a gagging sensation. They also can bock a cross arch approach to the mandibular inferior alveolar block injection. An inappropriately small prop may be an aspiration risk, so blocks should be secured with floss for easy retrieval [19]. In an extremely uncooperative patient, this block may have to be secured by an assistant or additional head holder. This practice increases the risk for biting injuries, but newer models of this mouth prop style have an attachment for extraoral head holding as shown in Fig. 7c (Open Wide® Reusable Mouth Prop, Specialized Care Company, Inc., Hampton, New Hampshire, USA) [19].
- Foam mouth props (Open Wide® Mouth Rests, Specialized Care Company, Inc., Hampton, New Hampshire, USA) are available for use in the office and for home care as shown in Fig. 7d. They are made from a disposable pliable but firm foam-like material and come in a regular and thick version [19]. This mouth prop may be a safer alternative to achieve initial opening, but it still has the potential to avulse mobile primary teeth. These mouth props can be deformed, or a patient can bite through them, resulting in injury from dental instruments and handpieces. Therefore, in patients who bite forcefully, they should be used for limited procedures or initial opening and replaced with a McKesson bite block for restorative treatment or lengthy scaling procedures. These can be very effective when used for daily home care [19].

Assessment

Regardless of the type of protective stabilization, ongoing assessment of the patient must be performed and the technique adjusted appropriately [24]. Struggling against restraint may not be solely due to oppositional behavior. It may be a natural response to pain or the feeling of being unable to breathe and exchange air [15]. Personnel must be able to recognize and respond to signs of physical and psychological distress such as positional asphyxia [22]. Monitoring the physical and psychological well-being of the patient is necessary including but not limited to respiratory and circulatory status, skin integrity, and vital signs [22]. In a worst-case scenario, if a patient ceases struggling after prolonged inappropriate restraint, he may be in respiratory distress with a poor prognosis for resuscitation [15]. The need for protective stabilization should be reevaluated throughout the procedure. As behavior permits, elements of the stabilization device can be removed as discussed in more detail in the case-based scenario.

Documentation

Documentation requirements vary by location and setting. However, basic elements of documentation involve the following [5, 24]:

- Indication for stabilization
- Type of stabilization

Informed Consent

- Reason for parent exclusion (if applicable)
- Duration of stabilization
- Behavior evaluation/rating during stabilization
- Untoward outcomes
- Plans for management at future appointments

It is also prudent to document the reason for a specific stabilization type. Typically, adverse outcomes related to medical immobilization are minor scratches or bruising [11, 24]. Regardless of the severity, adverse outcomes should be documented. If protective stabilization is implemented but was unplanned, the reason for its use and method of obtaining consent should be documented along with plans for future treatment [24]. The overall effectiveness of stabilization should be documented after the appointment [21].

Outcomes and Parental Acceptance

Contemporary behavioral approaches to assisting people with intellectual disabilities and challenging behavior call for the implementation of preventative procedures [43]. In contrast, protective stabilization is a reactive support strategy that does not generally support development of skills that enable the patient to receive care. Al Humaid et al. found that standard behavior guidance techniques including passive immobilization did not improve the behavior of children with autism compared to an Applied Behavior Analysis program (D-TERMINED) [30]. However, protective stabilization may still be needed even with the most successful treatment interventions, because for some children the complete elimination of severe challenging behavior is rare [43]. While protective stabilization is not focused on helping the patient develop dental skills, Marshall et al. reported a calming effect associated with a stabilization device occurred for 20% of patients observed [4]. The type of restraint used may also have implications for effectiveness. Parents have reported parental restraint (46%) and stabilization devices (44%) were the most effective forms of protective stabilization where staff restraint was only felt to be effective 27% of the time [4].

de Castro et al. found that parents of children with and without developmental disability accepted basic techniques more than advanced ones [44]. Parents of children with disabilities were significantly more likely than those of typically developing peers to accept protective stabilization with a restrictive device [44]. The authors hypothesized that these parents may have already been familiar with the technique or had a better understanding of the need for its use [44]. Marshall et al. evaluated parental acceptance of a variety of different behavior management techniques and found that among the varying methods of protective stabilization, parental restraint was most accepted (84%), followed by staff restraint (63%) and stabilization device (54%) [4]. Stabilization by dental staff was rated as more acceptable and effective when limited to holding a patient's hands versus holding the arms, trunk, or legs [4]. Many children in this study had previously received care with protective stabilization. Nearly all parents of those children who had received it in the past rated the technique as very acceptable for their child.

Training

Dentist and staff training is important for implementation of protective stabilization [27]. US federal law states that the patient has the right to safe implementation of restraint by trained staff [22]. However in the United States, few dentists receive training on either active or passive stabilization during their predoctoral education [24, 45]. Advanced training is advised prior to implementing protective stabilization. Currently at least one state (Colorado) requires training beyond basic dental education through a residency program, graduate program, or an extensive continuing education course that involves didactic and experiential mentored training prior to the use of medical immobilization [31].

Case-Based Scenario

Semaj is a 13-year-old teenager with autism. He has been a patient of a hospital-based dental clinic that sees a significant number of CSHCN since he was 8. When he initially presented for care, he had never seen a dentist because his mother had not been able to find a dentist willing to treat him. He was nonverbal and combative and had severe dental caries and generalized gingivitis. He required medical immobilization for his initial exam and general anesthesia for dental rehabilitation.

Semaj has been returning for preventive care semiannually. His mother has been trained to use foam mouth props at home to help Semaj stay open, and his oral hygiene has improved dramatically. His mother has altered his diet, and he has remained caries-free. Semaj has continued to be uncooperative for his preventive visits, so medical immobilization has been used, but improved behavior was noted at his last visit.

Today Semaj is brought by his mother, and she reports he has started a new school and is making significant progress with his new Individualized Education

Plan (IEP) and in therapy. His communication skills have improved which has led fewer outbursts and improved behavior. Her goal has always been for him to be treated at the dentist office without protective stabilization, but she is concerned about his safety if he becomes uncooperative during the procedure. After discussion, the dentist and mom agree to begin the appointment using a stabilization device since that has become Semaj's routine. If behavior is cooperative and treatment can be delivered safely, they will progressively remove the straps on the device. Mom provides written consent to this plan.

The stabilization device is laid on in Semaj's typical treatment room. He is helped into the device by the dentist and a familiar assistant with his mother there for support. An exam with a mirror and explorer is performed with a McKesson mouth prop to maintain opening. Semaj tentatively accepts treatment with repeated requests and positive reinforcement but has minimal movement. After the exam is completed, the Velcro strap over his legs is removed – the team does not draw attention to this change but praises Semaj for holding still. After scaling of the mandibular anterior teeth, the larger strap covering the torso is removed, again with praise. Semaj's teeth are polished, and the wrist straps are removed so that the device is fully removed for application of fluoride varnish. After the procedure is completed Semaj is praised and given a ball as a reward. His mother is very happy with the visit. Before dismissal, the dentist and Semaj's mom make a plan that for the next visit, the protective stabilization device will be placed on the chair, but the goal will be to complete the visit without the need to use the device. Mom says she is looking forward to bringing Semaj to his next visit under these circumstances.

Conclusions

- Protective stabilization can be a useful adjunct to other behavior guidance techniques or a last resort when they fail.
- Due to the history of the improper use of restraint in individuals with CSHCN, dentists should understand the rationale behind protective stabilization in dentistry and indications for its use.
- Proper informed consent and documentation are essential when implementing protective stabilization.

References

1. Newton JT. Restrictive behaviour management procedures with people with intellectual disabilities who require dental treatment. J Appl Res Intellect Disabil. 2009;22(2):128–5.
2. Romer M. Consent, restraint, and people with special needs: a review. Spec Care Dentist. 2009;29(1):58–66.
3. United States Department of Health and Human Services. Oral health in America: a report of the Surgeon General. Rockville: U.S. Department of Health and Human Services. National Institute of Dental and Craniofacial Research, National Institutes of Health; 2000.

4. Marshall J, Sheller B, Manci L, Williams BJ. Parental attitudes regarding behavior guidance of dental patients with autism. Pediatr Dent. 2008;30(5):400–7.
5. Fenton SJ, Fenton LI, Kimmelman BB, Shellhart WC, Sheff MC, Scott JP, Staggers JA, Purtugal BV. ADH ad hoc committee report: the use of restraints in the delivery of dental care for the handicapped—legal, ethical, and medical considerations. Spec Care Dentist. 1987;7(6):253–6.
6. American Dental Association. Principles of ethics & code of professional conduct. Available from https://www.ada.org/~/media/ADA/Publications/Files/ADA_Code_of_Ethics_2018.pdf?la=en. Accessed 13 Mar 2018.
7. Matson JL, Boisjoli JA. Restraint procedures and challenging behaviors in intellectual disability: an analysis of causative factors. J Appl Res Intellect Disabil. 2009;22(2):111–7.
8. Sturmey P. It is time to reduce and safely eliminate restrictive behavioural practices. J Appl Res Intellect Disabil. 2009;22(2):105–10.
9. McGill P, Murphy G, Kelly-Pike A. Frequency of use and characteristics of people with intellectual disabilities subject to physical interventions. J Appl Res Intellect Disabil. 2009;22(2):152–8.
10. Luiselli JK. Physical restraint of people with intellectual disability: a review of implementation reduction and elimination procedures. J Appl Res Intellect Disabil. 2009;22(2):126–34.
11. Spreat S, Lipinski D, Hill J, Halpin ME. Safety indices associated with the use of contingent restraint procedures. Appl Res Ment Retard. 1986;7(4):475–81.
12. Jones P, Kroese BS. Service users' views of physical restraint procedures in secure settings for people with learning disabilities. Br J Learn Disabil. 2006;35(1):50–4.
13. US General Accounting Office. Mental health: improper restraint or seclusion use places people at risk. (GAO publication HEH-99-176). Washington, DC: USGAO;1999.
14. Weiss EM. Deadly restraint: a nationwide pattern of death. Hartford Courant, 11–15 Oct. Available at: http://articles.courant.com/1998-10-11/news/9810090779_1_mental-health-deaths-restraint-policy/2. Accessed 13 Mar 2018.
15. Mohr WK, Petti TA, Mohr BD. Adverse effects associated with physical restraint. Can J Psychiatr. 2003;48(5):330–7.
16. Association for Behavioral Analysis. Statement on restraint and seclusion; 2010. Available at https://www.abainternational.org/about-us/policies-and-positions/restraint-and-seclusion,-2010.aspx. Accessed 13 Mar 2018.
17. Association for Behavioral Analysis. Statement on the right to effective behavioral treatment; 1989. Available at https://www.abainternational.org/about-us/policies-and-positions/right-to-effective-behavioral-treatment,-1989.aspx. Accessed 13 Mar 2018
18. British Society for Disability and Oral Health. Principles on intervention for people unable to comply with routine dental care; 2004 Apr. Available at http://www.bsdh.org/documents/PIDocument.pdf. Accessed 13 Mar 2018.
19. Southern Association of Institutional Dentists. Managing maladaptive behaviors—the use of dental restraints and positioning devices. Self-study course. Module 6:1–24. Available from http://saiddent.org/admin/images/03567700_1339447006.pdf. Accessed 13 Mar 2018.
20. United States Department of Health and Human Services Centers for Medicare & Medicaid Services Glossary. Available from http://www.cms.hhs.gov/apps/glossary/. Accessed 13 Mar 2018.
21. NYS Office for People with Developmental Disabilities. Administrative Memorandum—#2010-02. Medical immobilization/protective stabilization (MIPS) and sedation for medical/dental appointments. 2010;1–7. Available from https://opwdd.ny.gov/sites/default/files/documents/adm2010-02_121917.pdf. Accessed 13 Mar 2018.
22. Office of the Federal Register. Code of federal regulations. Title 42 public health, 482.13;2011. Available from https://www.gpo.gov/fdsys/pkg/CFR-2011-title42-vol5/pdf/CFR-2011-title42-vol5-sec482-13.pdf. Accessed 13 Mar 2018.
23. American Academy of Pediatric Dentistry. Management of Dental Patients with Special Health Care Needs. Pediatr Dent. 2017;39(6):229–34.

24. American Academy of Pediatric Dentistry. Protective Stabilization for Pediatric Dental Patients Pediatr Dent 2017;39(6): 229-234.
25. Hallonsten AL, Jensen B, Raadal M, Veerkamp J, Hosey MT, Poulsen S. European Academy of Pediatric Dentistry (EAPD) guidelines on sedation in paediatric dentistry. Available at: https://www.eapd.eu/uploads/5CF03741_file.pdf. Accessed 13 Mar 2018.
26. Royal College of Nursing. Restrictive physical intervention and therapeutic holding for children and young people. Guidance for nursing staff. London: RCN; 2010. Available at https://www.rcn.org.uk/professional-development/publications/pub-003573. Accessed 13 Mar 2018.
27. Nunn J, Foster M, Master S, Greening S, British Society of Pediatric Dentistry. British Society of Paediatric Dentistry: a policy document on consent and the use of physical intervention in the dental care of children. Int J Paediatr Dent. 2008;18(Suppl 1):39–46.
28. British Society for Disability and Oral Health. Guidelines for 'Clinical Holding' Skills for dental services for people unable to comply with routine oral health care; 2009 June. Available at http://www.bsdh.org/documents/BSDH_Clinical_Holding_Guideline_Jan_2010.pdf. Accessed 13 Mar 2018.
29. Scottish Intercollegiate Guideline Network. Safe sedation of children undergoing diagnostic and therapeutic procedures. Edinburgh; 2002. http://www.sign.ac.uk/guidelines/fulltext/58/index.html
30. Al Humaid J, Tesini D, Finkelman M, Loo CY. Effectiveness of the D-TERMINED program of repetitive tasking for children with autism spectrum disorder. J Dent Child. 2016;83(1):16–21.
31. State of Colorado Department of Regulatory Agencies. Board of dental examiners. 3CCR709-1. Rules and regulations; Medical immobilization/protective stabilization. 2011;37–8. Available at http://www.sos.state.co.us/CCR/GenerateRulePdf.do?ruleVersionId=4423. Accessed 13 Mar 2018.
32. Marshall J, Sheller B, Williams BJ, Manci L, Cowan C. Cooperation predictors for dental patients with autism. Pediatr Dent. 2007;29(5):369–76.
33. Yang SY, Boniello AJ, Poorman CE, Change AL, Wang S, Passias PG. A review of the diagnosis and treatment of atlantoaxial dislocations. Global Spine J. 2014;4(3):197–210.
34. Frankel RI. The Papoose Board and mothers' attitudes following its use. Pediatr Dent 1991;13(5):284–288.
35. Sfikas PM. A duty to disclose: issues to consider in securing informed consent. JADA. 2003;134:1329–33.
36. Roberts JF. Conscious sedation. Br Dent J. 2004;196(12):731–3.
37. Valler-Jones T, Shinnick A. Holding children for invasive procedures: preparing student nurses. Pediatr Nurs. 2005;17(5):20–2.
38. Kelly JR. The use of restraints in pedodontics. J Pedod. 1976;1(1):57–68.
39. Beaver HA. Control mechanisms for the special care pediatric patient. J Mich State Dent Assoc. 1970;52:34–6.
40. Shapiro M, Sgan-Cohen HD, Parush S, Melmed RN. Influence of adapted environment on the anxiety of medically treated. J Pediatr. 2009;154(4):546–50.
41. Chen H, Yang H, Chi H, Chen H. Physiologic and behavioral effect of papoose board on anxiety in dental patients with special needs. J Formos Med Assoc. 2014;113(2):94–101.
42. Mullen B, Champagne T, Krishnamurty S, Dickson D, Gao RX. Exploring the safety and therapeutic effects of deep pressure stimulation using a weighted blanket. Occup Ther Ment Health. 2008;42(1):65–89.
43. Allen D, Lowe K, Brophy S, Moore K. Predictors of restrictive reactive strategy use in people with challenging behavior. J Appl Res Intellect Disabil. 2009;22(2):159–68.
44. de Castro AM, de Oliveira FS, de Paiva Novaes MS, Araujo Ferreira DC. Behavior Guidance technique in pediatric dentistry: attitudes of parents of children with disabilities and without disabilities. Spec Care Dentist. 2013;33(5):213–7.
45. Adair SM, Schafer TE, Rockman RA, Waller JL. Survey of behavior management teaching in predoctoral pediatric dentistry programs. Pediatr Dent. 2004;26(2):143–50.

Orthodontic Treatment for Children with Intellectual Disabilities

Marc B. Ackerman

Introduction

Success in orthodontic treatment for a child with an intellectual disability (ID) is the extent to which the treatment rendered fulfills the parent's expectation. How close you come to delivering the experience and treatment outcome that the parent was promised the day of the initial examination will determine orthodontic success [1]. In many cases, a definitive assessment of the child's ability to tolerate treatment cannot be made during first contact [2]. All children survey new surroundings differently, and their first reaction to you and your office may not be indicative of their candidacy for orthodontic treatment. So, the concept of under-promise and over-deliver is usually a good policy. Each patient/parent interaction along the way matters. First impressions are lasting impressions especially in the eyes of the child with an ID. Direct communication is essential. The child is trying out for the lead in a show, and they deserve our full attention and a laser focus on the story they are trying to tell. Mindset is more important than technical ability.

Mindset

The goal of orthodontic treatment of the child with an ID is not the creation of an "ideal" dentoform occlusion. In many cases, this is impossible due to missing teeth, misshapen teeth, skeletal discrepancy, and/or soft tissue limitations. Treatment objectives and treatment plans may not resemble what you were taught in school. Orthodontics is a branch of dentistry that aims primarily to enhance human appearance affecting psychosocial fitness and in a small subset of cases improve physical oral health as it is affected by congenital or acquired pathology [3]. Orthodontic

M. B. Ackerman (✉)
Boston Children's Hospital, Boston, MA, USA
e-mail: marc.ackerman@childrens.harvard.edu

T. M. Nelson, J. R. Webb (eds.), *Dental Care for Children with Special Needs*,
https://doi.org/10.1007/978-3-030-10483-2_12

practice much like cosmetology exists to satisfy parent's and patient's desire to become normal or even better than normal to whatever degree they wish, e.g., teeth being straighter versus straight. The type and extent of orthodontic treatment rendered are guided by the parent and patient and delivered by the clinician. Parents are usually seeking a noticeable enhancement of the child's dentofacial appearance with the hope of improving their child's integration into mainstream society. However, the child with an ID must assent to treatment at some level. If the child cannot comprehend anything related to why they "need" treatment, what that treatment is, and how it will be delivered, treatment is not indicated. In fact, it is unethical to initiate treatment without assent. Even in the case of children with surrogate decision-makers, the ethical principles of patient autonomy and non-maleficence still apply [4].

Mode of Practice

There are two approaches to treating patients with ID. First, there is the isolationist method which employs separate office protocols administratively and clinically for treating these patients. Children with intellectual disabilities are seen at different times of the day, placed in private rooms, etc. Second, there is the mainstreaming method which integrates these patients into the standard office workflows. Children with intellectual disabilities are treated exactly like any other patient, albeit the appointment durations can be modified as needed. The mainstreaming method is preferable to the isolationist method from both an efficiency, effectiveness, and socialization standpoint [5].

The Initial Examination

It is important to develop communication scripts and a systematized method of clinical examination when treating children with intellectual disabilities [6]. Past dental history is important to know, but this information should not render a child guilty before proven innocent. Whether the child was referred by their dental home to the orthodontic office or whether the parent self-referred should not bias the clinician in the appropriateness of the examination. It will become clear very early on in the encounter who and what are driving the desire for an orthodontic intervention as well as the child's potential to tolerate an orthodontic intervention.

In terms of scripting, there are several questions that should be posed to the child prior to asking them to open their mouth. How these questions are answered and by whom will give the clinician a sense for how to examine the patient. Speaking to the parent as though the child is not present in the room is never a good idea as you don't know the child's listening skills and their ability to comprehend the conversation they overhear. One common scripting sequence that can be employed is:

- [Child's name], it is very nice to meet you. I'm Dr. [your first name], and I'm the person who looks at the teeth around here. Did you know we are going to look at your teeth today?
- Do you like to brush your teeth?
- I'm going to use this little mirror to look at your teeth. Would you be my helper by holding it for a minute?

How engaged the child is in the discussion above is the first indicator of their comfort in the clinic setting and their level of anxiety, and it gives you a general sense of their level of engagement. It should be noted that the first question tells the patient that their teeth will be looked at. The use of phrases like "do you mind if I" or "will you let me" will give *any* child the idea that they are entering into a negotiation. There are certainly times for negotiating with children, and I strongly recommend employing it in many clinical situations; however I would not recommend starting off by providing an early opportunity for the child to "opt" out of the visit.

An important facet of this initial conversation is who does the answering. If a parent completely speaks for a child, this could be a red flag. If the child has a verbal communication difficulty, then it is understandable that the parent may need to intervene in the discussion. However, if the parent takes the view that "this child is going to do whatever I want them to do, so it doesn't matter what they say," discretion is the better part of valor. Our natural instinct is to make a snap judgment about why the parent is taking an aggressive stance on their child's candidacy for orthodontic treatment. From experience, many times this behavior is driven by frustration and hope. Imagine how many times the child has been denied participation in school activities, sports, social activities, and perhaps standard medical/dental treatment. Parents of children with intellectual disabilities may be coming to you fresh from a negative experience, and their frustration tolerance may be very low. On average, the parent of the child with an ID may have been subjected to multiple orthodontic opinions before arriving in your office [7]. Parents have told me that previous experiences have ranged from not even getting beyond the waiting room due to the child's ID all the way to having comprehensive orthodontic records taken only to be told by the orthodontist that they do not have the "training or skill set" to treat the child. The second thing that may color the parent's behavior at the initial examination is their level of hope for a positive outcome. A parent with unbridled hope for their child will often react to a clinician's negative determination with anger or resentment if it echoes what the previous clinician might have said in another opinion. The human condition is such that hope will often drive us to repeat our actions over and over again in spite of the high probability that we will not get the result that we are looking for. In general, some would call this behavior insanity. However, as an agent of the healing arts, we must understand where the parent of the child with ID is coming from and at least try to have a dialogue that is caring but honest.

Once it becomes clear that a clinical examination is going to be possible, the clinician needs to explain the sequence to the child. By and large, children with or without intellectual disabilities tend to be overwhelmed by too much information. Breaking down the exam into parts with explanations prior to each segment will help the child understand what you are doing. There are several choices for how you can physically examine the child. First, some clinicians prefer to use a straight-back chair and to examine the patient in a sitting-up position. The proponents of this method argue that the normal chair is less threatening to the child since they surely have had the experience of sitting in a chair. Second, some clinicians prefer to have the child sit upright in the dental chair. The clinicians who use this method believe that this method allows the child to experience the feel of the dental chair but at the same time feel less vulnerable by sitting upright. Third, some clinicians believe in examining the child in the dental chair in a fully reclined position. The clinicians who advocate for this method are of the opinion that the child should be exposed to exactly what the environment will be like during orthodontic treatment. I strongly believe that the first two methods are preferable to the third. Each child with an ID is different and the assumption that a cookie cutter examination sequence can be applied to all patients is a fallacy. That is to say, sometimes it is better to evaluate some characteristics of the patient's dentofacial complex rather than none. There are many instances in which the clinician may spread the examination over two visits in order to desensitize the patient to the new environment and their new doctor.

Communication

The goal of the clinical examination is to characterize a patient's dentofacial condition in as few descriptive terms as possible [8]. The categories in which every patient's dentofacial complex can be characterized are:

- Profile and smile
- Alignment (crowding, spacing, missing teeth, etc.)
- Class (angle classification both dentally and skeletally)
- Bite depth (vertical components)
- Transverse (crossbites)

It is important to note that all of the features listed in the examination are descriptive and not necessarily indicative of pathology. Communication in all parent/patient interactions is paramount. Parents of children with intellectual disabilities are well aware that their child is not neurotypical. In fact, many of these parents are very sensitive to the notion of "normal" and "ideal." In advance of discussing the findings of the clinical examination, it is best to preface your diagnostic summary with "I am going to tell you what I have seen in the exam and want you to know that each of these findings are merely descriptive and not necessarily bad things in need of correction." This strategy works for all orthodontic consultations. Overemphasis on any particular finding may cause the parent or child to solely focus on it.

Once the parent has processed the findings, the clinician can proceed to a discussion of which particular characteristics the parent and/or patient is concerned with and what the possible orthodontic interventions that could be employed to treat them. Orthodontists have traditionally considered anything less than comprehensive (full) treatment as a "compromise." [9] This is a terrible conceptual framework from which to operate, in particular with children who have ID. Depending on the clinical situation, there are always going to be multiple treatment options, including no treatment. So, if a parent decides that they only want to address one particular finding and it is possible to treat it without creating other more significant problems, it is perfectly reasonable. At this point, it is still early in the evolving relationship between the clinician and parent/child. It is essential that the clinician explains what is required of the patient in order to achieve success in all of the options presented. As was mentioned earlier in the chapter, orthodontic treatment of the child with ID is an iterative feedback loop. Each step along the way will affect the following one, and patient response both clinically and behaviorally will determine the trajectory of treatment.

Data Gathering

Traditionally, all orthodontic patients have the same diagnostic record set taken [10]. This would include photos, a panoramic radiograph, a cephalometric radiograph, and study models. Some orthodontic records may not be appropriate based on the nature of the problem treated. In the case of study models, there are currently two methods for taking this record. First, there is the alginate impression method. This requires the patient to have an impression tray placed in their mouth with alginate for several minutes. Patients with an elevated gag reflex have great difficulty with impressions and are prone to vomiting during the procedure. Many clinicians have used the alginate impression as the single test for whether or not a child with ID can tolerate or have orthodontic treatment. This is somewhat of an unfair test. Orthodontic treatment in many instances can be initiated without study models. If it appears that a child with ID seems to be a positive, but borderline candidate for some orthodontic intervention, it might be wise to forgo impressions. However, all orthodontic interventions require some type of retention. Most retainers require an impression to be taken for fabrication. The best-case scenario is that the child progresses through orthodontic treatment with increasing confidence and will at the end be able to tolerate an impression. The second method of acquisition for study models is the intraoral scanner [11–13]. This involves a relatively small wand placed in the mouth and moved around the arches to capture the desired anatomy. A well-trained assistant can take a scan in a matter of a few minutes. The intraoral scan is preferable to the alginate impression for patient comfort and speed with which the clinician obtains the data. In many cases, not all of the traditional orthodontic records are needed. If the child presents with non-skeletal issues or if the initial exam discerns that a limited treatment of the teeth is most desirable, then a cephalometric radiograph may not be required. It is up to the individual clinician to decide on what records they are going to take.

Treatment Planning and Orthodontic Treatment

The treatment planning exercise largely occurs in the initial examination. Clinical findings determine the options which were discussed with the parent and child. At the conclusion of the dialogue discussed earlier, the clinician and parent will have arrived at a mutually agreeable plan. However, the real treatment planning has to do with placement of appliances and patient management. More often than not, the child with ID requires a staged approach to appliance placement. Shorter appointments with well-circumscribed goals work very well. Placing just a few brackets and allowing the patient to get used to the feel of them may produce a better behavioral response than placing a whole arch of braces. As well, placing several brackets with no wire and colored ligature ties only is another way of easing a child into orthodontic treatment. Some clinicians will recommend that the parent, school aid, or therapist create a Social Story™ about orthodontic procedures. Although the orthodontist can provide accurate photographs of what they do in the office, the script that the storyteller uses can negatively affect behavior. For example, if the storyteller calls acid etch "blue jelly," but the clinician refers to it as "tooth shampoo," the child may become confused about what is going to happen. In some circumstances, the tell-show-do technique at each visit can be more effective than any preparation at home [14].

Each child will respond differently to clinical orthodontic procedures. In general, it is better to schedule an appointment of slightly longer duration than is actually needed. This will give the clinician flexibility in performing the planned treatment as well as time for any unforeseen issues such as repairing breakage, solving behavioral issues at the appointment, or dealing with being behind in the overall clinic schedule. It should be emphasized that there are no hard and fast rules when it comes to performing any of the technical orthodontic procedures for the child with ID.

Case-Based Scenario

An 11-year-old male with pervasive developmental disability and autism spectrum disorder presented to the orthodontic clinic with his parents. The patient had a history of acute stress reaction in the dental chair and had previously been taken to the operating room for dental care under general anesthesia. Mom's orthodontic chief complaint was "his front teeth are crooked and we don't like them that way."

Since the patient had not been able to withstand routine treatment in the dental chair, the parents were cautioned about his ability to withstand a short course of fixed appliance orthodontic treatment. Several appointments were undertaken to desensitize the patient to the clinic. Photographs and X-rays were taken, but no impressions for study casts were made. It was determined that at the end of Phase I treatment, one impression would be required for fabrication of a clear thermoplastic retainer. By that point in treatment, an educated guess was made that the patient would be able to tolerate the alginate impression procedure. The original plan was to place two of the six brackets on the teeth and then slowly work toward bonding the remaining four. The first archwire was to be placed when the six brackets were in place. However, the oral and maxillofacial surgeon who was planning to perform the frenectomy suggested that the braces be placed during the surgical operating room visit for efficiency and patient tolerance. It is not generally advisable to routinely take patients with intellectual disabilities to the operating room for appliance placement, since the majority of treatment has to take place in the dental chair, and the patient must be able to tolerate treatment in an ambulatory setting. However, an exception was made in this case, and braces were placed in the operating room.

Phase I Clinical Findings (Mixed Dentition, Delayed Dental Age) (Fig. 1a, b)

Profile/smile: straight, gummy smile
Alignment: maxillary midline diastema with incisor rotations, mandibular incisor spacing
Class: I with anterior crossbite
Other: large maxillary labial frenum attachment

Treatment Objectives, Phase I Orthodontics

Frenectomy
Level and align maxillary incisors and close space

Mechanotherapy

Direct bond brackets teeth #s: 3, 7, 8, 9, 10, 14
Successive leveling archwires
Elastomeric chain
Removable clear thermoplastic retainer

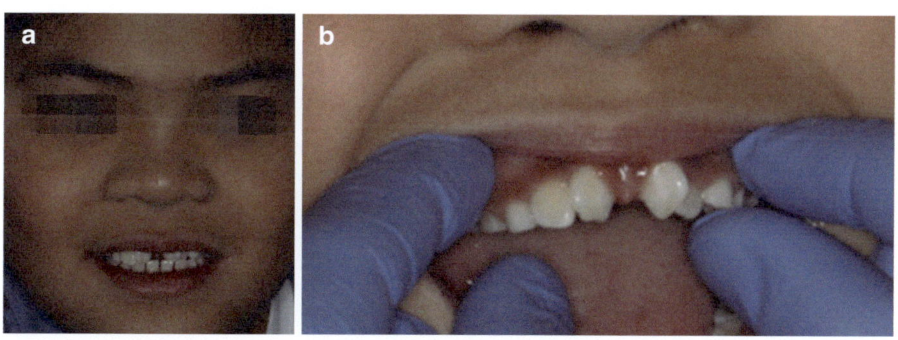

Fig. 1 (**a**) Facial smiling view pre-treatment. (**b**) Intraoral view of the large diastema with large frenum attachment

The patient was successfully bonded in the operating room. Six weeks later the patient returned for his first adjustment. Oral hygiene was good and there was no breakage. Tell-show-do technique was used to teach the patient about changing archwires, and he was cooperative during the first visit. The patient was seen on 6-week intervals for orthodontic adjustments (Fig. 2). After a total of 6 months, treatment was complete, and the patient was scheduled for debond. A disposable plastic impression tray was customized to only capture the anterior portion of the dentition (Fig. 3). An acceptable impression was achieved on the second attempt and a clear thermoplastic retainer was given to the patient for nighttime (sleeping) use only (Fig. 4).

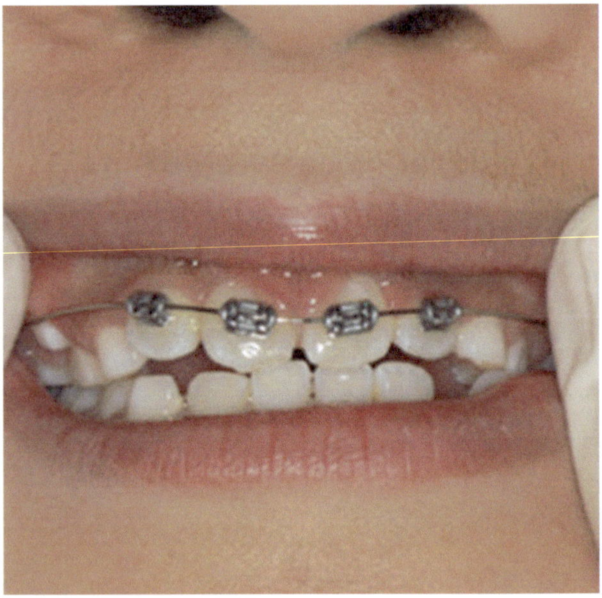

Fig. 2 Maxillary utility arch (2 × 4) with light nickel titanium archwire

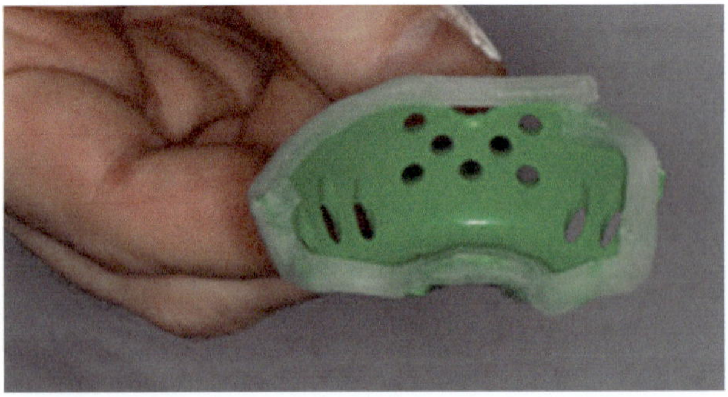

Fig. 3 Modified plastic disposable impression tray

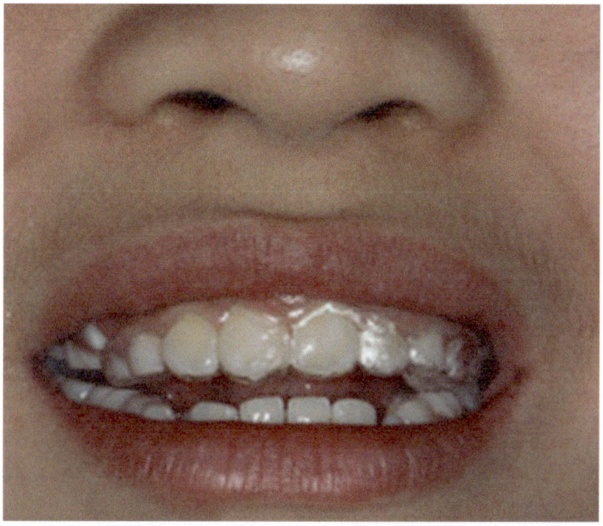

Fig. 4 Post-Phase I treatment with clear thermoplastic retainer over anterior teeth

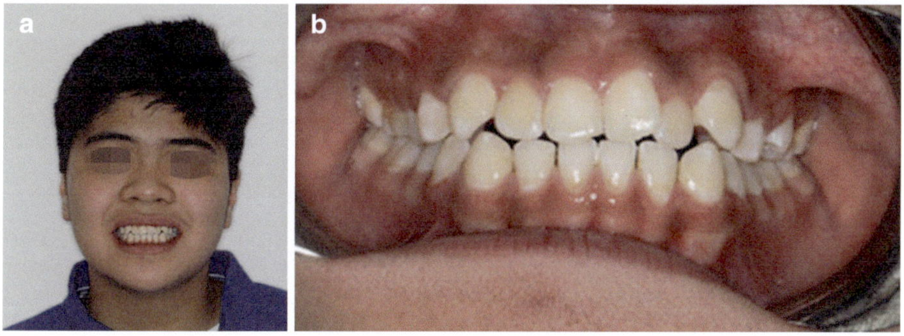

Fig. 5 (**a**) Alignment issues related to anterior tooth display. (**b**) Intraoral view

The patient's dentitional development was tracked on 6-month intervals for roughly 1.5 years. Upon exfoliation of the maxillary primary canines, the removable retainer was discontinued. The patient returned in the late mixed dentition at age 15 (teeth #A,J present).

At this point, the parents were again concerned about the esthetics of maxillary anterior tooth display. Although there was some spacing in the anterior portion of the mandibular arch, the parents did not wish to address this characteristic. A second phase of orthodontic treatment was initiated to only address the maxillary anterior tooth display.

Phase 2 Clinical Findings (Late Mixed Dentition) (Fig. 5a, b)

Max crowding with labial ectopic canines

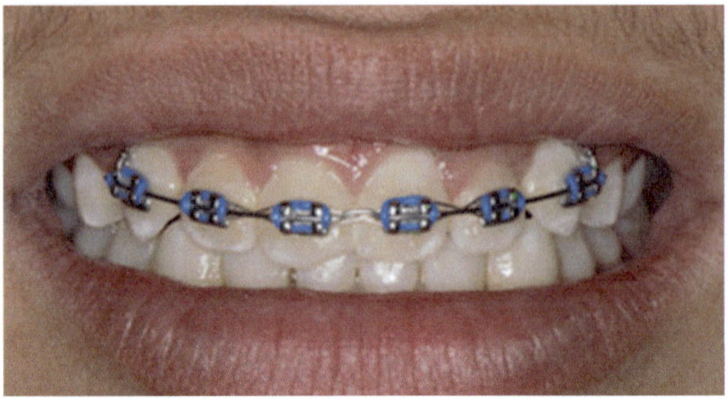

Fig. 6 Maxillary anterior fixed appliance

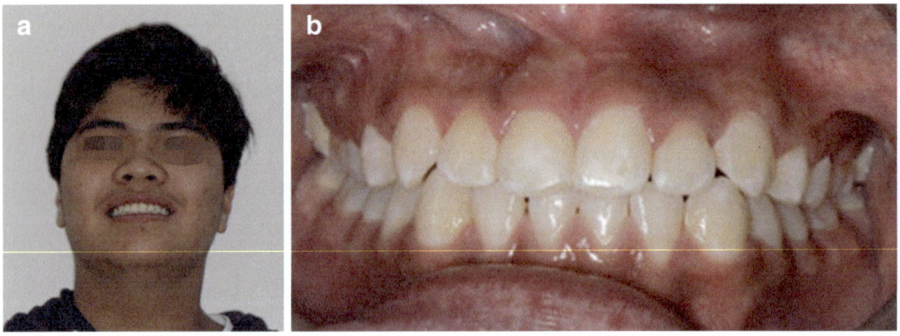

Fig. 7 (**a**) Facial view posttreatment. (**b**) Intraoral view posttreatment

Treatment Objectives, Phase II Orthodontics

Level and align max arch

Mechanotherapy

Direct bond brackets teeth #s: 6, 7, 8, 9, 10, 11
Successive leveling archwires
Removable clear thermoplastic retainer

A very straight forward 4-month course of orthodontic treatment was undertaken (Fig. 6) and completed (Fig. 7a, b).

Conclusion

- Orthodontic treatment of the child with ID is the art of the achievable and not the science of the improbable. With the correct mindset, any clinician can orthodontically treat children with intellectual disabilities.

- Open and honest communication with parents is essential for treatment success.
- It isn't possible to treat every child with ID for a myriad of reasons. Although it's awkward and difficult having to tell a parent that their child is not a good candidate for treatment, it must be done in some cases.
- Orthodontic treatment of children with intellectual disabilities is very rewarding and with a little practice is really no different than treating a neurotypical child.

References

1. Ackerman M, Burris B. Straighter: the rules of orthodontics. Orlando, FL: Ackerman-Burris Publishing; 2017.
2. Ackerman JL, Proffit WR. Treatment response as an aid in diagnosis and treatment planning. Am J Orthod. 1970;57:490–6.
3. Ackerman MB. Enhancement orthodontics: practice and theory. Ames, IA: Blackwell Publishing; 2007.
4. Ackerman JL, Proffit WR. Communication in orthodontic treatment planning: bioethical and informed consent issues. Angle Orthod. 1995;65:253–61.
5. Huck S, Kemp C, Carter M. Self-concept of children with intellectual disability in mainstream settings. J Intellect Develop Disabil. 2010;35:141–54.
6. Sarver DM, Ackerman MB. Dynamic smile visualization and quantification: part 1. Evolution of the concept and dynamic records for smile capture. Am J Orthod Dentofac Orthop. 2003;124:4–12.
7. Musich DR. Orthodontic intervention and patients with Down syndrome. Angle Orthod. 2006;76:734–5.
8. Ackerman JL, Proffit WR. The characteristics of malocclusion: a modern approach to classification and diagnosis. Am J Orthod. 1969;56:443–54.
9. Ackerman MB, Rinchuse DJ, Rinchuse DJ. ABO certification in the age of evidence and enhancement. Am J Orthod Dentofac Orthop. 2006;130:133–40.
10. Rischen RJ, Breuning KH, Bronkhorst EM, Kuijpers-Jagtman AM. Records needed for orthodontic diagnosis and treatment planning: a systematic review. PLoS One. 2013;12:e74186.
11. Jacob HB, Wyatt GD, Buschang PH. Reliability and validity of intraoral and extraoral scanners. Prog Orthod. 2015;16:38.
12. Lecocq G. Digital impression-taking: fundamentals and benefits in orthodontics. Int Orthod. 2016;14:184–94.
13. Burzynski JA, Firestone AR, Beck FM, Fields HW Jr, Deguchi T. Comparison of digital intraoral scanners and alginate impressions: Time and patient satisfaction. Am J Orthod Dentofac Orthop. 2018;153:534–54.
14. Schindel RH, Chahine A, Anderson N, Banville M, Eaton-Bove J, Weidenbaum N. Behavior modification of children with autism spectrum disorder in an orthodontic setting. J Clin Orthod. 2014;48:285–91.

Shifting the Dental Care Paradigm for CSHCN

Travis M. Nelson and Jessica R. Webb

Introduction

In recent years, much has changed in our understanding of disability. Older notions and assumptions about disability have fallen by the wayside, and the inherent dignity and value of people with disabilities are now widely accepted. There is currently a much better understanding of disability and health than there has ever been, with unprecedented inclusion of people with disabilities in all aspects of society. Additionally, fundamental values that have been gleaned from all aspects of healthcare now inform best practices for dental treatment for children with disabilities.

However, challenges still exist. Healthcare systems, training of healthcare providers, and research practices have yet to catch up to this paradigm shift. Straightforward solutions do not exist, but it is possible to change the paradigm of care for this population by steadily building upon a foundation of respect and equality.

Shifting the Dental Care Paradigm

Disability Is Not Synonymous with Poor Health

By definition, disability results in impairments and differences that impact health. Medications and therapies are frequently employed to help manage the physical and

T. M. Nelson (✉)
Department of Pediatric Dentistry, University of Washington, Seattle, WA, USA
e-mail: tmnelson@uw.edu

J. R. Webb
Children's Village, Yakima, WA, USA
e-mail: Jessica.DeBord@nyulangone.org

T. M. Nelson, J. R. Webb (eds.), *Dental Care for Children with Special Needs*,
https://doi.org/10.1007/978-3-030-10483-2_13

intellectual conditions that affect CSHCN. While these health interventions may impact oral health and delivery of oral health services, disability is not synonymous with poor oral health.

Oral health providers with expertise and dedication to the care of CSHCN can reduce the impact of disability on patient health through appropriate support and accommodations.

All Children Deserve Access to High-Quality Dental Care

The lives of CSHCN are complicated by a wide variety of physical and behavioral conditions that compete for caregiver attention. In the context of these daily challenges, oral care can be overlooked, and the patient's overall well-being may suffer. The dental professional can support patient health by working with the family and the medical team to assure appropriate access to professional and home dental care. Best practices indicate that all children should have access to comprehensive family-centered oral healthcare in the context of a dental home [1]. This is particularly important for CSHCN who may require more support than unaffected peers. The paradigm has shifted from attempting to fit the child into a standard dental care delivery model. Instead we must focus on recognizing the child's unique strengths and adapting the care approach to best suit her needs. Quality care for this population means:

- Adopting a patient- and family-centered approach, taking into account the individual's specific health needs with a focus on the emotional and social experience of the condition
- Focusing on the patient's strengths, instead of her weaknesses
- Respecting autonomy and soliciting input from the patient when possible
- Providing treatment in the least restrictive environment, meaning that when possible CSHCN receive care without medical immobilization/protective stabilization (MIPS) and pharmacological methods
- Prioritizing safety by making an effort to understand the patient's unique mental and physical characteristics

Breaking Down Barriers

High cost, poor insurance reimbursement, inadequate transportation, and behavioral challenges are frequently cited barriers to CSHCN receiving needed dental care [2, 3]. Lack of providers with the appropriate skill set and interest in caring for this population also impedes access. Many oral health providers receive inadequate training in care of CSHCN, which decreases confidence in their ability to offer services to these children [4]. The aims of this book are to improve access to quality care and to help CSHCN achieve health that is similar to a typically developing children. These can be accomplished by:

- Providing perspective on the culture and language of disability
- Building on the individual's strengths, rather than her limitations
- Finding ways to mitigate physical and behavioral challenges the patient experiences
- Becoming acquainted with common conditions encountered by CSHCN
- Learning about treatment modifications that may be required to safely care for the children with medical complexities (CMC)
- Understanding communication differences and implementing strategies for more effective communication
- Adapting the dental environment to better suit the patient's strengths
- Implementing behavioral strategies that are used to teach life skills outside the dental context
- Recognizing differences in habits, home environment, and feeding that can affect the patient's risk for disease and dental management
- Using pharmacologic and non-pharmacologic approaches to provide compassionate and effective care
- Developing a curiosity for each patient's unique experience
- Being flexible to address each patient's individual circumstances

Fundamental Values: What We Aspire to as Providers

As clinicians who devote our time and energy to the service of CSHCN, we approach care from a unique perspective. We appreciate diversity in the human experience and recognize that emotional intelligence can be more important than technical expertise. We must challenge ourselves to perpetually seek knowledge and to learn more about the culture and unique circumstances of CSHCN. Most importantly, we must strive to be patient, humble, and curious about each patient as an individual.

Cultural Awareness and Sensitivity Is a Baseline

Culturally sensitive care starts from a position of respect. We show patients and families respect by using language that demonstrates that we value them as a *person first*. We demonstrate our commitment to them by learning more about the circumstances of their lives and by soliciting input when making care decisions.

Success Is Relative and Creativity Is Mandatory

We understand that patient progress is incremental, so success cannot be measured on a binary scale. When approaching dental problems, providers who care for CSHCN think outside the box. For example, we may consider a nontraditional approach such as fitting a Hall crown, or we might delay treatment using silver diamine fluoride until a patient can learn to accept it through desensitization.

Seasoned practitioners understand that outcomes must be patient focused. Therefore, it may be better to accept a fair treatment result than to force the child to accomplish what is traditionally considered ideal.

The Family Is the Key to Success

Healthcare providers are important figures in the lives of CSHCN, but their roles pale in comparison with that of the family. Interactions with providers are episodic, whereas the family is continuously involved in the patient's care throughout the life course. Parents and caregivers are responsible for setting appointments, arranging transportation to medical visits, and for playing the role of patient advocate at each encounter. They synthesize information from multiple healthcare providers and often make decisions on behalf of the patient. Caregivers may not be experts in each particular medical discipline, but they are the foremost experts on their child. The family is primarily responsible for long-term health maintenance efforts such as home hygiene and establishing healthy dietary habits. Therefore, it is critical that we engage them to ensure that an intervention is practical and meaningful. We listen to caregiver concerns and desires and are flexible and practical with recommendations. Logistical factors such as availability of preferred appointment times and the family's home routines may not be the first thing that comes to mind as a provider, but they may be key to caregiver satisfaction and engagement. It is also important to note that we as providers often have significant limitations on the time we are able to devote to behavioral interventions such as teaching dental skills. Many behavioral accomplishments therefore occur as a result of practice outside the dental clinic. Engaging the child at school, the behavioral therapy office, and in the home environment can be instrumental in achieving long-term dental successes.

Oral Health Is Impacted by Many Variables

With typically developing patients, there is a relatively discrete set of factors that affect oral health. In contrast, a wide variety of additional conditions impact the oral health status of CSHCN. Lengthy lists of medications, medical diets, feeding tubes, altered physiology, and behavioral limitations can have significant effects on the patient's risk for caries, periodontal disease, and dental trauma. It is important to be aware of these factors and to mitigate them whenever possible.

Different Is OK: CSHCN and Their Unaffected Peers Will Have Different Dental Experiences

Our goal is for CSHCN to have oral health that is similar to unaffected peers; however that doesn't mean that the patient's experience with dental care should be the same. In fact, attempting to provide the same types of dental experiences for typically developing children and CSHCN may make dental encounters more challenging and decrease the chances of long-term success. For example, it may not be realistic for a CSHCN to willingly accept the same type of dental cleaning as her typically developing sibling. Forcing the child to endure this procedure can overwhelm her and make it more difficult to accept it when she is older. Instead, it may be prudent to desensitize the patient to the procedure over time or to alter the dental environment to help facilitate success. It may also be necessary to adjust treatment plans according to the patient's individual medical needs (e.g., the CSHCN may need to be seen for more frequent recall visits and require antibiotic premedication prior to invasive procedures, or she may not be able to undergo invasive procedures outside of a hospital environment). For some children to receive needed dental services, it may be necessary to employ MIPS, mouth props, and additional dental staff. For others care may not be possible without advanced pharmacologic behavior guidance such as sedation or general anesthesia. Parents often want their child to receive the same types of services as typically developing peers, so it is important to determine their expectations for the visit and to reach consensus on the care approach.

Caring for CSHCN Means Reaching Out Beyond the Dental Office

It isn't possible to provide effective care to this population without reaching out to other professionals. To ensure that each patient receives medically necessary care, we need to communicate with experts in many areas of the patient's life. We must be comfortable:

- Consulting regularly with medical colleagues regarding the patient's fitness to receive procedures
- Working with occupational and behavioral therapy on home hygiene measures and dental visit preparation
- Coordinating transportation and consent for dental and medical visits through social work colleagues
- Discussing therapy and individualized educational plans (IEP) with educators
- Relying on experts in sedation and anesthesia to provide safe pharmacological care when indicated

Future Directions

- The number of individuals with disabilities will continue to rise as medical technology improves longevity and quality of life.

  The need for clinicians who are interested and able to care for CSHCN will continue to increase.

- Historically, training in the care of people with disabilities has not been a dental education priority. Clinicians today are faced with more complicated treatment scenarios than ever before.

  Increased focus and training in the care of CSHCN is needed to equip providers to care for future generations.

- There is a lack of evidence regarding best practices for care of CSHCN.

  Well-designed research studies are needed to help delineate best practices for diagnosis, treatment, and preventive efforts involving these children.

- We have moved away from paternalistic care and shifted to a model that values developing therapeutic relationships with patients.

  People with disabilities must be engaged and included in their own healthcare.

- It is not possible to care for CSHCN in isolation.

  Providing an effective dental home for this population requires interactions with families, educators, and medical colleagues.

- CSHCN experience barriers that impede access to dental care.

  Dental providers can reduce care barriers by learning more about CSHCN and advocating for improved resources to care for this population.

Final Thoughts

It is our hope that the concepts within this text provide a framework for the thoughtful treatment of CSHCN. There is truly no group of people more deserving of our focus, study, and devotion. We envision a future where every child is recognized for her unique and diverse contributions and each individual receives dental care that enables her to enjoy all that life has to offer.

References

1. American Academy of Pediatric Dentistry. Definition of dental home. Pediatr Dent. 2017;39(6):12.
2. McKinney CM, Nelson T, Scott JM, et al. Predictors of unmet dental need in children with autism spectrum disorder: results from a national sample. Acad Pediatr. 2014;14(6):624–31.
3. Lewis C, Robertson AS, Phelps S. Unmet dental care needs among children with special health care needs: implications for the medical home. Pediatrics. 2005;116(3):e426–31.
4. Casamassimo PS, Seale NS, Ruehs K. General dentists' perceptions of educational and treatment issues affecting access to care for children with special health care needs. J Dent Educ. 2004;68(1):23–8.

MIX
Papier aus verantwortungsvollen Quellen
Paper from responsible sources
FSC® C105338

If you have any concerns about our products,
you can contact us on
ProductSafety@springernature.com

In case Publisher is established outside the EU,
the EU authorized representative is:
Springer Nature Customer Service Center GmbH
Europaplatz 3, 69115 Heidelberg, Germany

Printed by Libri Plureos GmbH
in Hamburg, Germany